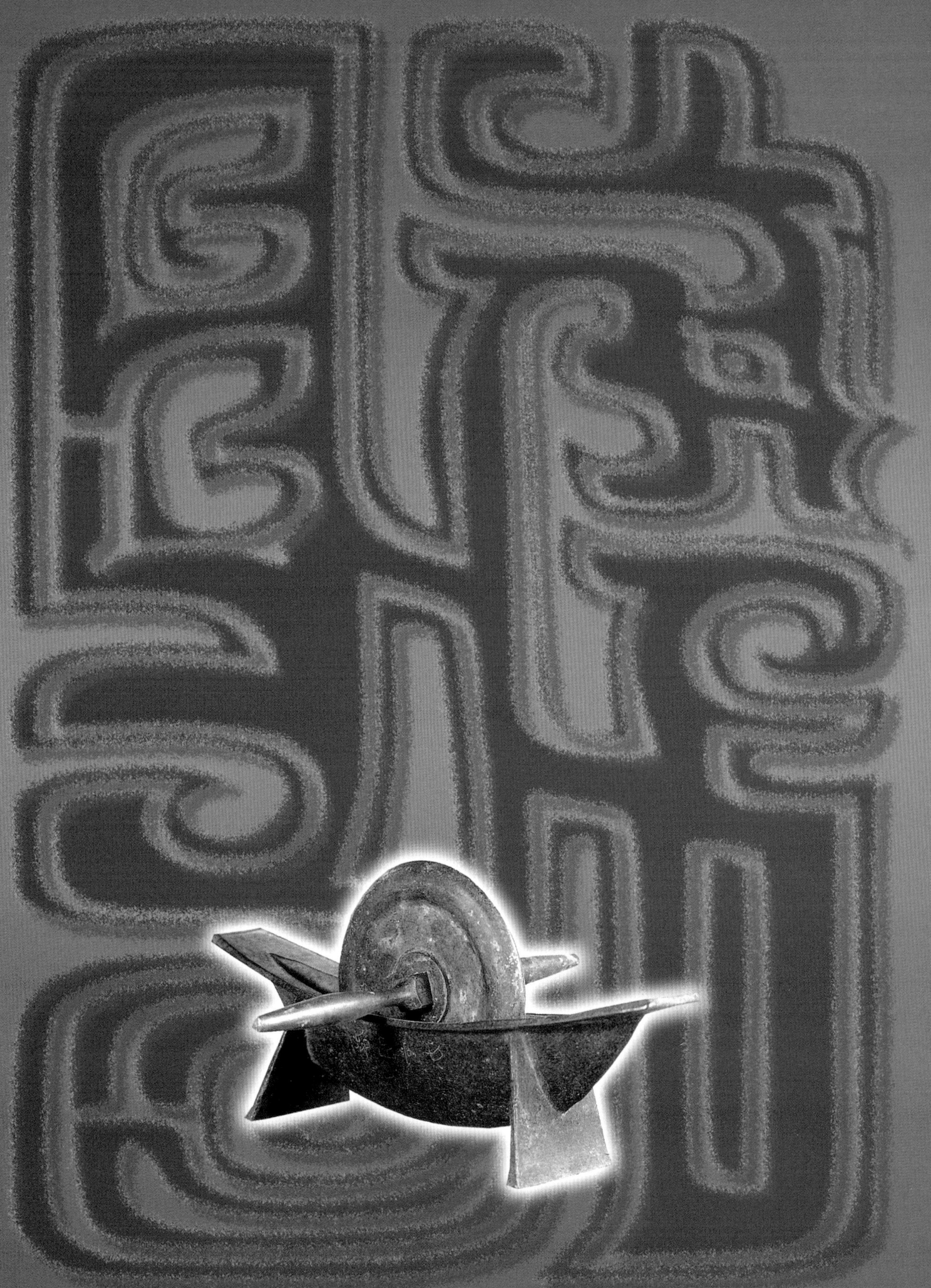

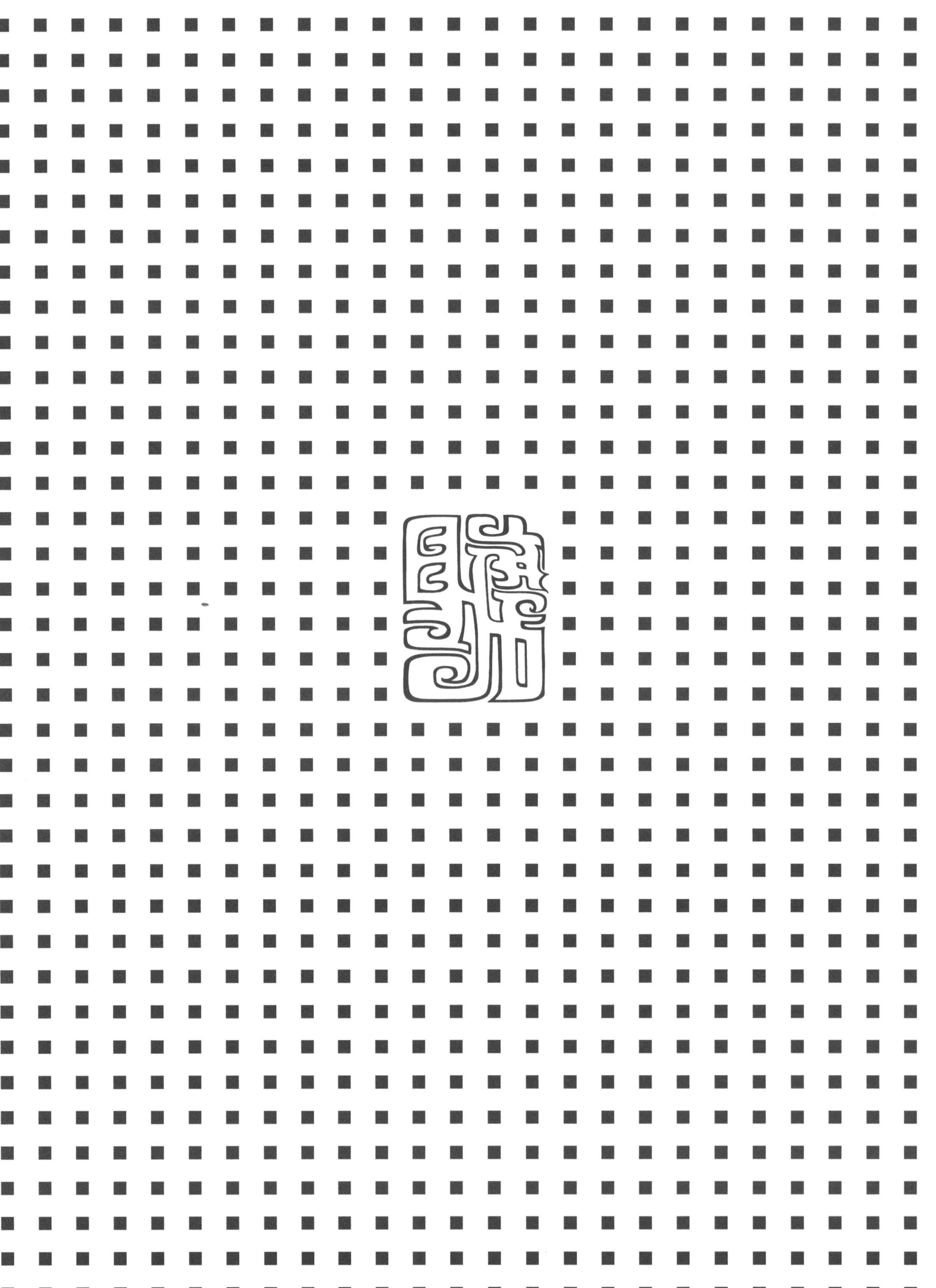

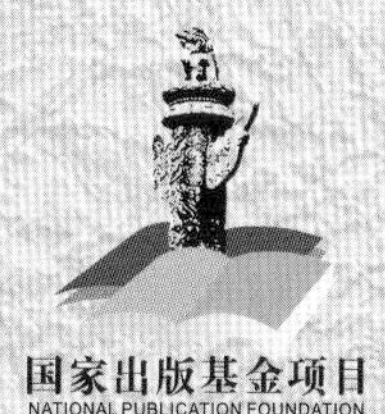

中华医药卫生

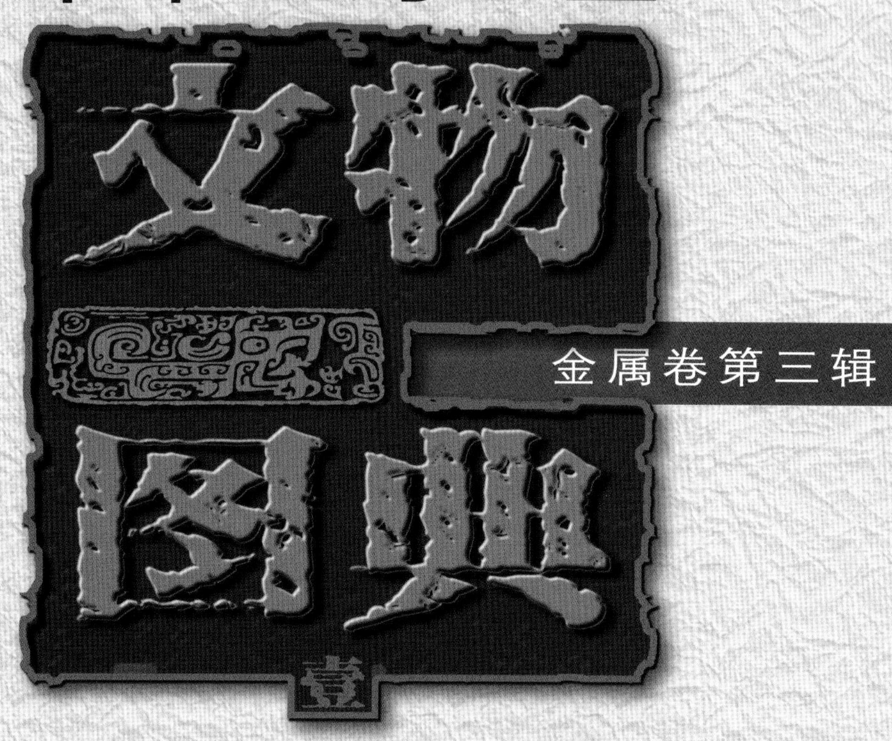

金属卷第三辑

主　编　李经纬　梁　峻　刘学春
总主译　白永权
主　译　李小棉

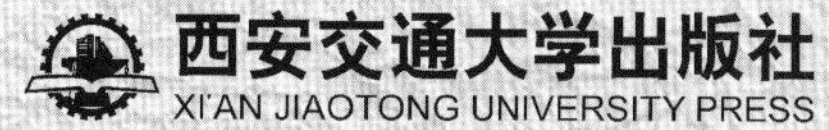
西安交通大学出版社
XI'AN JIAOTONG UNIVERSITY PRESS

图书在版编目 (CIP) 数据

中华医药卫生文物图典 . 1. 金属卷 . 第 3 辑 . / 李经纬，梁峻，刘学春主编 . — 西安：西安交通大学出版社，2016.12

ISBN 978-7-5605-7025-9

Ⅰ . ①中… Ⅱ . ①李… ②梁… ③刘… Ⅲ . ①中国医药学—金属器物—古器物 - 中国—图录 Ⅳ . ① R-092 ② K870.2

中国版本图书馆 CIP 数据核字（2015）第 013548 号

书　　名　中华医药卫生文物图典（一）金属卷第三辑

主　　编　李经纬　梁　峻　刘学春

责任编辑　王　磊　李　晶

出版发行　西安交通大学出版社

（西安市兴庆南路 10 号　邮政编码 710049）

网　　址　http://www.xjtupress.com

电　　话　（029）82668805　82668502（医学分社）

（029）82668315（总编办）

传　　真　（029）82668280

印　　刷　中煤地西安地图制印有限公司

开　　本　889mm × 1194mm　1/16　**印张**　28.75　**字数**　428 千字

版次印次　2017 年 12 月第 1 版　2017 年 12 月第 1 次印刷

书　　号　ISBN 978-7-5605-7025-9

定　　价　880.00 元

读者购书、书店添货、如发现印装质量问题，请通过以下方式联系、调换。

订购热线：（029）82665248　（029）82665249

投稿热线：（029）82668805　（029）82668502

读者信箱：medpress@126.com

銘記感受歷史
自信自重自強
書賀
中華醫藥衛生文物圖典問世
陳可冀謹題
二〇一七年春

陈可冀 中国科学院院士、国医大师

精修醫藥衛生文物
圖典功著當代
深究岐黄学術思想
渊源惠澤千秋

中華醫藥衛生文物圖典出版誌慶

丁酉孟秋　孫光荣敬題於北京

孙光荣　国医大师

中華醫藥衛生文物圖典出版

彰顯中醫藥
文化精神
体現中醫藥
歷史價值

歲次丁酉夏　王琦

王琦　国医大师

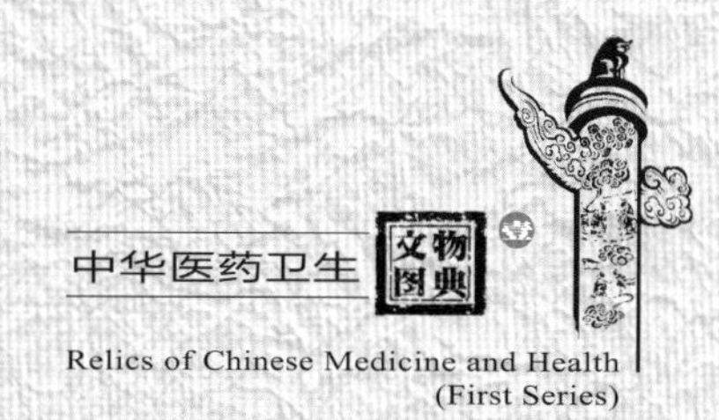

中华医药卫生文物图典（一）
丛书编撰委员会

译　者（按姓氏音序排列）

迟征宇　邓　甜　付一豪　高　琛　高　媛　郭　宁
韩　蕾　何宗昌　胡勇强　黄　鋆　蒋新蕾　康晓薇
李静波　刘雅恬　刘妍萌　鲁显生　马　月　牛笑语
唐云鹏　唐臻娜　田　多　铁红玲　佟健一　王　晨
王　丹　王　栋　王　丽　王　媛　王慧敏　王梦杰
王仙先　吴耀均　席　慧　肖国强　许子洋　闫红贤
杨姣姣　姚　晔　张　阳　张　鋆　张继飞　张梦原
张晓谦　赵　欣　赵亚力　郑　青　郑艳华　朱江嵩
朱瑛培

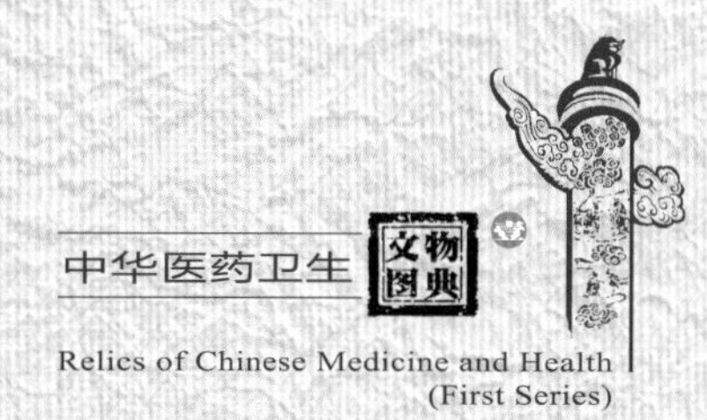

本册编撰委员会

主　编　李经纬　梁　峻　刘学春

副主编　廖　果　吴鸿洲　康兴军　和中浚　刘小斌　杨金生
郑怀林　徐江雁　白建疆　黄　煌

编　委　李洪晓　梁永宣　王强虎　董树平　马　健　王　霞
张雅宗　朱德明　包哈申　张建青　郑　蓉　庄乾竹
李宏红　刘哲峰　王宏才　陈润东

总主译　白永权

主　译　李小棉

副主译　詹菊红

译　者　唐臻娜　王慧敏　迟征宇　张梦原　高　琛　王　媛
牛笑语　吴耀均　黄　鋆　杨姣姣　蒋新蕾　席　慧

丛书策划委员会

丛书总策划 王强虎 王宏才 李 晶 秦金霞

统 筹 人 员 王强虎

丛 书 外 审 王宏才

编辑委员会 王强虎 李 晶 赵文娟 张沛烨 秦金霞 王 磊

郭泉泉 郅梦杰 田 滢 张静静

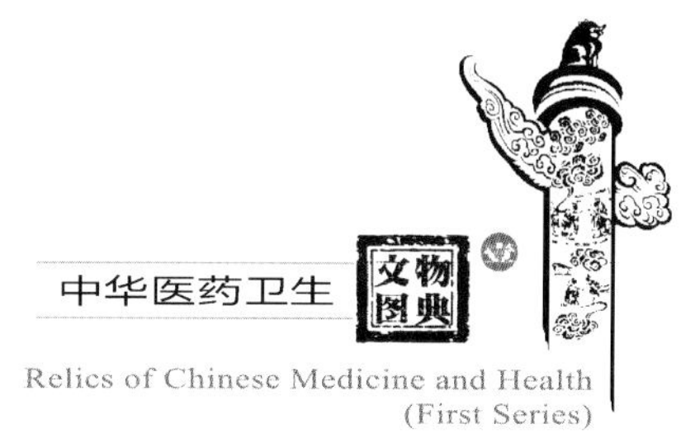

序 言

探索天、地、人运动变化规律以及“气化物生”过程的相互关系，是人类永恒的课题。宇宙不可逆，地球不可逆，人生不可逆业已成为共识。天地造化形成自然，人类活动构成文化。文物既是文化的载体，又是物化的历史，还是文明的见证。

追求健康长寿是人类共同的夙愿。中华民族之所以繁衍昌盛，健康文化起了巨大的推动作用。由于古人谋求生存发展、应对环境变化产生的智慧，大多反映在以医药卫生为核心的健康文化之中，所以，习总书记说:“中医药学是中国古代科学的瑰宝,也是打开中华文明宝库的钥匙”。

秉持文化大发展、大繁荣理念，中国中医科学院李经纬、梁峻等为负责人的科研团队在完成科技部“国家重点医药卫生文物收集调研和保护”课题获 2005 年度中华中医药学会科技二等奖基础上，又资鉴“夏商周断代工程”“中华文明探源工程”等相关考古成果，用有重要价值的新出土文物置换原拍摄质量较差的文物，适当补充民族医药文物，共精选收载 5000 余件。经西安交通大学出版社申报，《中华医药卫生文物图典（一）》（以下简称《图典》）于 2013 年获得了国家出版基金的资助，并经专业翻译团队翻译，使《图典》得以面世。

文物承载的信息多元丰富，发掘解读其中蕴藏的智慧并非易事。医药卫生文物更具有特殊性，除文物的一般属性外，还承载着传统医学发展史迹与促进健康的信息。运用历史唯物主义观察发掘文物信息，善于从生活文物中领悟卫生信息，才能准确解读其功能，也才能诠释其在民生健康中的历史作用，收到以古鉴今之效果。“历史是现实的根源”，任何一个民族都不能割断历史，史料都包含在文化中。“文化是民族的血脉，是人民的精神家园”，文化繁荣才能实现中华民族的伟大复兴。值本《图典》付梓之际，用“梳理文化之脉，必获健康之果”作为序言并和作者、读者共勉！

中央文史研究館館員
中国工程院院士　王永炎
丁酉年仲夏

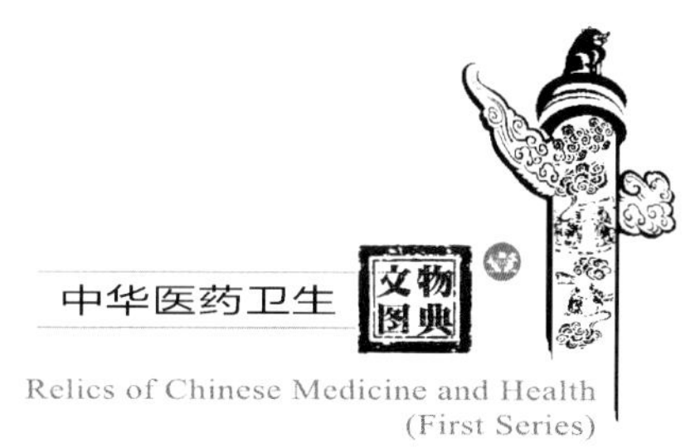

前 言

文化是相对自然的概念，是考古界常用词汇。文物是文化的重要组成部分，既是文明的物证，又是物化的历史。狭义医药卫生文物是疾病防治模式语境下的解读，而广义医药卫生文物则是躯体、心态、环境适应三维健康模式下的诠释。中华民族是56个民族组成的多元一体大家庭，中华医药卫生文物当然包括各民族的健康文化遗存。

天地造化如造山、板块漂移、气候变迁、生物起源进化等形成自然。气化物生莫贵于人，即整个生物进化的最高成果是人类自身。广义而言，人类生存思维留下的痕迹即物质财富和精神财富总和构成文化，其一般的物化形式是视觉感知的文物、文献、胜迹等。其中质变标志明晰的文化如文字、文物、城市、礼仪等可称作文明。从唯物史观视角观察，狭义文化即精神财富，尤其体现人类精、气、神状态的事项，其本质也具有特殊物质属性，如量子也具有波粒二相性，这种粒子也是物质，无非运动方式特殊而已。现代所谓可重复验证的“科学”，事实上也是从文化中分离出来的事项，因此也是一种特殊文化形式。追求健康长寿是人类共同的夙愿。中华民族之所以繁衍昌盛，是因为健康文化异彩纷呈。中华优秀传统医药文化之所以博大精深，是因为其原创思维博大、格物致知精深，所以，习总书记说：“中医药学是中国古代科学的瑰宝，也是打开中华文明宝库的钥匙”。

文化既反映时代、地域、民族分布、生产资料来源、技术水平等信息，又反映人类认知水平和生存智慧。发掘解读文物、文献中蕴藏的健康知识和灵动智慧，首先是从事健康工作者的责任和义务。《易经》设有“观”卦，人类作为观察者，不仅要积极收藏展陈文物，而且要善于捕捉文物倾诉的信息，汲取养分，启迪思维，收到古为今用之效果。墨子三表法，首先一表即“本之于古者圣王之事”，也是强调古代史实的重要性。“历史是现实的根源”，现实是未来的基础。任何一个国家、地区、民族都不能割断历史、忽略基础，这个基础就是文化。“文化是民族的血脉，是人民的精神家园”。文化繁荣才能驱动各项事业发展，才能实现中华民族的伟大复兴。

人类从类人猿分化出来。“禄丰古猿禄丰种”是云南禄丰发现的类人猿化石，距今七八百万年。距今200万年前人类进入旧石器时代，直立行走，打制石器产生工具意识，管理火种，是所谓“燧人氏”时代。中国留存有更新世早、中期的元谋、蓝田、北京人等遗址。距今10万—5万年前，人类进入旧石器时代中期，即早期智人阶段，脑容量增加，和欧洲、非洲人种相比，原始蒙古人种颧骨前突等，是所谓“伏羲氏”时代。中国发现的马坝、长阳、丁村人等较典型。距今5万—1万年前，人类进入旧石器时代晚期，即晚期智人阶段，细石器、骨角器等遍布全国，山顶洞、柳江、资阳人等较典型。

中石器时代距今约1万年，是旧石器时代向新石器时代的短暂过渡期，弓箭发明，狗被驯化。河南灵井、陕西沙苑遗址等作为代表。距今1万—公元前2600年前后，人类进入新石器时代，磨光石器、烧制陶器，出现农业村落并饲养家畜，是所谓“神农氏”时代。公元前7000年以来，在甲、骨、陶、石等载体上出现契刻符号、七音阶骨笛乐器等，反映出人文气息趋浓。公元前6000—公元前3500年的老官台、裴李岗、河姆渡、马家浜、仰韶等文化遗址，彰显出先民围绕生存健康问题所做的各种努力。

公元前4800年以来，以关中、晋南、豫西为中心形成的仰韶文化，是中原史前文化的重要标志。以半坡、庙底沟类型为典型，自公元前3500年走向繁荣，属于锄耕粟黍稻兼营渔猎饲养猪鸡经济方式，彩陶尤其发达。公元前4400—公元前3300年，长江中游的大溪文化，薄胎彩陶和白陶发达。公元前4300—公元前2500年山东丰岛的大汶口文化，红陶为主。公元前3500年前后，辽东的红山文化原始宗教发展。公元前 3300 年以来，长江下游由河姆渡、马家浜文化衍续的良渚文化和陇西的马家窑文化、江淮间的薛家岗文化时趋发达。

公元前 2600—公元前 2000 年，黄河中下游龙山文化群形成，冶铸铜器，制作玉器，土坯、石灰、夯筑技术开始应用。公元前 2697 年，轩辕战败炎帝（有说其后裔）、蚩尤而为黄帝纪元元年。黄帝西巡访贤，“至岐见岐伯，引载而归，访于治道”。其引归地“溱洧襟带于前，梅泰环拱于后”，即今河南新密市古城寨。岐黄答问，构建《黄帝内经》健康知识体系，中华文明从关注民生健康起步。颛顼改革宗教，神职人员出现；帝喾修身节用，帝尧和合百国，舜同律度量衡，大禹疏导治水，中华民族不断繁衍昌盛。

公元前 2070 年，禹之子启以豫西晋南为中心建立夏王朝，二里头青铜文化为其特征，半地穴、窑洞、地面建筑并存。饮食卫生器具、酒器增多。朱砂安神作用在宫殿应用。公元前 1600 年，商灭夏。偃师商城设有铸铜作坊。公元前 1300 年，盘庚迁殷，使用甲骨文。武丁时期青铜浑铸、分铸并存。公元前 1056 年，相传周“文王被殷纣拘于羑里，演《周易》，成六十四卦”。公元前 1046 年，武王克商建周，定都镐京。青铜器始铸长篇铭文，周原发掘出微型甲骨文字。公元前 770 年，平王东迁。虢国铸铜柄铁剑。公元前 753 年，秦国设置史官。公元前 707 年出现蝗灾、公元前 613 年出现“哈雷彗星”，均被孔子载入《春秋》。公元前 221 年，秦始皇统一中国，多元一体民族大家庭形成，中华医药卫生文物异彩纷呈。

中国是治史大国，历来重视发展文化博物事业，1955 年成立卫生部中医研究院时就设置医史研究室，1982 年中国医史文献研究所成立时复建中国医史博物馆研究收藏展陈文物。2000—2003 年，经王永炎院士、姚乃礼院长等呼吁，科技部批准立项，由李经纬、梁峻为负责人的团队完成“国家重点医药卫生文物收集调研和保护”项目任务，受到科技部项目验收组专家的高度评价，获中华中医药学会科技进步二等奖。2013 年，在国家出版基金资助下，课题组对部分文物重新拍摄或必要置换、充实民族医药文物后，由西安交通大学出版社编辑、组聘国内一流翻译团队英译说明文字付梓，受到国家中医药博物馆筹备工作领导小组和办公室的高度重视。

“物以类聚”，《图典》主要依据文物质地、种类分为 9 卷，计有陶瓷，金属，纸质，竹木，玉石、织品及标本，壁画石刻及遗址，少数民族文物，其他，备考等卷。同卷下主要根据历史年代或小类分册设章。每卷下的历史时段不求统一。遵循上述规则将《图典》划分为21册，总计收载文物5000余件。对每件文物的描述，除质地、规格、馆藏等基本要素外，重点描述其在民生健康中的作用。对少数暂不明确的事项在括号中注明待考。对引自各博物馆的材料除在文物后列出馆藏外，还在书后再次统一列出馆名或参考书目，以充分尊重其馆藏权，也同时维护本典作者的引用权。

21世纪，围绕人类健康的生命科学将飞速发展，但科学离不开文化，文化离不开文物。发掘文物承载的信息为现实服务，谨引用横渠先生四言之两语："为天地立心，为生民立命"，既作为编撰本《图典》之宗旨，也是我们践行国家"一带一路"倡议的具体努力。希冀通过本《图典》的出版发行，教育国人，提振中华民族精神；走向世界，为人类健康事业贡献力量。

李经纬　梁峻　刘学春

2017年6月于北京

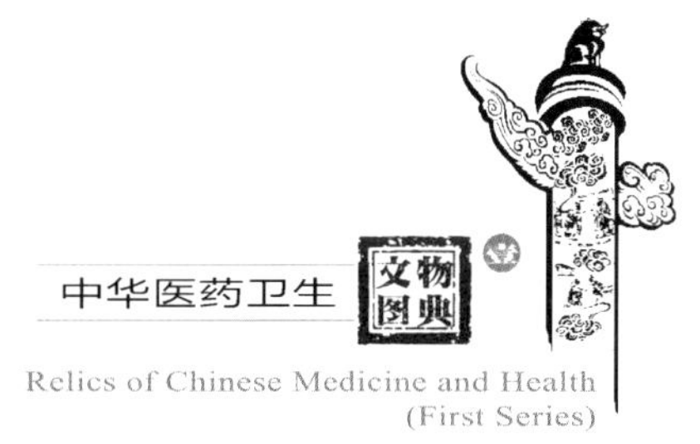
中华医药卫生
文物
图典
Relics of Chinese Medicine and Health
(First Series)

目 录

秦汉时期

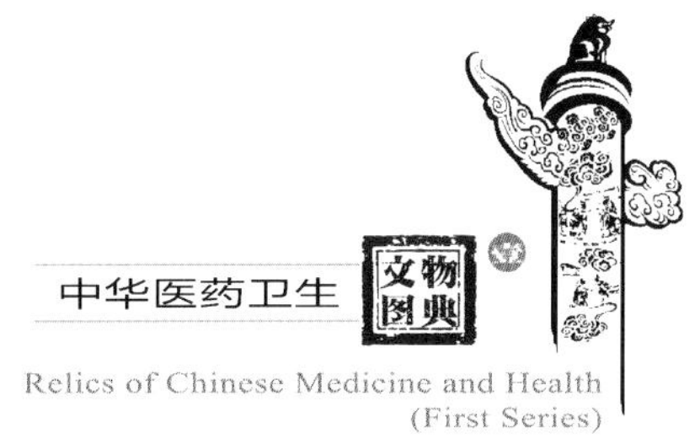

Contents

Qin and Han Dynasties

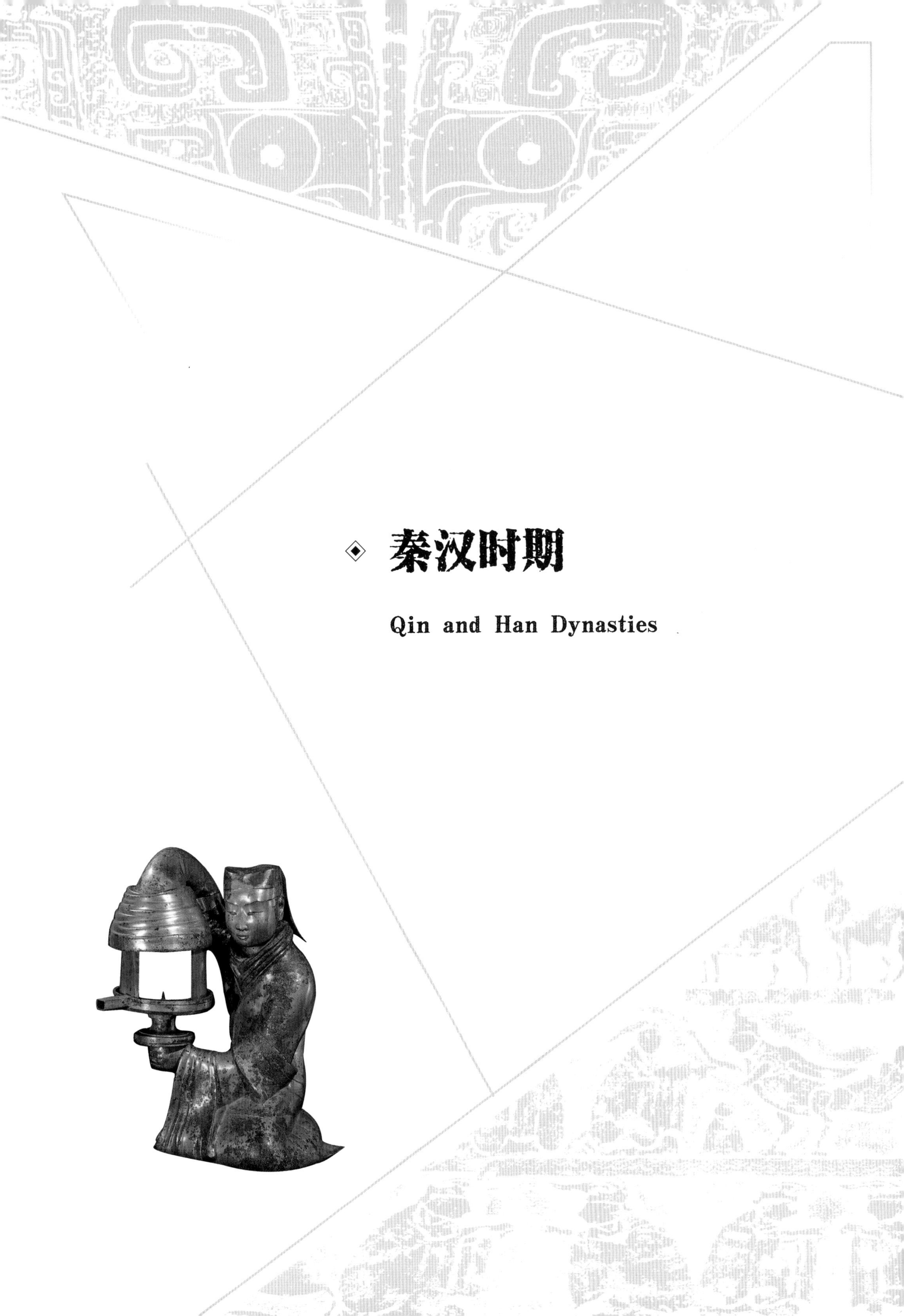

◈ 秦汉时期

Qin and Han Dynasties

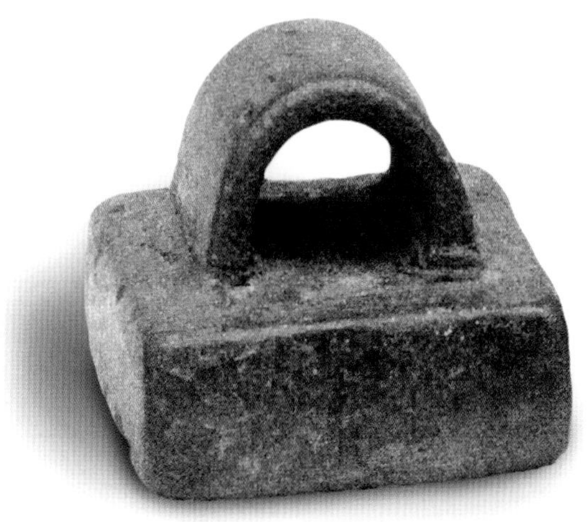

汉太医丞印

汉

铜质

宽 2.5 厘米，通高 3 厘米 ，重 59 克

Seal of Imperial Physician of Han Dynasty

Han Dynasty

Copper

Width 2.5 cm/ Total Height 3 cm/ Weight 59 g

方形，互钮。《后汉书》曾载郭玉“和帝时为太医丞”，可与此印相印证。图右为其印蜕。

故宫博物院藏

The piece is square with a seal knob. It is recorded in Book of the Late Han Dynasty: “Guo Yu was the Imperial Physician of Emperor He of the Han Dynasty”, which is accordance with the seal. The right figure shows its imprint.

Preserved in the Palace Museum

華

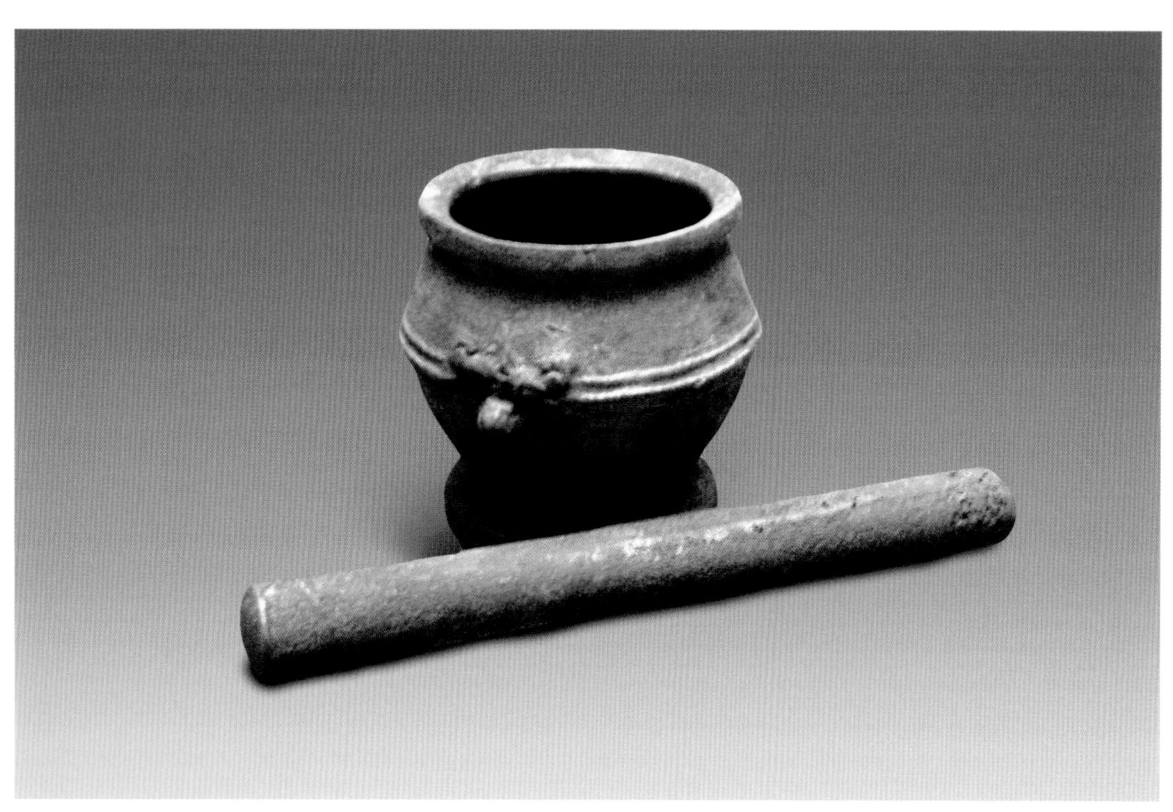

“医工”铜盆

西汉

铜质

口径 27.6 厘米，底径 14 厘米，高 8.3 厘米

Bronze Basin with Characters “Yi Gong” (which means medical workers)

Western Han Dynasty

Copper

Caliber 27.6 cm/ Base Diameter 14 cm/ Height 8.3 cm

此盆口沿两处、器壁一处均刻有“医工”两字，前者镌刻工整。口沿和底部有修补痕迹。1968年河北满城中山靖王刘胜墓出土。

河北省文物研究所藏

On both the mouth and the wall of the basin are inscribed two Chinese characters “Yi Gong”, The former is inscribed more neatly and orderly. There are repairing traces on the mouth and the base. This piece was unearthed from the mausoleum of King Jing—Liu Sheng, a Feudatory King of the Western Han Dynasty, in Hebei Province in 1968.

Preserved in Cultural Relics Institute of Hebei Province

華

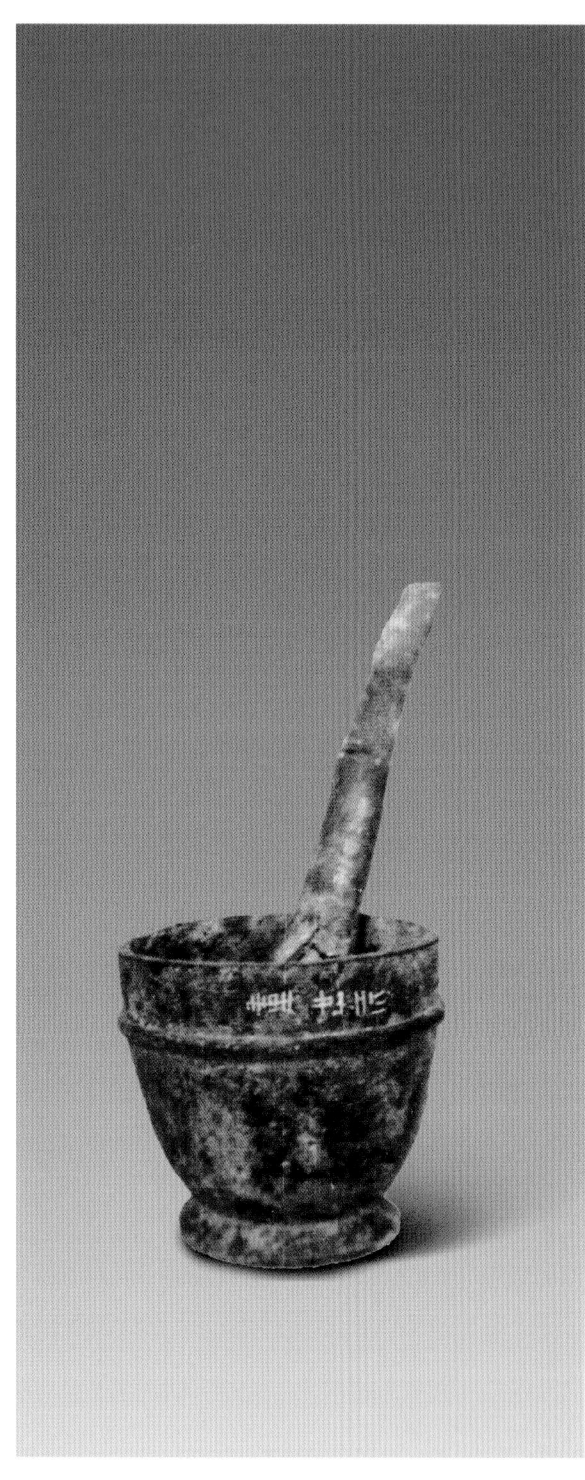

药臼、药杵

西汉

铜质

口径 15 厘米，口厚 5.7 厘米，底径 11 厘米；臼高 13.6 厘米，臼重 5200 克

杵长 36 厘米，一端直径 3.6 厘米，另一端直径 2.4 厘米，杵重 2250 克

Mortar and Pestle for Medicine Processing

Western Han Dynasty

Copper

Mortar Caliber 15 cm/ Thickness of Mouth 5.7 cm/ Base Diameter 11 cm/ Height 13.6 cm/ Weight 5,200g

Pestle Length 36 cm/ Diameter of One End 3.6 cm/ Diameter of The Other End 2.4 cm/ Weight 2,250g

臼为圆筒形，方唇，腹下部渐收平底，底缘外折呈假圈足状，腹上部有凸棱一圈，口沿一侧铭刻“重廿一斤”4 字。杵龟裂变形，棒状，中刻铭文“重八斤一两”5 字。山东巨野出土。

山东省巨野县文化馆藏

The mortar is in the shape of a cylinder with a square edge. The lower part of the belly gradually decreases to a flat base. The edge of the base is folded outward in the shape of a circular foot. There is a circle of convex ridge on the upper part of the belly. On one side of the rim is inscribed with four Chinese Characters: “Zhong Nian Yi Jin” which tells the weight of the mortar. The rodlike pestle is impaired due to fracturing, with five characters inscribed on it: “Zhong Ba Jin Yi Liang” which tells the weight of the pestle. They were unearthed in Juye, Shandong.

Preserved in Juye Cultural Center of Shandong Province

華

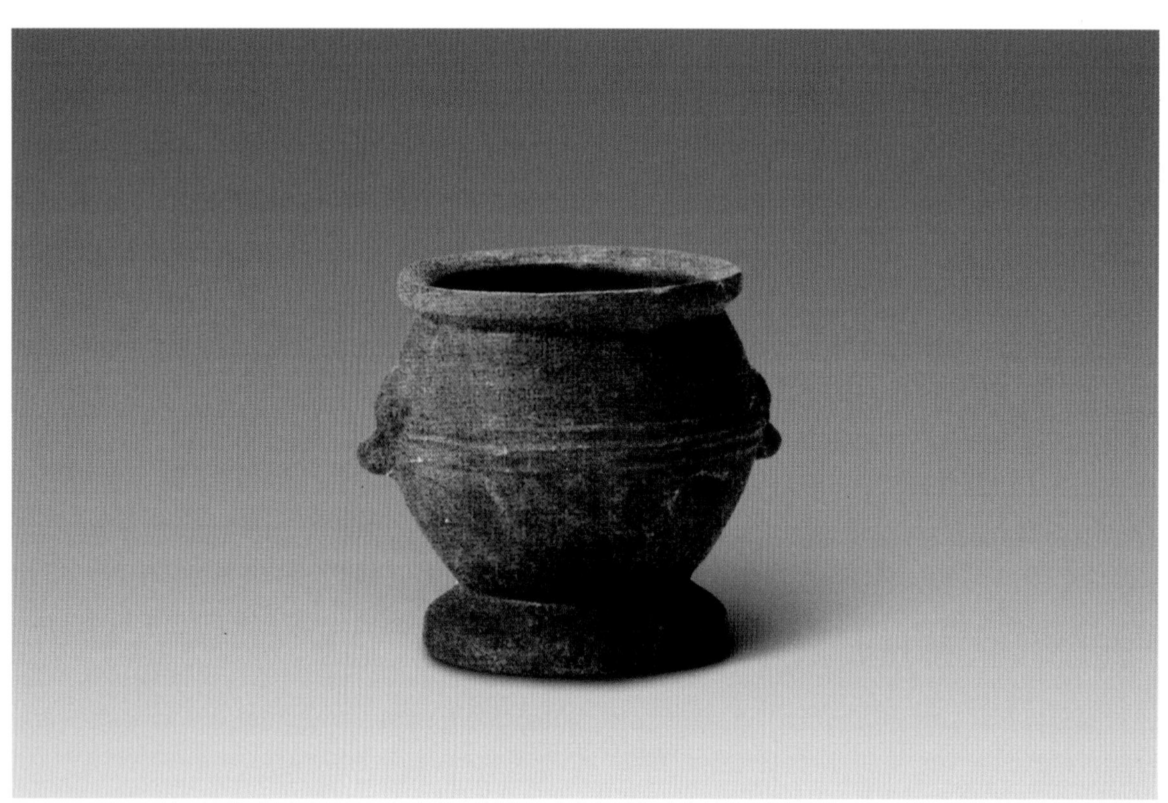

药臼、药杵

西汉

铜质

口径 9.9 厘米，腹径 11 厘米，高 11 厘米

Mortar and Pestle for Medicine Processing

Western Han Dynasty

Copper

Caliber 9.9 cm/ Belly Diameter 11 cm/ Height 11 cm

侈口鼓腹，复盘型假圈足，腹部饰凸纹三道，并有兽头形铺首二个，左右对称。紫红色，外形厚重朴拙。1988 年四川成都天回镇大湾汉墓出土。

成都中医药大学中医药传统文化博物馆藏

The object has a wide mouth, a swelling belly, and a double-plate circular foot. The belly is ornamented with three lines of convex pattern as well as two sculptures of animal's heads with bilateral symmetry. It is purple in color and has an appearance of massiness and naturalness. This piece was unearthed from Dawan Han Mausoleum in Chengdu, Sichuan Province, in 1988.

Preserved in Museum of Traditional Chinese Medicine Culture, Chengdu University of Traditional Chinese Medicine

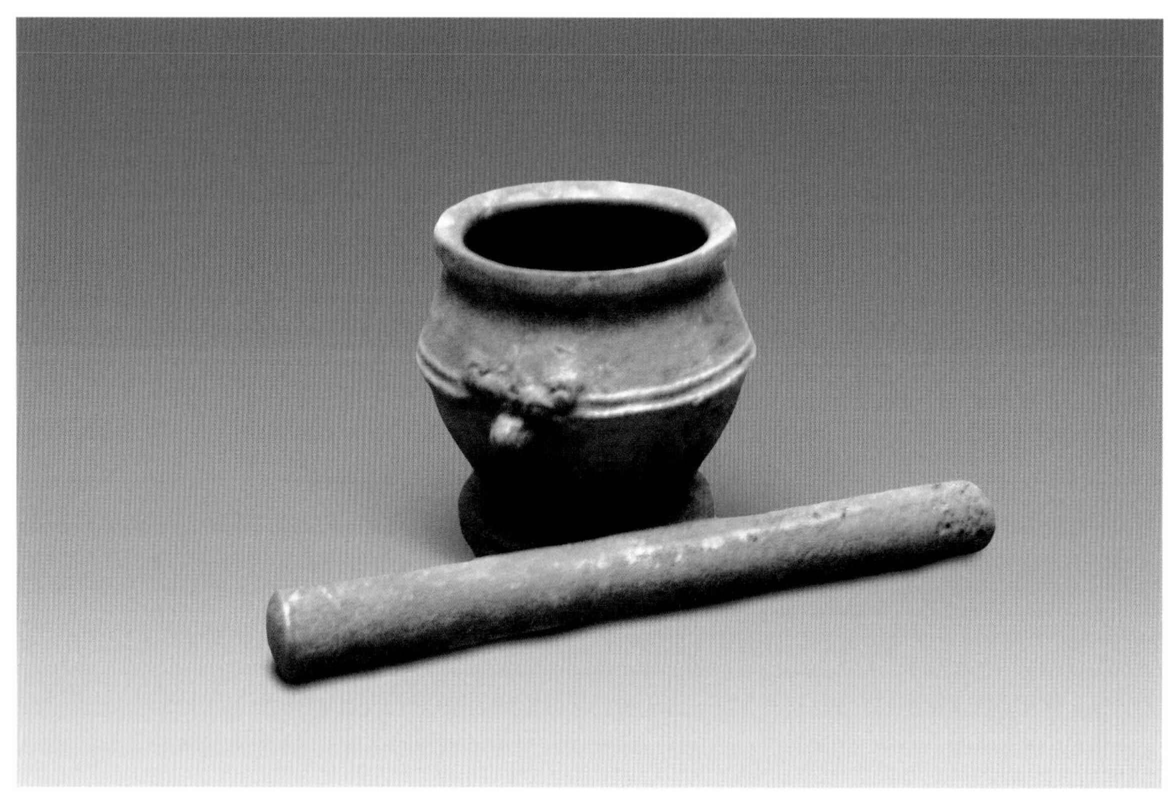

药臼

汉

铁质

高 9.5 厘米

Mortal for Medicine Processing

Han Dynasty

Iron

Height 9.5 cm

直口束颈，腹微鼓，中部有两根凸旋纹，环绕一周，其上有两个铺首纹，饼形足。器物造型端庄，线条简捷流畅，色泽沉稳，是件珍贵的药用文物和艺术精品。从成都市考古队征集。

成都中医药大学中医药传统文化博物馆藏

The mortal has an upright mouth, a tightened neck, and a slightly swelling belly circled by two convex lines of vortex pattern. On the convex patterns are decorated with two animal head appliques. It has a pie-shaped foot. The shape is dignified with simple smooth lines, steady color, and luster which present it as a precious relic of medical culture and art. It was collected from Chengdu Municipal Archaeological Team.

Preserved in Museum of Traditional Chinese Medicine Culture, Chengdu University of Traditional Chinese Medicine

華

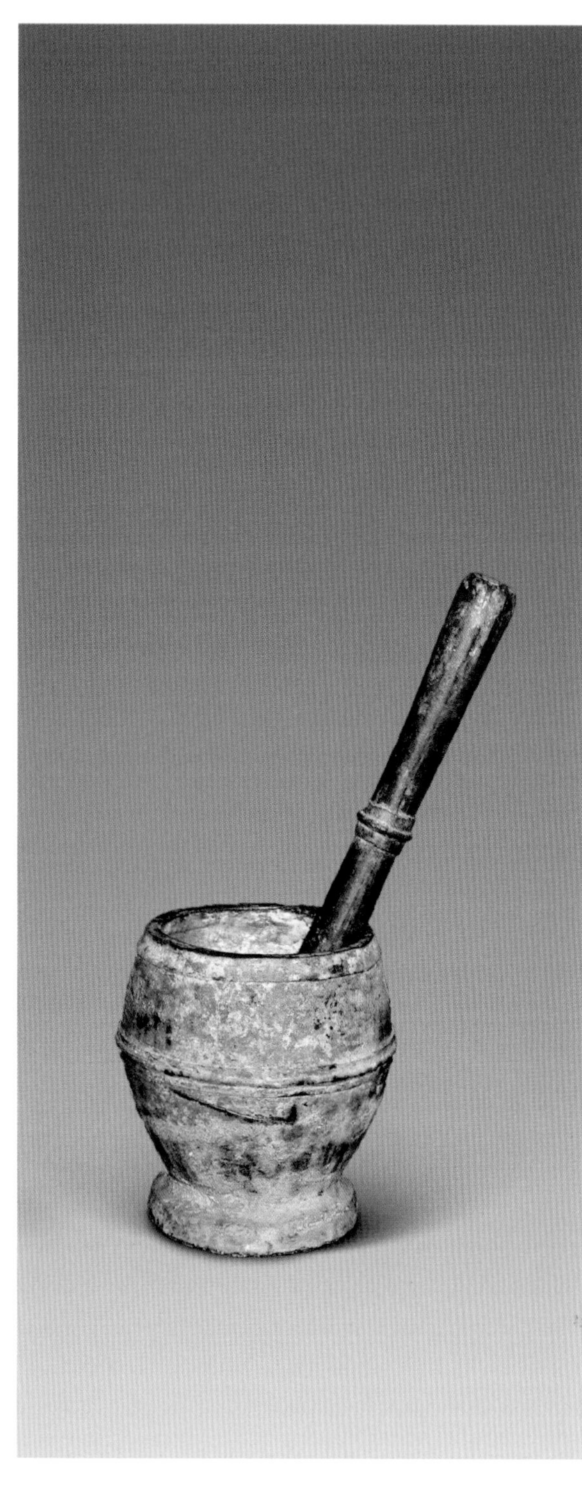

铜药臼

汉

铜质

口径 11 厘米，腹围 43 厘米，底径 11 厘米，高 14.5 厘米，重 5900 克

杵长 30.5 厘米，直径 1~3.2 厘米

Copper Mortar for Medicine Processing

Han Dynasty

Copper

Caliber 11 cm/ Abdominal Perimeter 43 cm/ Base Diameter 11 cm/ Height 14.5 cm/ Weight 5,900 g

Pestle Length 30.5 cm/ Diameter 1-3.2 cm

敛口，彭腹，平底，平口沿，腹中间一圈凸棱，带一杵，杵中部一圈凸棱。三级文物，捣药工具。完整无损。1980 年入藏，陕西省咸阳市北杜乡征集。

陕西医史博物馆藏

The mortar has a tightened mouth with a flat edge, a swelling belly and a flat base. The belly is circled by a convex ridge around the middle part. The piece has a pestle with a circle of convex ridge around the middle part. They are Grade 3 cultural relics and in good shape. They are tools for porphyrizing medicinal herbs. They were collected from Beidu Township, Xianyang, Shaanxi Province, in 1980.

Preserved in Shaanxi Museum of Medical History

華

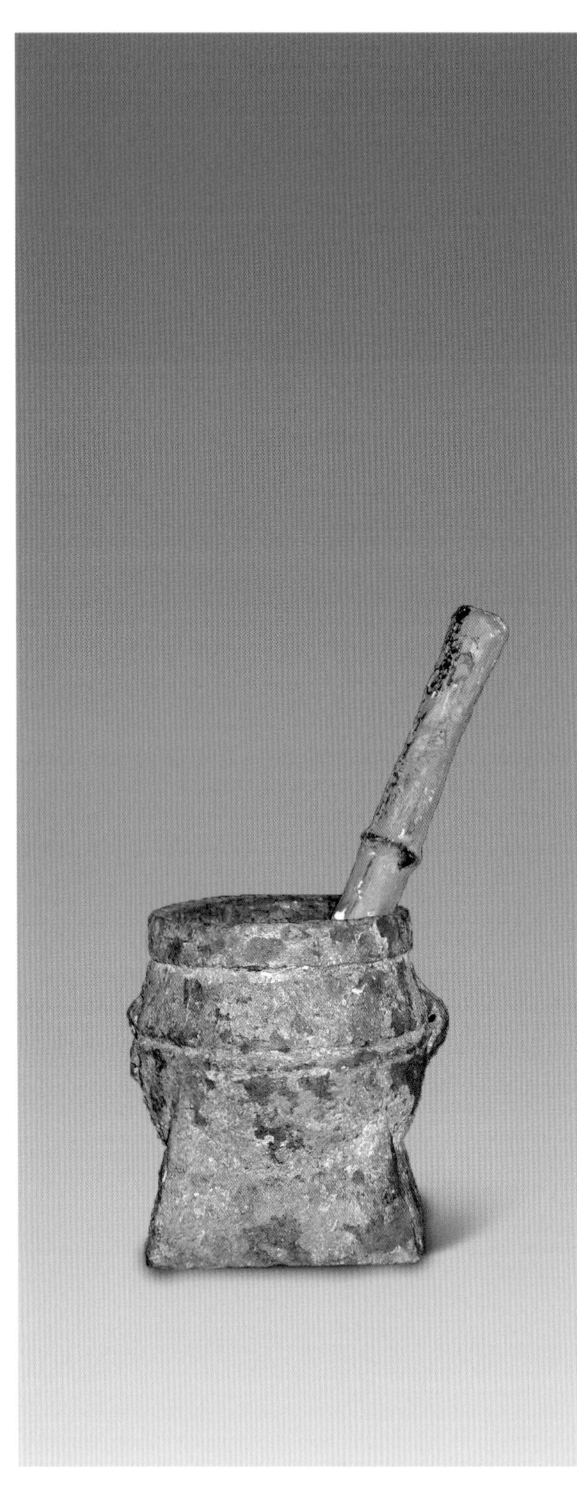

铁药臼

汉

铁质

口径 14.5 厘米，底径 15.6 厘米，通高 17.8 厘米，重 1240 克

Iron Mortar for Medicine Processing

Han Dynasty

Iron

Caliber 14.5 cm/ Base Diameter 15.6 cm/ Total Height 17.8 cm/ Weight 1,240g

敛口，彭腹，平底，平口沿，腹中间一圈凸棱，带一杵，杵中部一圈凸棱。三级文物，捣药工具。完整无损。1980 年入藏，陕西省咸阳市北杜乡征集。

陕西医史博物馆藏

The mortar has a tightened mouth, a swelling belly, and a square pedestal. The piece has a pestle with a circle of convex ridge around the middle, They are Grade 3 cultural relics and in good shape. They are tools for porphyrizing medicinal herbs. They were collected from Beidu Township, Xianyang, Shaanxi Province.

Preserved in Shaanxi Museum of Medical History

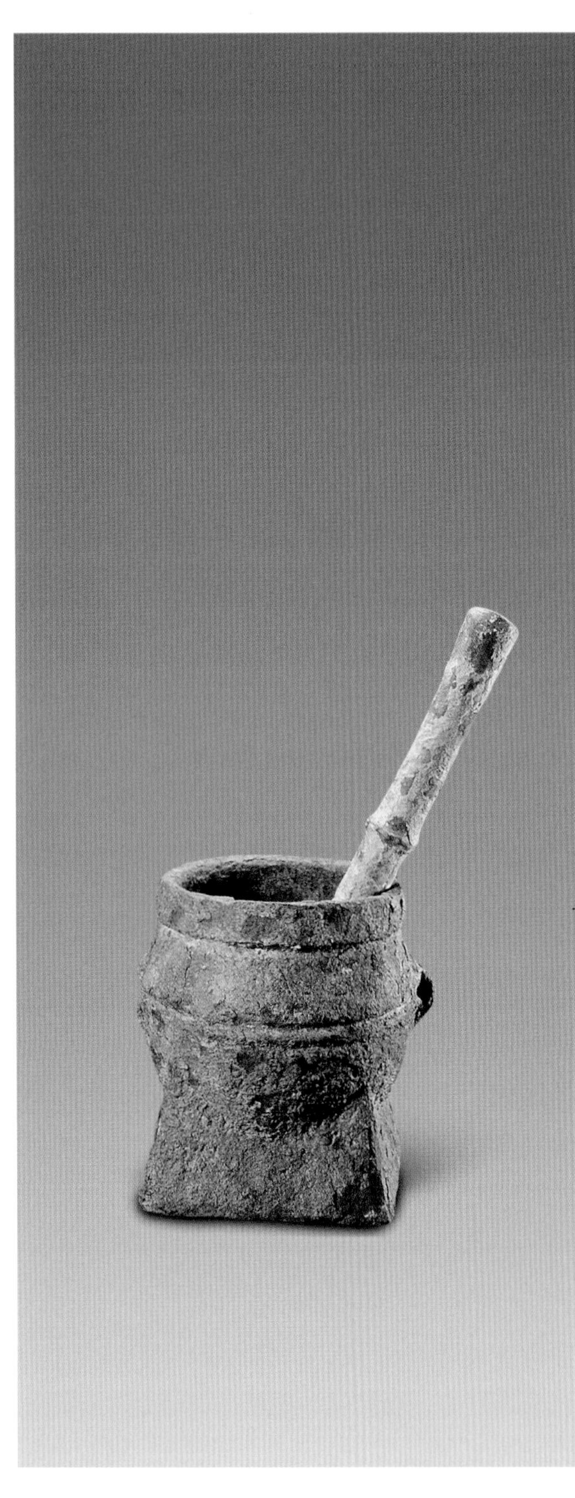

药臼

西汉

铁质

口外径 14.8 厘米，高 18 厘米

Mortar for Medicine Processing

Western Han Dynasty

Iron

Outer Diameter 14.8 cm/ Height 18 cm

圆口，鼓腹，方足。腹有两道线纹，两耳（一残）。陕西鄠邑区西汉遗址出土。

陕西医史博物馆藏

The mortar has a circular mouth, a swelling belly, and a squre foot. There are two line patterns around the belly part. The utensil has two ears (one is broken). This piece was unearthed in Heritage Site of the Western Han Dynasty in Huyi District County, Shaanxi Province.

Preserved in Shaanxi Museum of Medical History

華

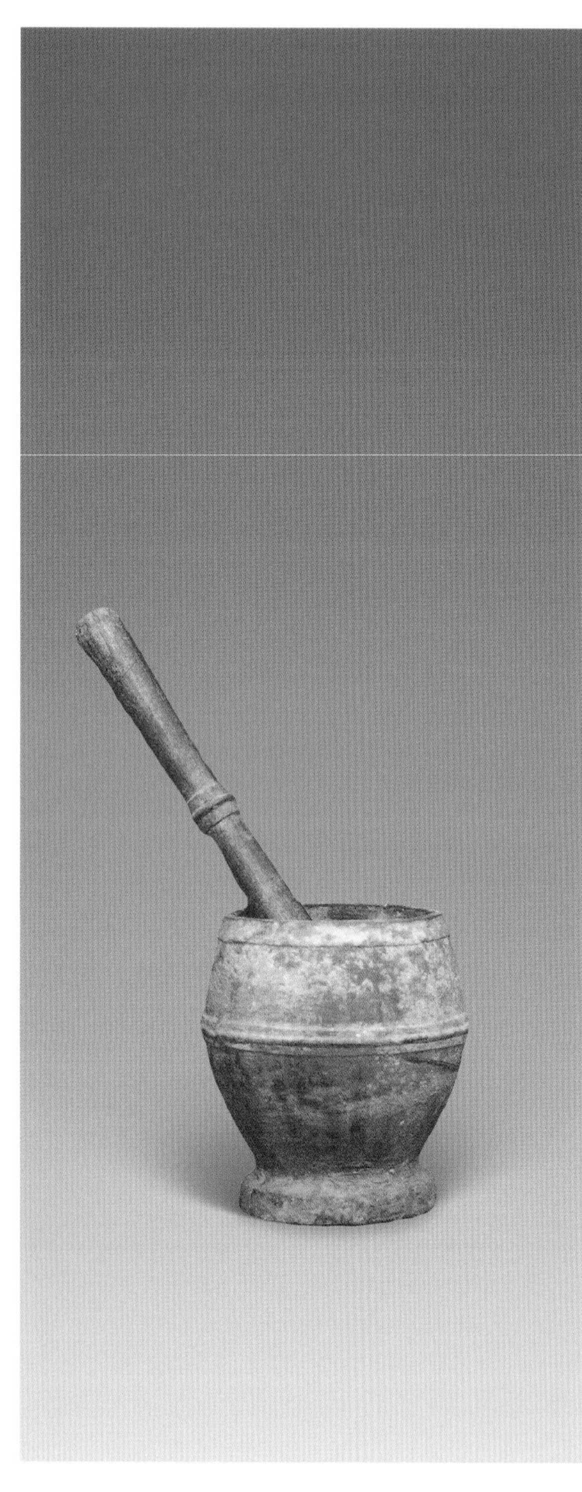

药臼（附杵）

西汉

铜质

口径 9.5 厘米，腹围 42 厘米，臼高 14.4 厘米；头径 3.3 厘米，杵长 30.8 厘米

Mortar and Pestle for Medicine Processing

Western Han Dynasty

Copper

Caliber 9.5 cm/ Belly Diameter 42 cm/ Height 14.4 cm; Head Diameter 3.3 cm/ Pestle Length 30.8 cm

臼腰有带状纹饰。杵上中部有带状纹。器物完整精致。20世纪70年代初于陕西咸阳北杜出土。

陕西医史博物馆藏

A strip pattern is ornamented on the waist of the mortar and on the upper middle part of the pestle. They are exquisite and intact. In the early 1970s, this piece was unearthed in Beidu Township, Xianyang, Shaanxi Province.

Preserved in Shaanxi Museum of Medical History

華

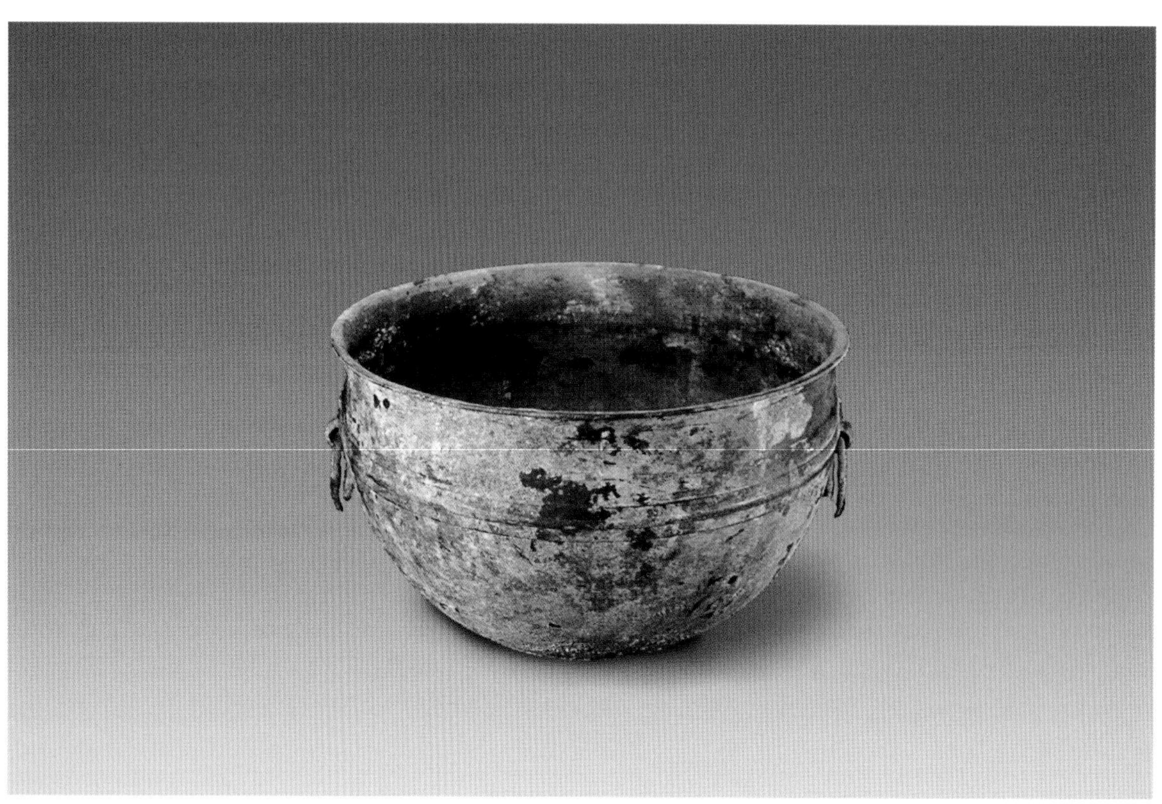

药釜

西汉

铜质

口径 21.7 厘米，底径 13 厘米，腹围 67 厘米，高 13 厘米

Cauldron for Medicine Processing

Western Han Dynasty

Copper

Caliber 21.7 cm/ Base Diameter 13 cm/ Belly Diameter 67 cm/ Height 13 cm

口微侈，腹有带状纹饰，两侧有兽面耳及提环。20 世纪 70 年代初于陕西咸阳北杜出土。

陕西医史博物馆藏

The cauldron has a slight wide mouth. A strip pattern is decorated around the belly and both sides are decorated with two animal-face ears and two lifting rings. In the early 1970s, this piece was unearthed in Beidu Township, Xianyang, Shaanxi Province.

Preserved in Shaanxi Museum of Medical History

華

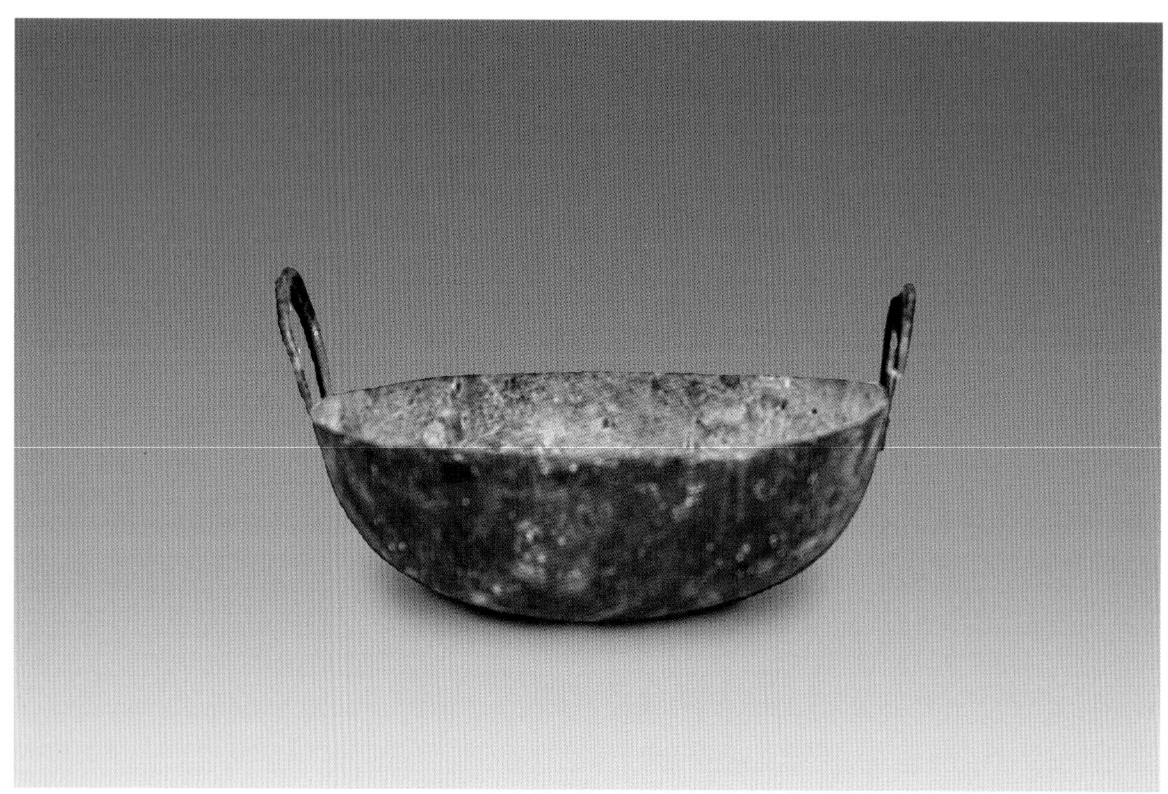

铜膏药锅

汉

铜质

口径 34 厘米，通高 18 厘米，锅高 12.5 厘米，重 2800 克

Copper Pot for Making Plaster

Han Dynasty

Copper

Caliber 34 cm/ Height 18 cm/ Depth 12.5 cm/ Weight 2,800 g

敞口，立耳，圜底。炊器，医药器具。有残。武子望后人捐赠。

陕西医史博物馆藏

The copper pot is a cooking vessel or a medicine-making vessel with an open mouth, two prick ears, and a circular base. It is partly damaged. It was donated by the descendant of Wu Ziwang.

Preserved in Shaanxi Museum of Medical History

華

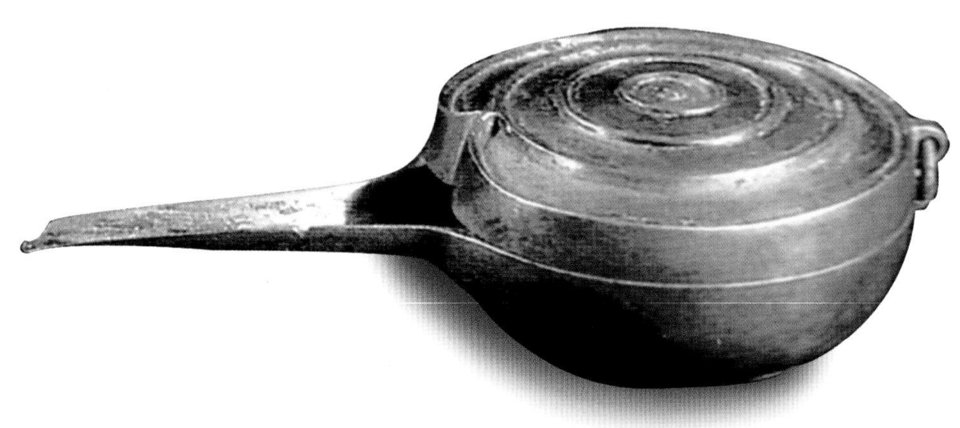

长流银匜

西汉

银质

口径 6.4 厘米，流长 6.6 厘米，高 3 厘米

Long Flow Silver Yi (ancient Chinese water vessel)

Western Han Dynasty

Silver

Caliber 6.4 cm/ Length of the spout 6.6 cm/ Height 3 cm

口沿有一细长流，流底与匜低相通。器上有盖，形似覆盘，盖面有凸弦纹四周，中心为一乳钉。盖与身间用活动环钮相连。银匜与银漏斗配合使用，为抢救危重病人的灌药器。1968 年，西汉满城陵钟山靖王刘胜墓出土。

河北博物院藏

The piece is a ladle. There is a long narrow spout on the edge of the mouth. The spout is connected with the base of the vessel. The vessel has a plate-like cover ornamented with convex string pattern centered with a small nail design. The cover is linked to the body by a mobilizable loop. The silver gourd-shaped ladle is used with a silver funnel as a drencher to save critical patients. In 1968, this piece was unearthed in the Mausoleum of Liu Sheng, a feudatory king of the Western Han Dynasty.

Preserved in Hebei Museum

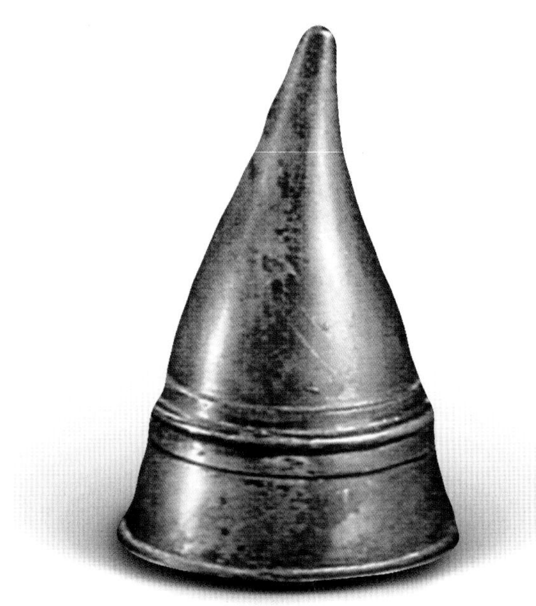

银漏斗

西汉

银质

口径 3.8 厘米，高 5.2 厘米

银漏斗侈口，口沿平折，漏口扁圆，尖底作漏，器身饰宽带纹一周。银漏斗与匜银配合使用，为抢救危重病人的灌药器。

河北博物院藏

Silver Funnel

Western Han Dynasty

Silver

Caliber 3.8 cm/ Height 5.2 cm

The silver funnel has a wide circular mouth with a flat-folded edge. The base is tightened into an oblate ventage. The body is decorated with a circle of wide strip pattern. It is used with a silver gourd-shaped ladle as a drencher to save critical patients.

Preserved in Hebei Museum

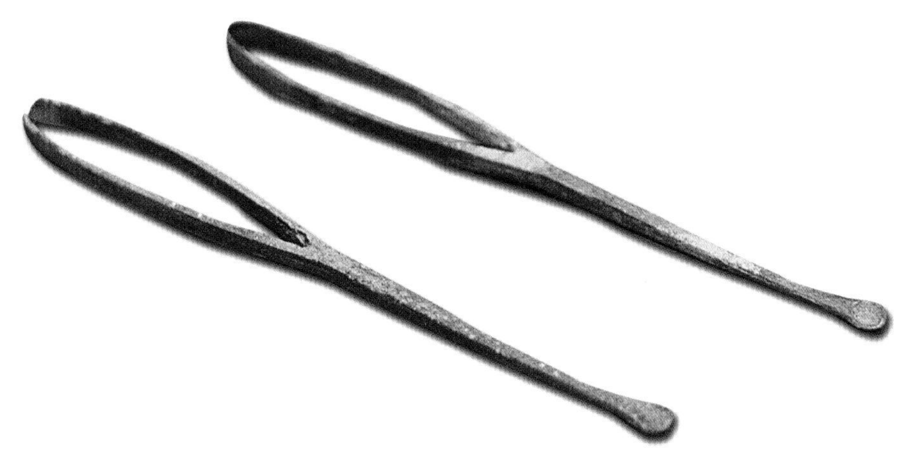

两用镊子

汉

铜质

长 13 厘米

一端为镊，另一端为药勺。镊子至今仍富有弹性。

首都博物馆藏

Dual-use Tweezer

Han Dynasty

Copper

Length 13 cm

The piece is a tweezer. One end of the tweezer is used to pick up medicine and the other end is used as a medicine spoon. The tweezer is still of high resilience.

Preserved in the Capital Museum

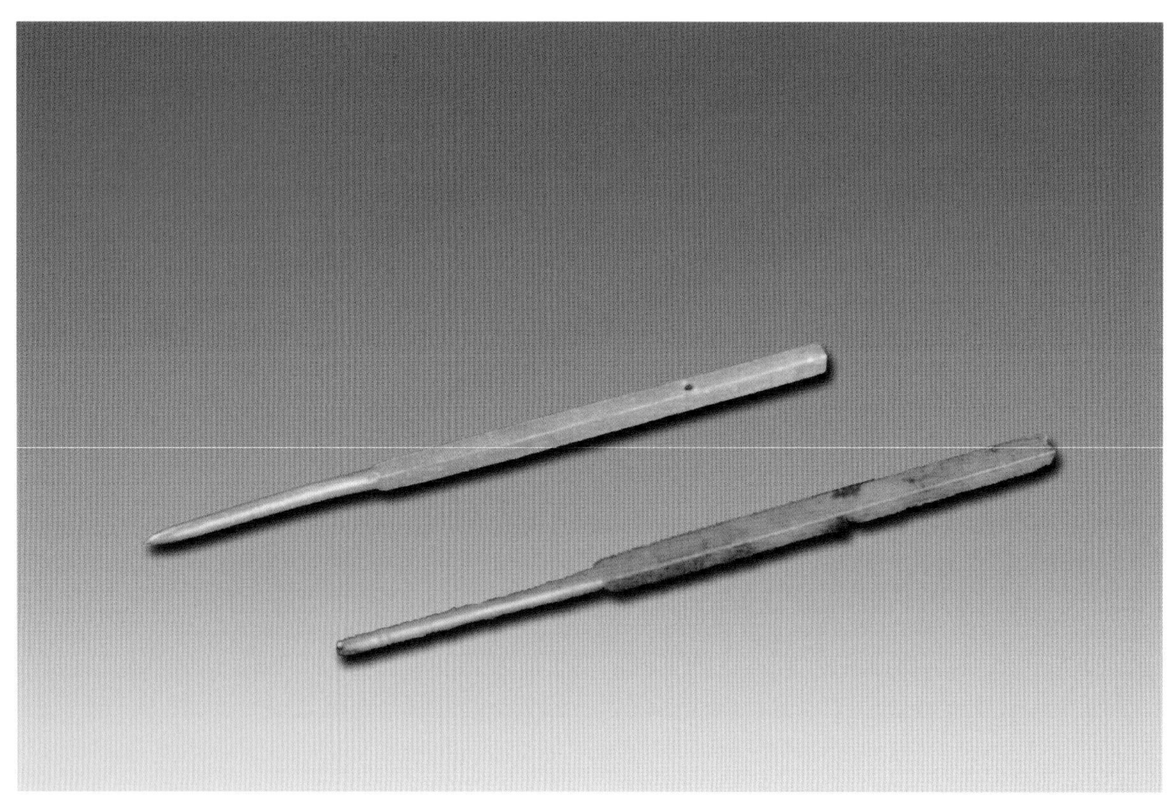

金医针、银医针

西汉

金质 / 银质

长 6.5~6.9 厘米

Gold and Silver Acupuncture Needles

Western Han Dynasty

Gold/Sliver

Length 6.5–6.9 cm

出土金针四枚，银针五枚。针上端呈方柱形柄，有一小孔，针尖稍钝，不同的针有不同用途，疗效也不同。此为我国目前发现的最早的医针。1968 年，西汉满城陵中山靖王刘胜墓出土。

河北博物院藏

Four gold acupuncture needles and five silver acupuncture needles were unearthed in the Mausoleum of Liu Sheng, a Feudatory King of the Western Han Dynasty in 1968. The needle handle is square in shape with a tiny hole. The needle tip is a bit dull. Different needles are used for different purposes with different curative effects. At present, they are the earliest medical needles found in our country.

Preserved in Hebei Museum

華

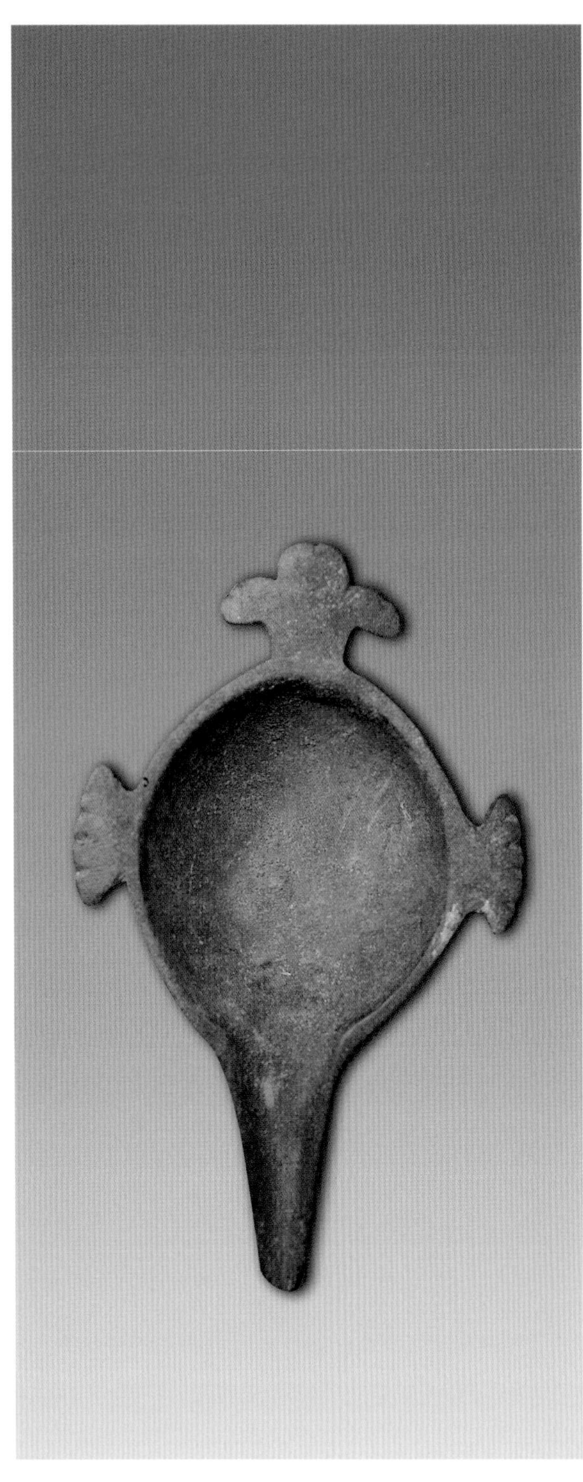

灌药器

秦汉

青铜质

长 8.4 厘米，宽 5.1 厘米

瓢形，平沿，云头纹执柄，羽翅状双耳，喙状短流。做工精细，器型厚重，急救器具。

张雅宗藏

Drench

Qin and Han Dynasty

Bronze

Length 8.4 cm/ Width 5.1 cm

The piece is in the shape of gourd ladle with a solid body. It has a flat edge, a cloud-patterned handle, two winged ears, and a short spout. It shows exquisite workmanship. It wsa used to save critical patients.

Collected by Zhang Yazong

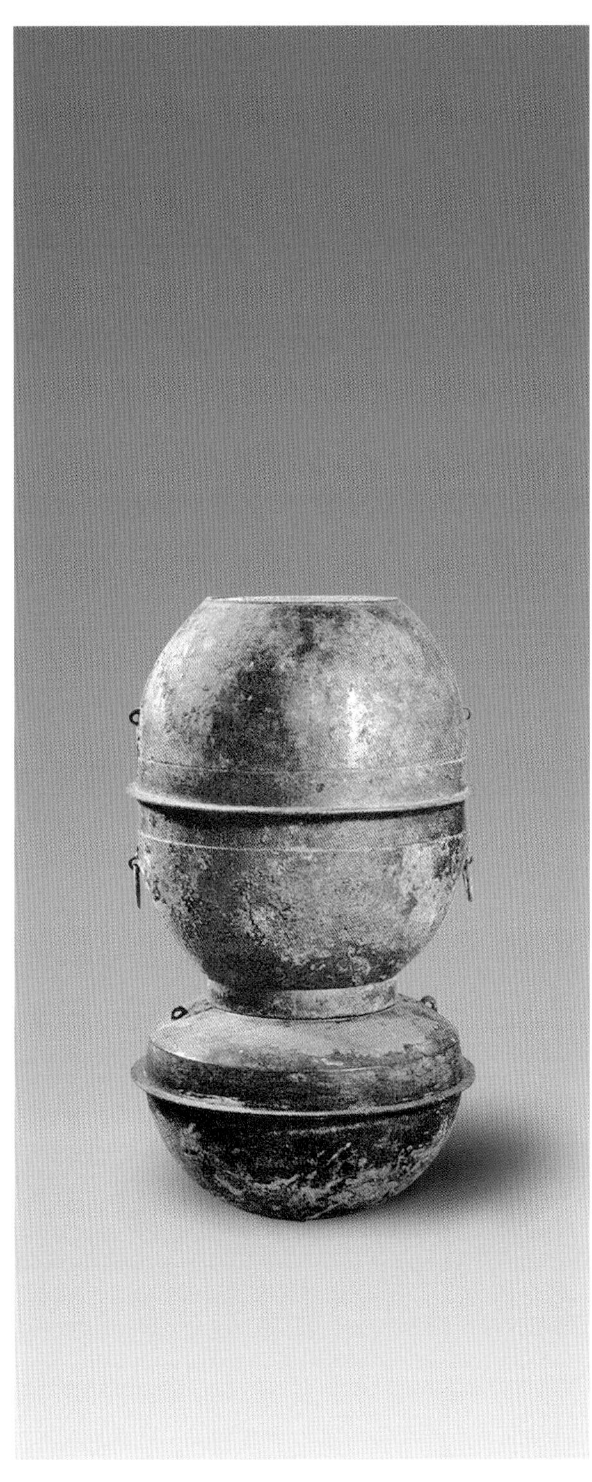

青铜甗

西汉

青铜质

通高 51 厘米

此件下部是圜底釜，釜上置甑，甑盖实系平底无孔之甑，显是一件盛贮器。由于釜是圆底无足之器，所以这套器具需与灶结合方可使用。山西省平朔供应公司出土。

山西省考古研究所藏

Bronze Yan

Western Han Dynasty

Bronze

Total Height 51 cm

Its lower part is a cauldron with a circular base. Above the base is a steamer whose cover actually is also a flat steamer without holes. There is no foot on the circular basel; thus, it must be used with a kitchen range. It was unearthed from the Pingshuo Supply Corporation in Shanxi Province.

Preserved in Shanxi Provincial Institute of Archaeology

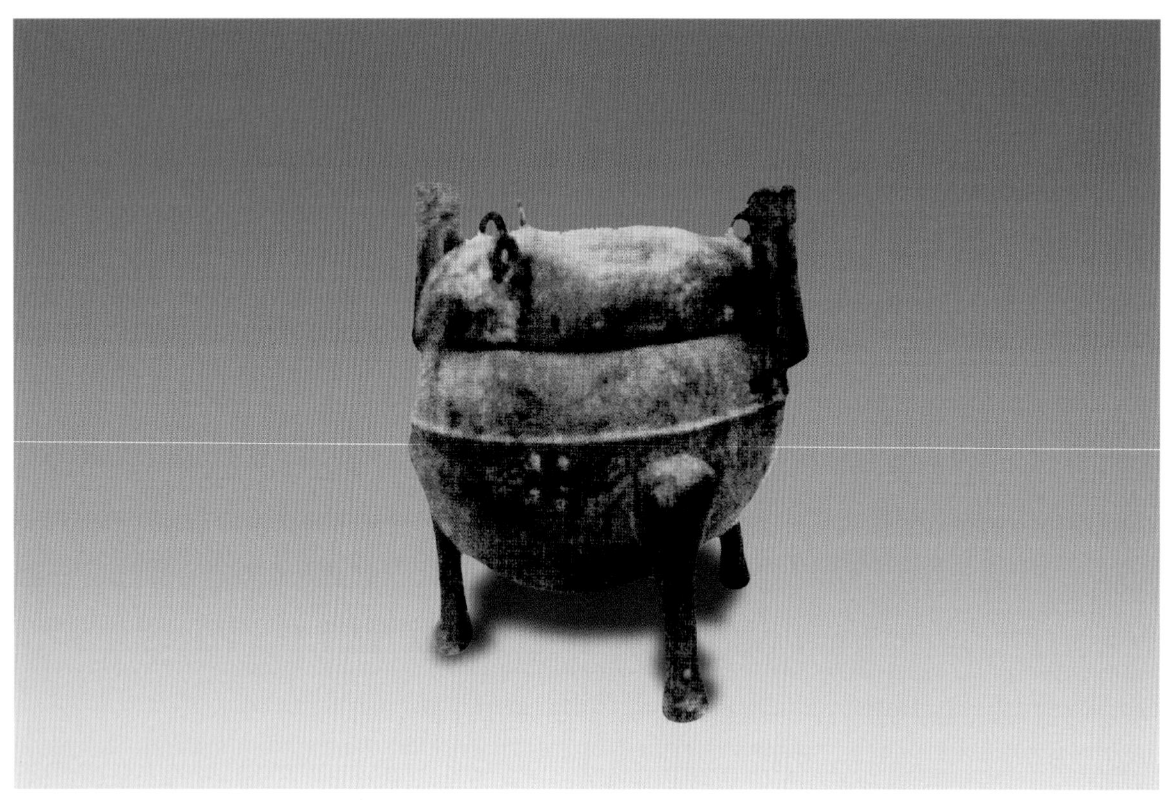

丹鼎

西汉

铜质

口径 26 厘米，耳宽 10.9 厘米，足高 16.5 厘米

Cinnabar Tripod

Western Han Dynasty

Copper

Caliber 26 cm/ Width of the ears 10.9 cm/ Height of the feet 16.5 cm

腹中部有一周凸棱。出土时内有丹药250多粒及朱砂、蚌壳等。山东巨野哀王刘髆墓出土。

山东省巨野县文化馆藏

The piece is a tripod. A convex ridge is circled around the middle part of the belly. There were more than 250 immortality pills, cinnabar, and clamshell as well. This piece was unearthed in the Mausoleum of Liu Bo, a baron in the Western Han Dynasty, in Juye County, Shandong Province.

Preserved in Juye Cultural Center of Shandong Province

華

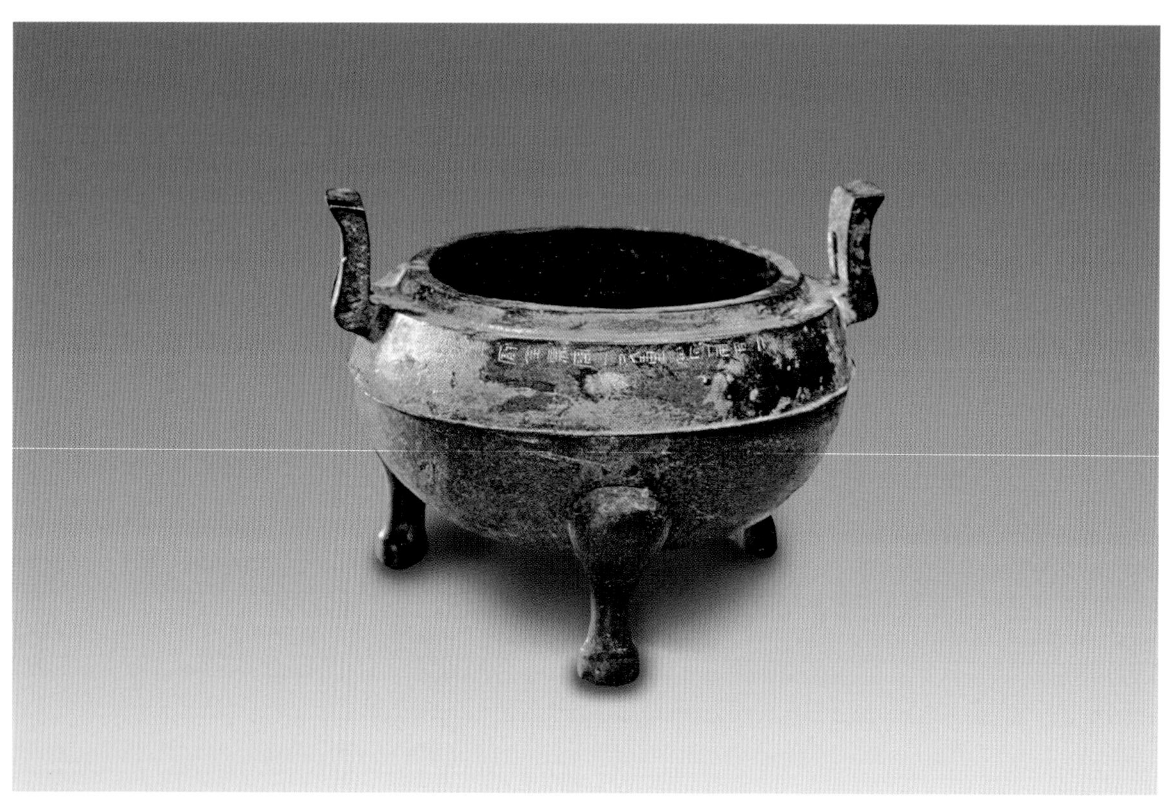

咸阳临平共厨鼎

秦

铜质

口径 14.5 厘米，通高 14.5 厘米

Xian Yang Linping Cooking Tripod

Qin Dynasty

Copper

Caliber 14.5 cm/ Height 14.5 cm

敛口平唇，鼓腹圆底，附耳，三蹄足，失盖。腹部有凸弦纹一周。

山西博物院藏

The tripod has a tightened mouth with a flat edge, a swelling belly, a circular base, two ears, and three horseshoe-shaped feet. Its cover was lost. The belly is patterned with a circle of convex string.

Preserved in Shanxi Museum

華

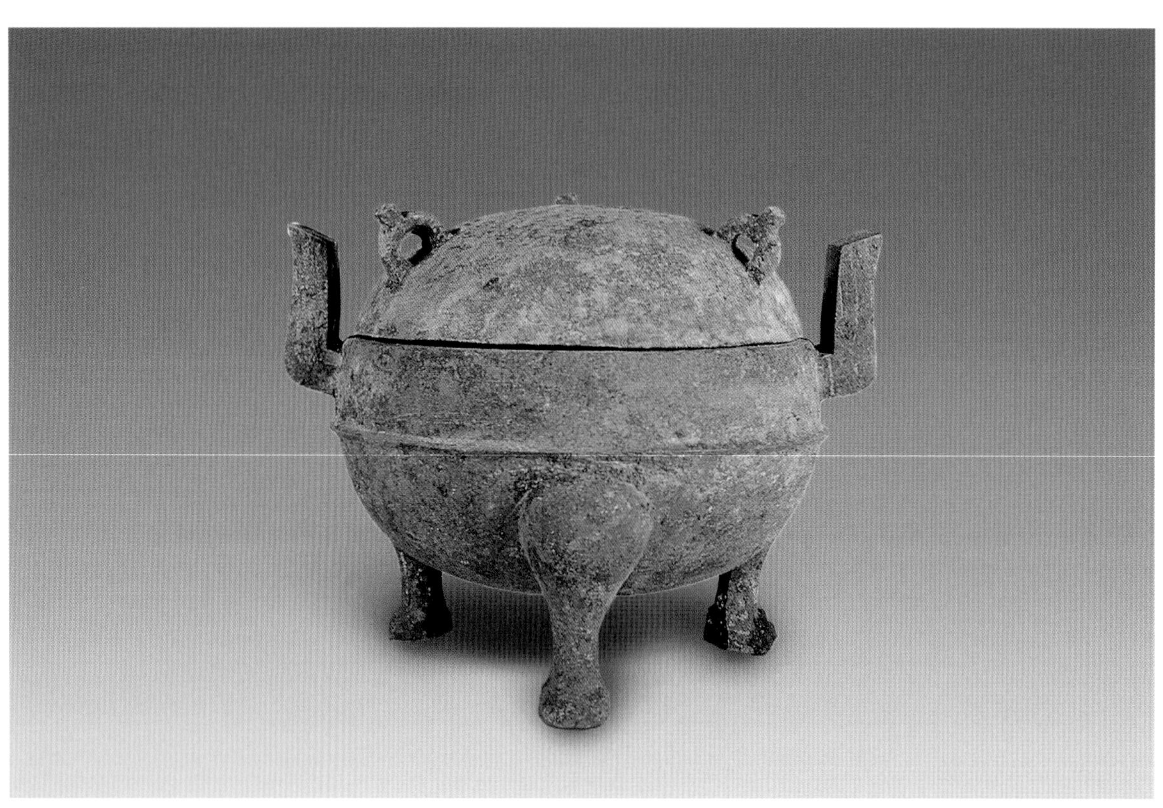

青铜盛羹鼎

秦至西汉初

青铜质

口径 15 厘米，高 16 厘米

Bronze Soup Tripod

From Qin Dynasty to Early Western Han Dynasty

Bronze

Caliber 15 cm/ Height 16 cm

出土时鼎内盛有半腹的食物，因年代久远，颜色已变为深绿或浅蓝。河南省济源市轵国故城桐花沟墓地出土。

河南省文物考古研究院藏

The piece is a tripod. Half of the belly was still filled with food when this piece was unearthed. The food has turned dark green or light blue due to age. This piece was unearthed from the Mausoleum in Tonghuagou Village, site of an ancient Country Zhi, in Jiyuan, Henan Province.

Preserved in Henan Provincial Institute of Cultural Heritage and Archaeology

華

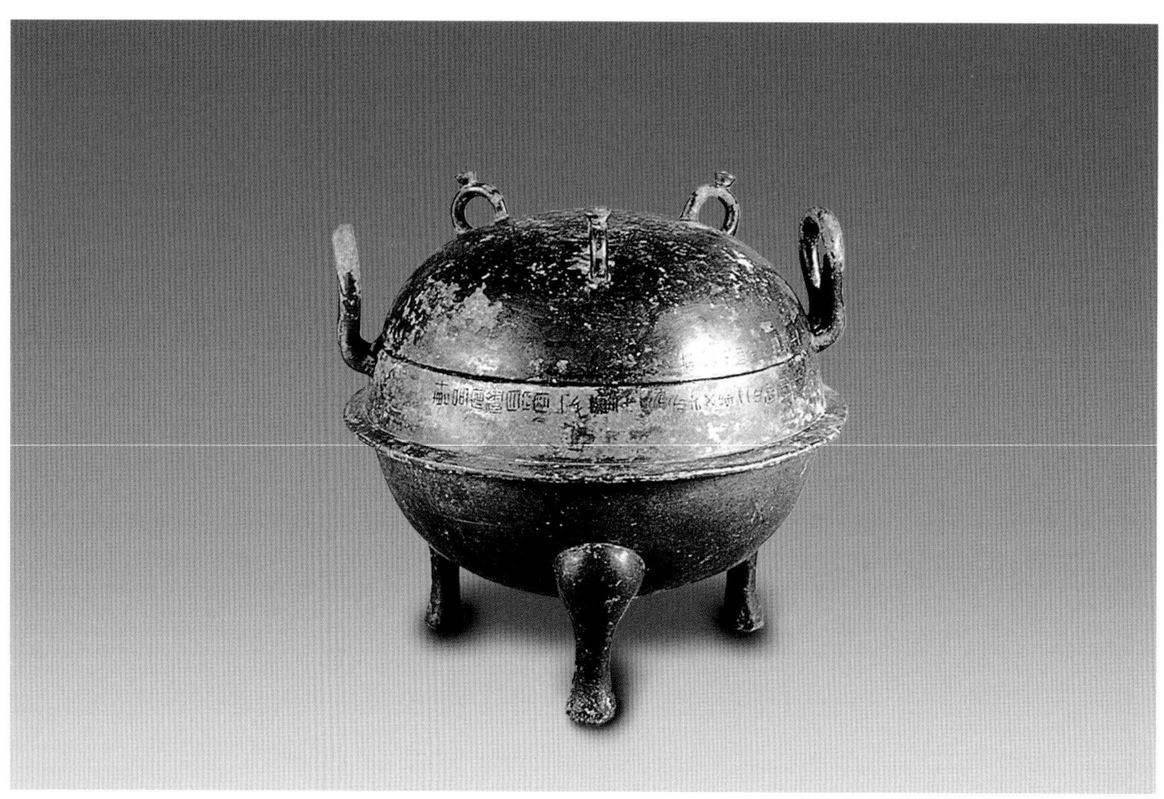

青铜盛羹鼎

西汉

青铜质

腹径 20.5 厘米，高 19.7 厘米

Bronze Soup Tripod

Western Han Dynasty

Bronze

Belly Diameter 20.5 cm/ Height 19.7 cm

这是一件传世的西汉铜器，其造型是典型的西汉风格，与考古发掘出土的汉代铜鼎非常相近。造型纹饰典雅古朴。鼎口和盖口上各有一行隶体的阴刻铭文，记载了有关鼎的身世，成为汉代考古研究的重要史料。鼎身的铭文共 23 字，曰“博邑家铜鼎容一斗重十一斤永光五年河东平阳造”。

北京大学赛克勒考古与艺术博物馆藏

The piece is a bronze vessel handed down from the Western Han Dynasty with a classic Western Han designing style. It is very similar to other unearthed archaeological bronze tripods of the Han Dynasty. The shape and the ornaments are elegant and simple in design. There is a line of engraved inscription in official script on both the mouth of the vessel and its cover which records its origin. This provides important historical data for archaeological study of the Han Dynasty. There are 23 words inscribed on the body, saying that “This vessel belongs to Boyi’s Family. Its capacity is one Dou. Its weight is one Jin. It was made in Pingyang, Hedong County, in 39 B.C.”

Preserved in Arthur M. Sackler Museum of Art and Archaeology at Peking University

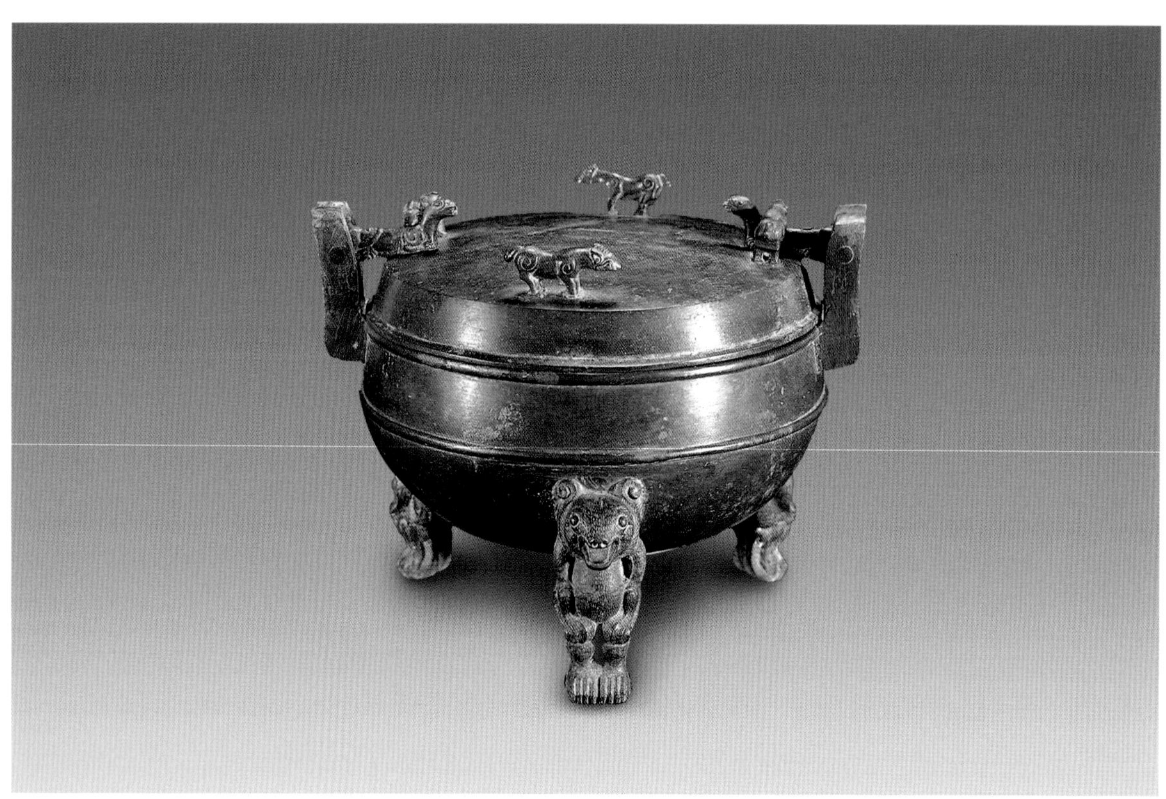

四兽组熊足铜鼎

西汉

铜质

口径 17.2 厘米，腹径 19.6 厘米，通高 18.1 厘米

Copper Tripod with Four Animal-shaped Buttons and Three Bear-shaped Feet

Western Han Dynasty

Copper

Caliber 17.2 cm/ Belly Diameter 19.6 cm/ Height 18.1 cm

鼎身作子口微敛，圆底，三熊足，熊作蹲立状。腹两侧附长方形耳，耳上有可翻转的小兽钮。腹有一周凸弦纹。鼎盖似覆盘，其上有四小兽作等距离环立。鼎盖扣合后，将鼎耳兽纽翻转于盖上，向左转动鼎盖，盖上小兽头部恰好卡于鼎耳兽钮上，使鼎盖闭锁。

河北博物院藏

The tripod has a slightly tightened mouth, a circular base, and three bear-shaped feet. The bears stand in a squatting down position. On each side of the belly are two rectangular ears with small turnover animal-shaped buttons. Meanwhile the belly is patterned with a circle of convex string. The plate-like cover is designed with four animal sculptures standing equidistantly in a circle. If the cover is rotated to left after it is put on the pod, the four animal sculptures will block the buttons, and thus the cover will be locked.

Preserved in Hebei Museum

華

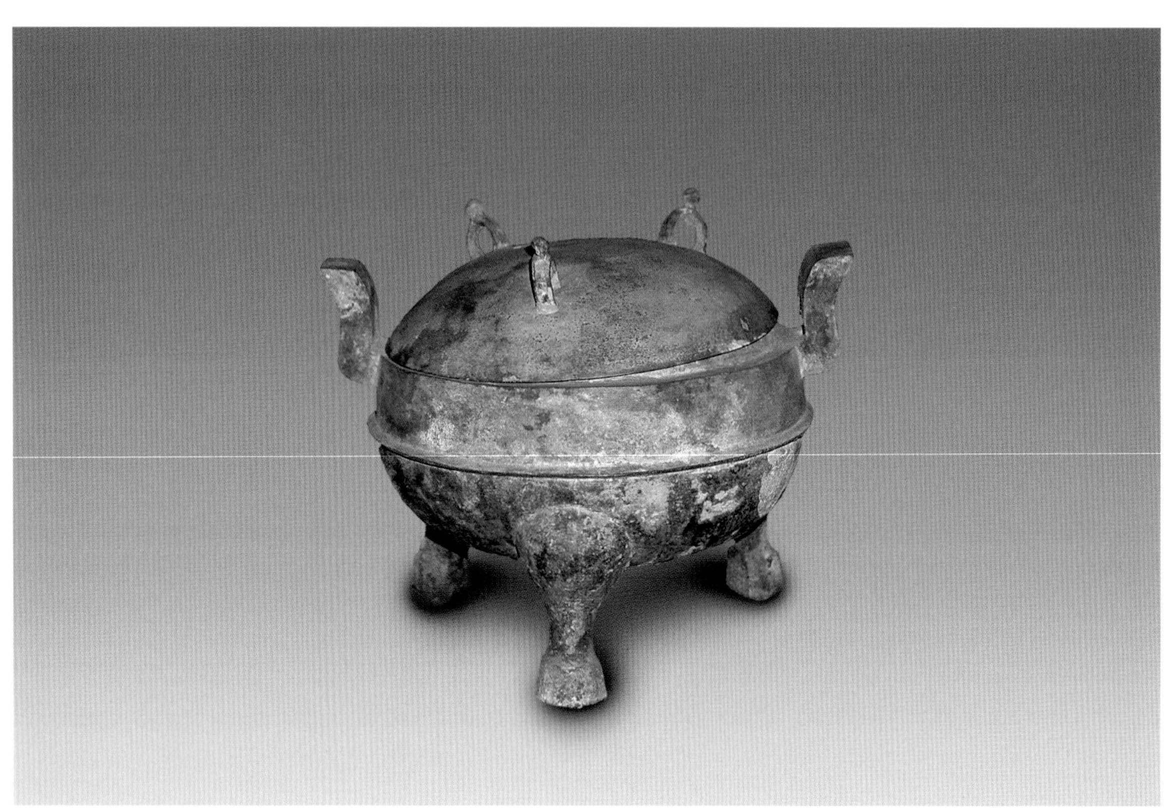

铜鼎

汉

铜质

口径 17.1 厘米，足高 9 厘米，通高 18.2 厘米，重 2510 克

Copper Tripod

Han Dynasty

Copper

Caliber 17.1 cm/ Height of the feet 9 cm/ Height 18.2 cm/ Weight 2,510g

子母口，附耳，三蹄足，带一盖，盖顶有三环。礼器。完整无损陕西省西安市征集。

陕西医史博物馆藏

The tripod has two matching mouths, two ears, three horseshoe-shaped feet, and a cover with three rings on its top. It is a sacrificial vessel and has been preserved intact. It was collected from Xi'an, Shaanxi Province.

Preserved in Shaanxi Museum of Medical History

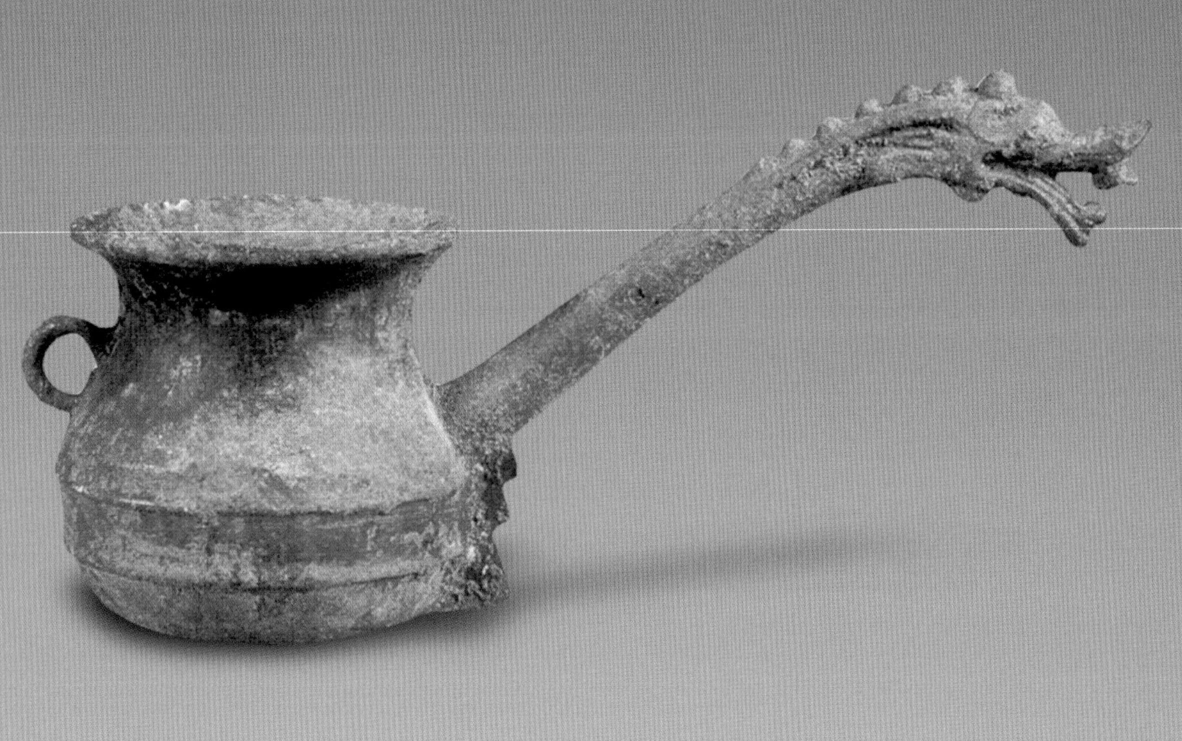

龙首柄青铜鏊

西汉

青铜质

在汉代的炊具系列中，釜是一种基本的形态。釜之有耳者即是鏊，亦为汉代常见的器形。而鏊之有柄者较少，其形制颇类釜之带柄而叫做“锜”的另一类炊具。因此，这件介于釜与锜之间的带柄鏊，可作为汉代炊具的中介形态。贵州省水城县黄土坡出土。

贵州省博物馆藏

Bronze Pot with a Dragon-head Handle

Western Han Dynasty

Bronze

Cauldron' was a common cooking vessel in the Han Dynasty. A cauldron with ear was a pot, another common vessel in the Han Dynasty. A pot with a handle was less common, whose shape is very similar to another cooking vessel called "Qi" (an ancient Chinese cauldron with a handle). This vessel is an inter-form between cauldron and "Qi". This piece was unearthed at Huangtupo, Shuicheng County, Guizhou Province.

Preserved in Guizhou Provincial Museum

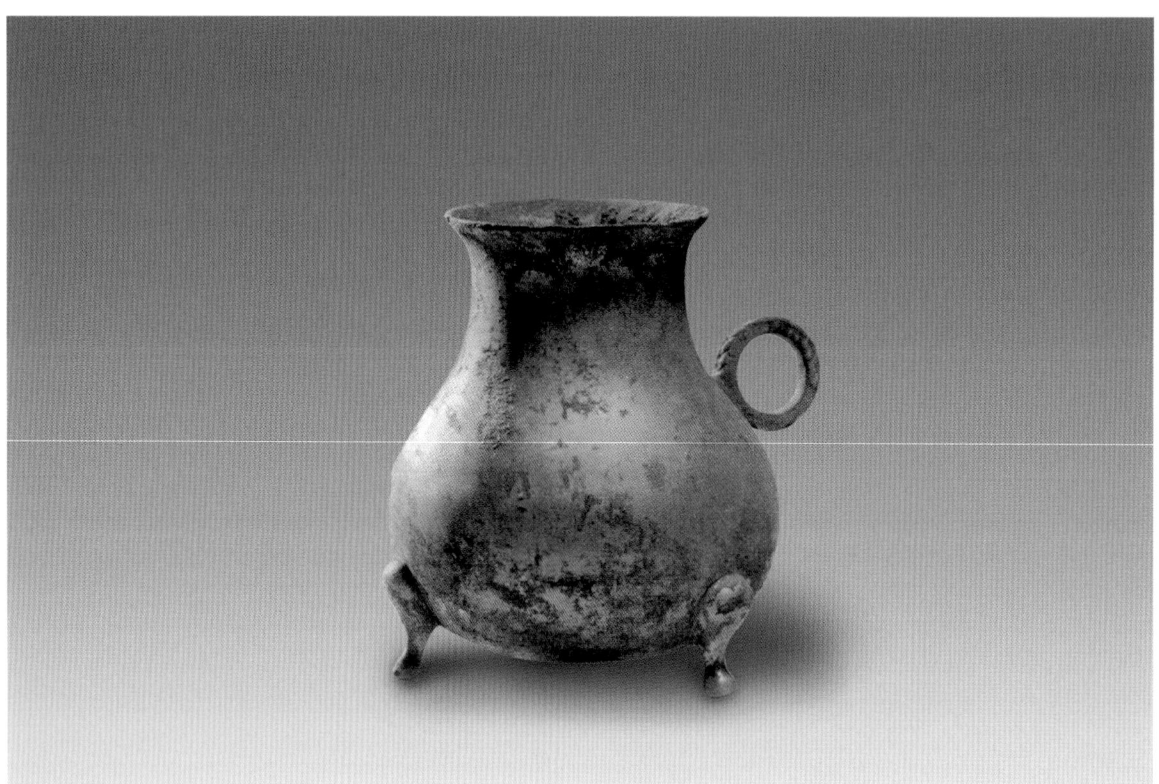

鎏金铜鍪

汉

青铜质

高 11 厘米

Gilded Copper Pot

Han Dynasty

Bronze

Height 11 cm

鍪是一种金属炊具，实际是釜的一种变体。此件敞口粗颈，腹部圆鼓而深，底下有三条较矮的兽蹄足，肩颈部有一只圆环形耳，系鍪的标准式样。表面通体鎏金，为汉代铜鍪中的精品。贵州赫章可乐出土。

贵州省博物馆藏

The piece is a metal cooking utensil, a variant of cauldron in nature. This pot has an open mouth and a thick neck. The belly is circular, swelling, and deep. Under the belly are three short horseshoe-shaped feet. On the shoulder is a circular ear which is the standard cauldron style. Gilded, it ranks high in the cauldron relics of the Han Dynasty. This piece was unearthed from Kele Mausoleum in Hezhang County, Guizhou Province.

Preserved in Guizhou Provincial Museum

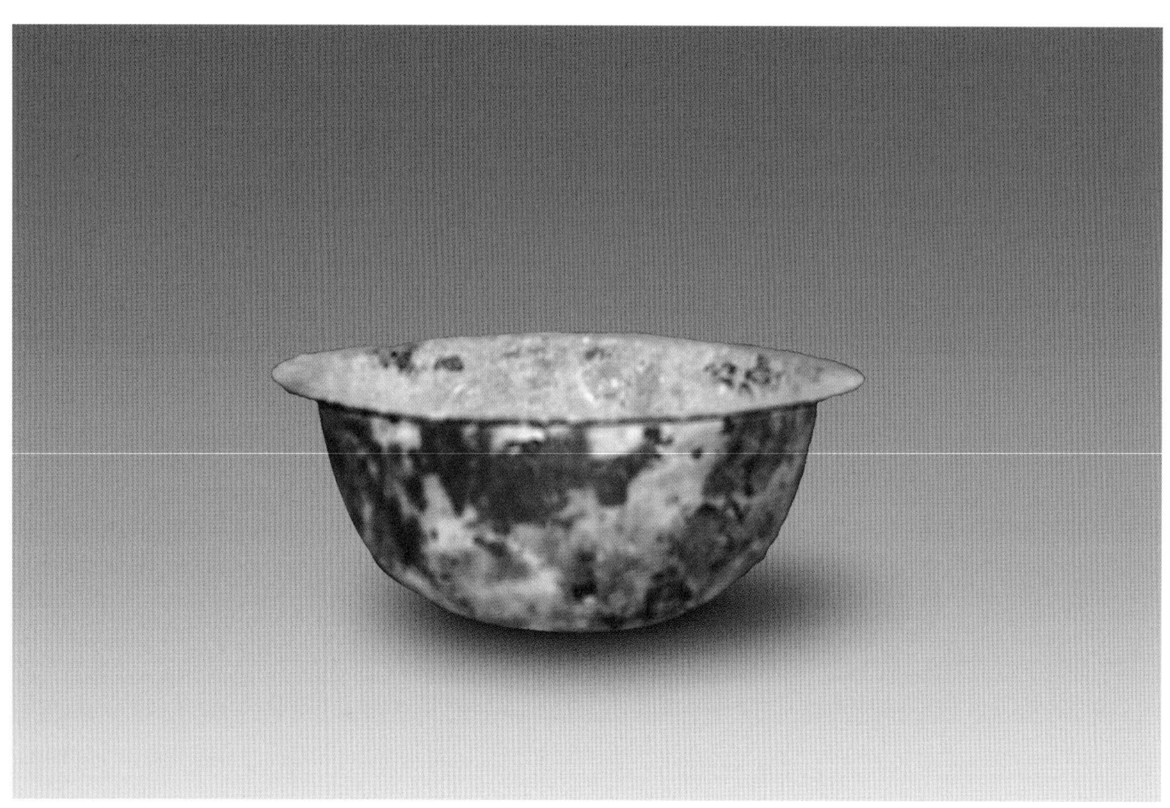

铜锅

汉

铜质

口径 21.5 厘米，口沿宽 1.6 厘米，通高 9 厘米，重 550 克

Copper Pot

Han Dynasty

Copper

Caliber 21.5 cm/ Width of the edge 1.6 cm/ Height 9 cm/ Weight 550 g

平口沿，斜腹，圆底。炊器。底有修补。

陕西医史博物馆藏

The object is a cooking utensil. The edge of the mouth is flat. It has an oblique belly and a circular base. The base was repaired.

Preserved in Shaanxi Museum of Medical History

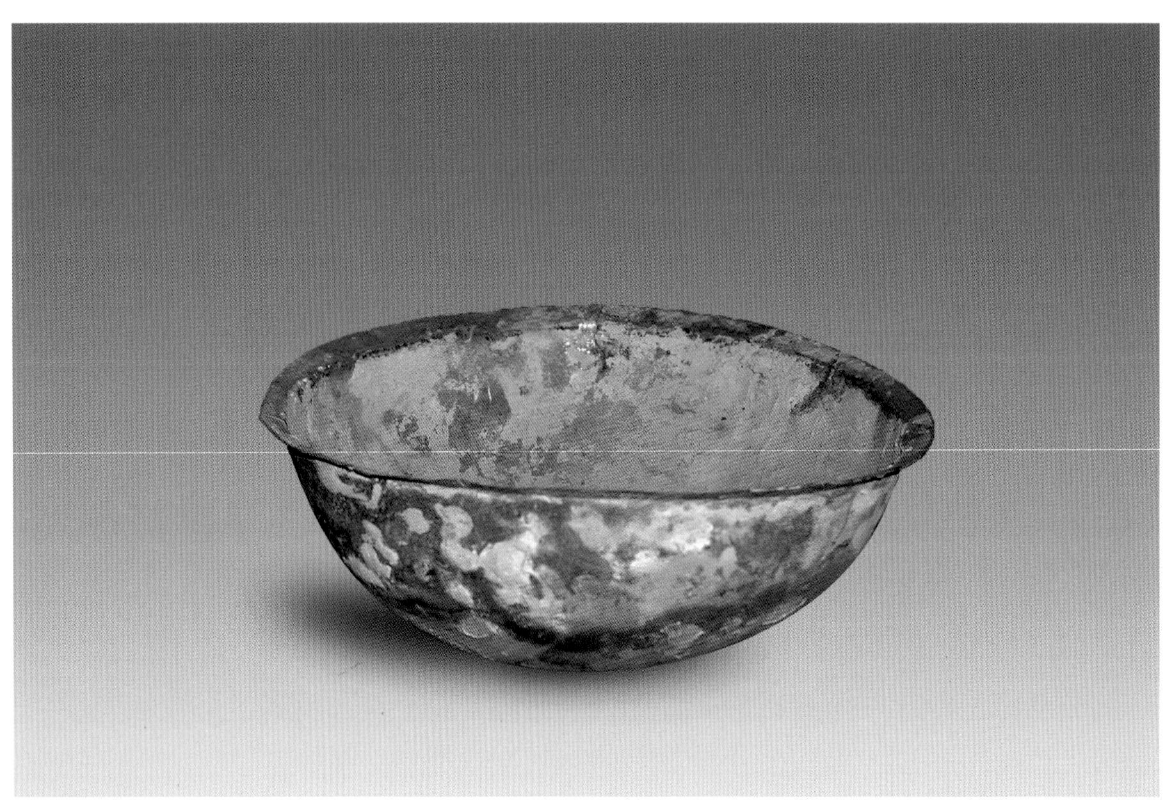

铜锅

汉

铜质

口径 22.2 厘米，通高 8.5 厘米，重 300 克

Copper Pot

Han Dynasty

Copper

Caliber 22.2 cm/ Height 8.5 cm/ Weight 300 g

平口沿，圆腹，圜底，无纹饰。炊器。口沿，底残。陕西省西安市鄠邑区征集。

陕西医史博物馆藏

The object is a cooking utensil. The edge of the mouth is flat. It has a circular belly and a circular base without ornaments. Part of the edge of the mouth and the base are damaged. It was collected from Huyi District, Xi'an, Shaanxi Province.

Preserved in Shaanxi Museum of Medical History

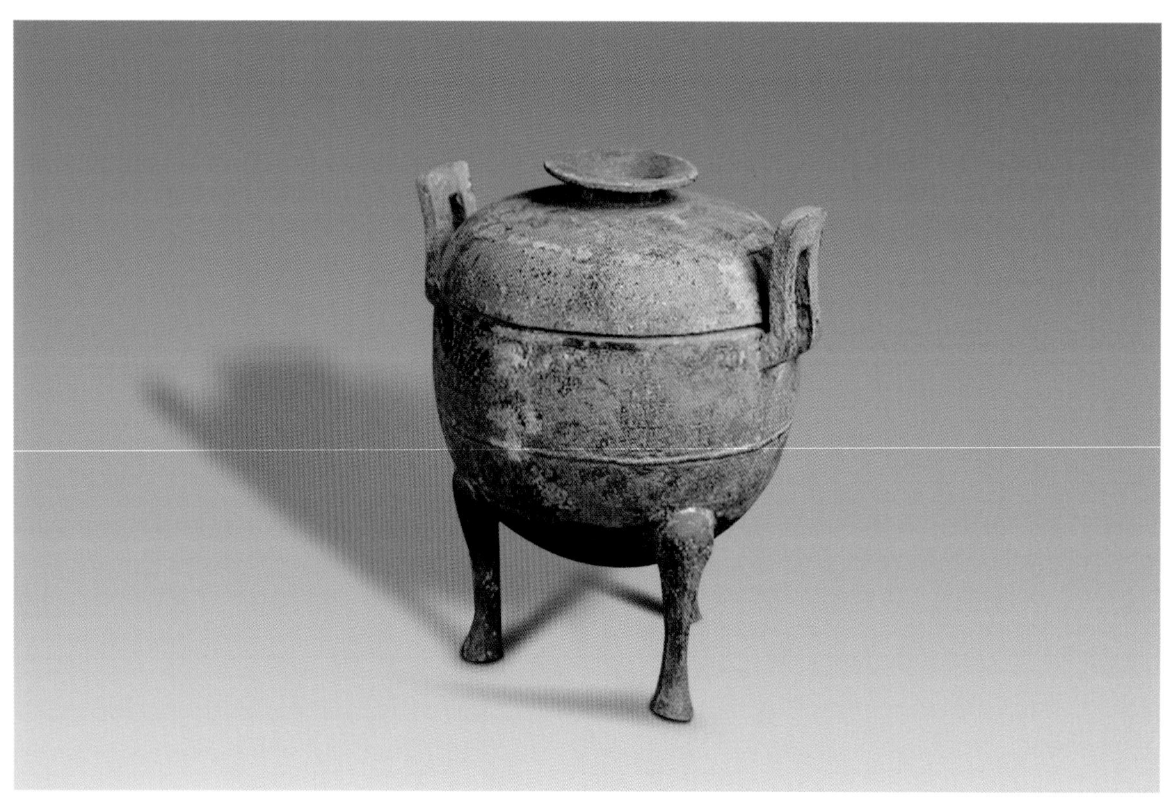

丹鼎

汉

青铜质

腹径 26 厘米，足高 10 厘米

Alchemy Ding Vessel

Han Dynasty

Bronze

Belly Diameter 26 cm/ Feet Height 10 cm

子母口，直腹，双直立桥形耳，圆底，三足，有盖，器身刻有精美的纹饰。

北京御生堂中医药博物馆藏

The vessel has a cluster mouth, a vertical belly, double straight bridge-shaped ears, a round base, three feet and a lid. The belly is carved with exquisite patterns.

Preserved in Chinese Medicine Museum of Beijing Yu Sheng Tang Drugstore

華

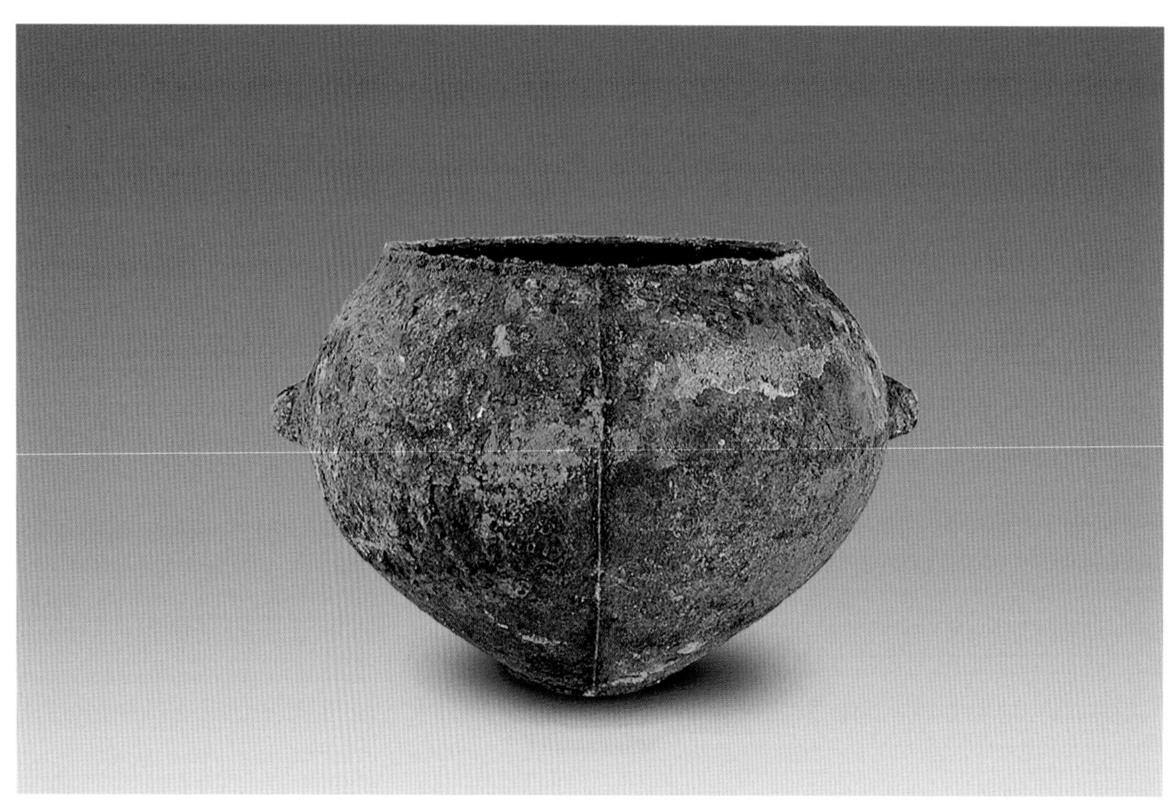

铁釜

西汉

铁质

口径 20.2 厘米，底径 8.5 厘米，高 23.2 厘米

Iron Cauldron

Western Han Dynasty

Iron

Caliber 20.2 cm/ Base Diameter 8.5 cm/ Height 23.2 cm

方唇鼓肩，腹部斜收成极小的平底。由于底部较小而难以在盛食情况下稳固自立，所以这种形态的铁釜是放置在灶上使用的。其上可以加盖，也可以置甑，与常见的汉代陶灶中的灶具组合与使用方式一致。河南省渑池县俱利城墓地出土。

河南省文物考古研究所藏

The cauldron has a square lip and protruding shoulders. The belly is tightened obliquely into a small flat base. Due to the small base, the vessel cannot stand by itself when it is filled with food. So it is used with a kitchen range. A cover or a steamer can be placed above it. This piece was unearthed from Julicheng Mausoleum in Mianchi County, Henan Province.

Preserved in Henan Provincial Institute of Cultural Heritage and Archaeology

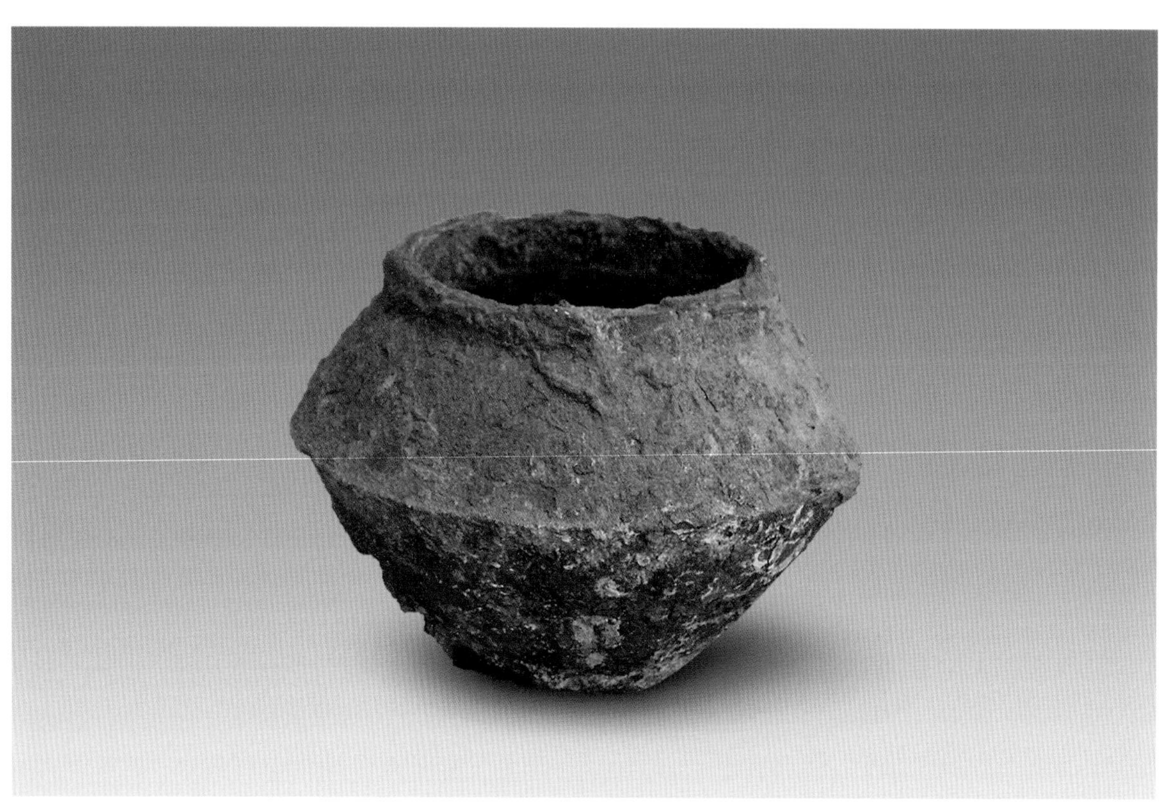

铁釜

汉

铁质

口径 8 厘米，底径 5.5 厘米，高 9 厘米，重 1000 克

Iron Cauldron

Han Dynasty

Iron

Caliber 8 cm/ Base Diameter 5.5 cm/ Height 9 cm/ Weight 1,000 g

直口鼓腹，平底，腹中间有一道凸棱，无纹饰，表面粗糙。炊器，完整无损。

陕西医史博物馆藏

The utensil has a straight mouth, a swelling belly, and a flat base. A convex ridge is around the middle part of the belly. There are no decorating patterns on the vessel. The surface is rough. It is a cooking utensil preserved well.

Preserved in Shaanxi Museum of Medical History

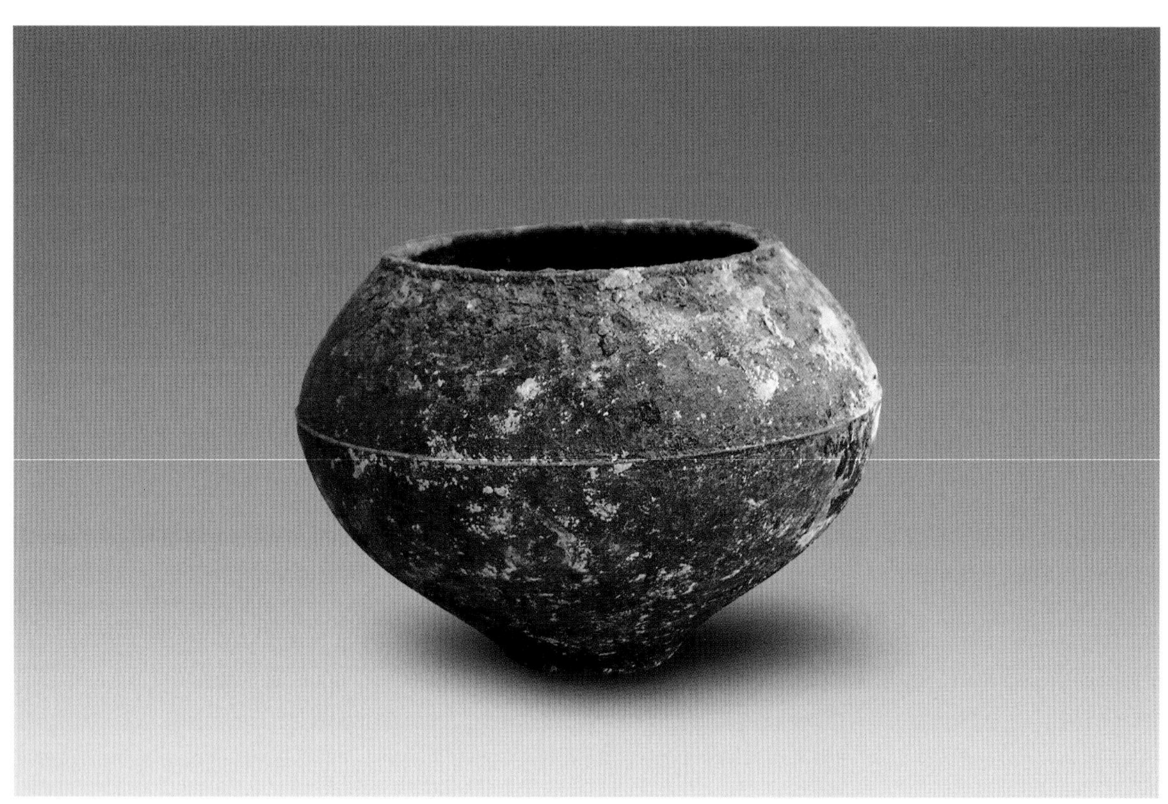

铁釜

汉

铁质

长口径 18.5 厘米，底径 9 厘米，高 19 厘米，重 4300 克

Iron Cauldron

Han Dynasty

Iron

Caliber 18.5 cm/ Base Diameter 9 cm/ Height 19 cm/ Weight 4,300 g

圆口，鼓腹，平底，腹中部有一道凸棱，无纹饰。炊具，完整无损。

陕西医史博物馆藏

The piece is a cooking utensil. It has a circular mouth, a swelling belly, and a flat base. There is a convex ridge on the middle part of the belly. There is no pattern decorating the vessel, which is well preserved.

Preserved in Shaanxi Museum of Medical History

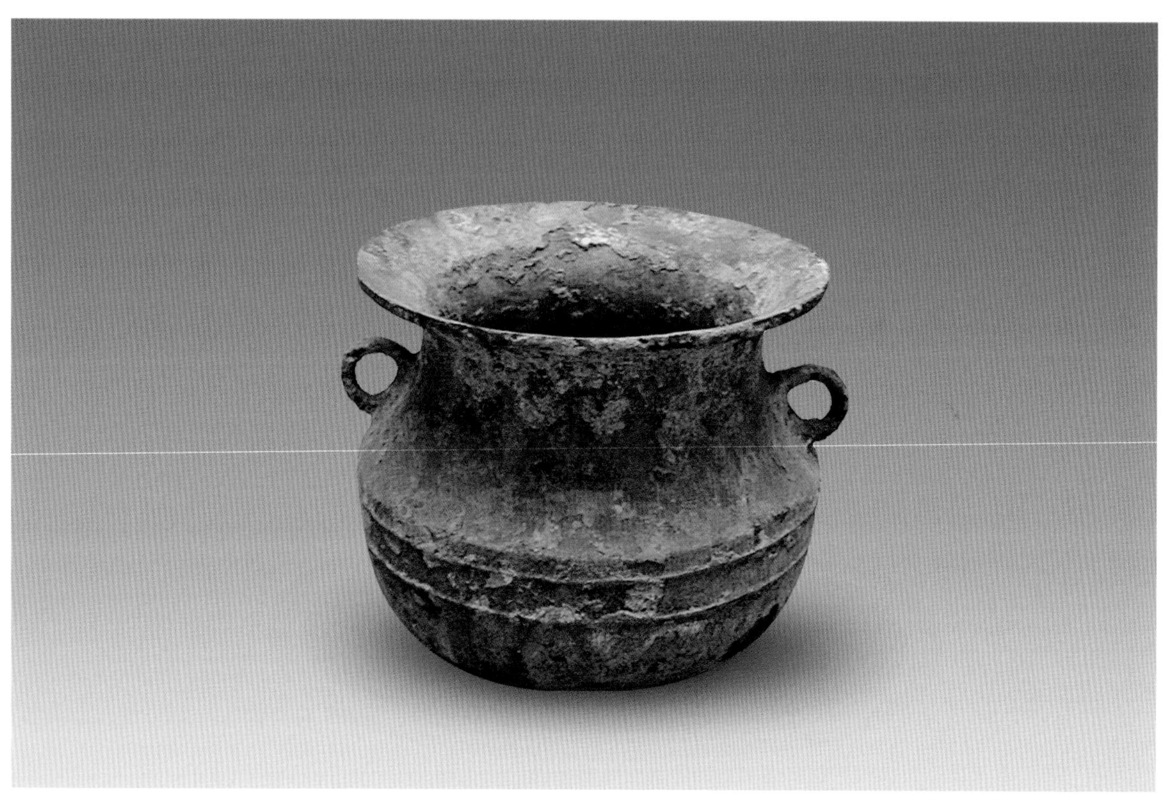

釜

汉

铜质

口径 19 厘米，高 22 厘米

Cauldron

Han Dynasty

Copper

Caliber 19 cm/ Height 22 cm

敞口，束颈，平底，腹部有三道旋纹，双环形耳，由民间征集。

成都中医药大学中医药传统文化博物馆藏

The cauldron has an open mouth, a tightened neck, a flat base, and two annular ears. There are three lines of vortex pattern around the belly. It was collected from the folks.

Preserved in Museum of Traditional Chinese Medicine Culture, Chengdu University of Traditional Chinese Medicine

華

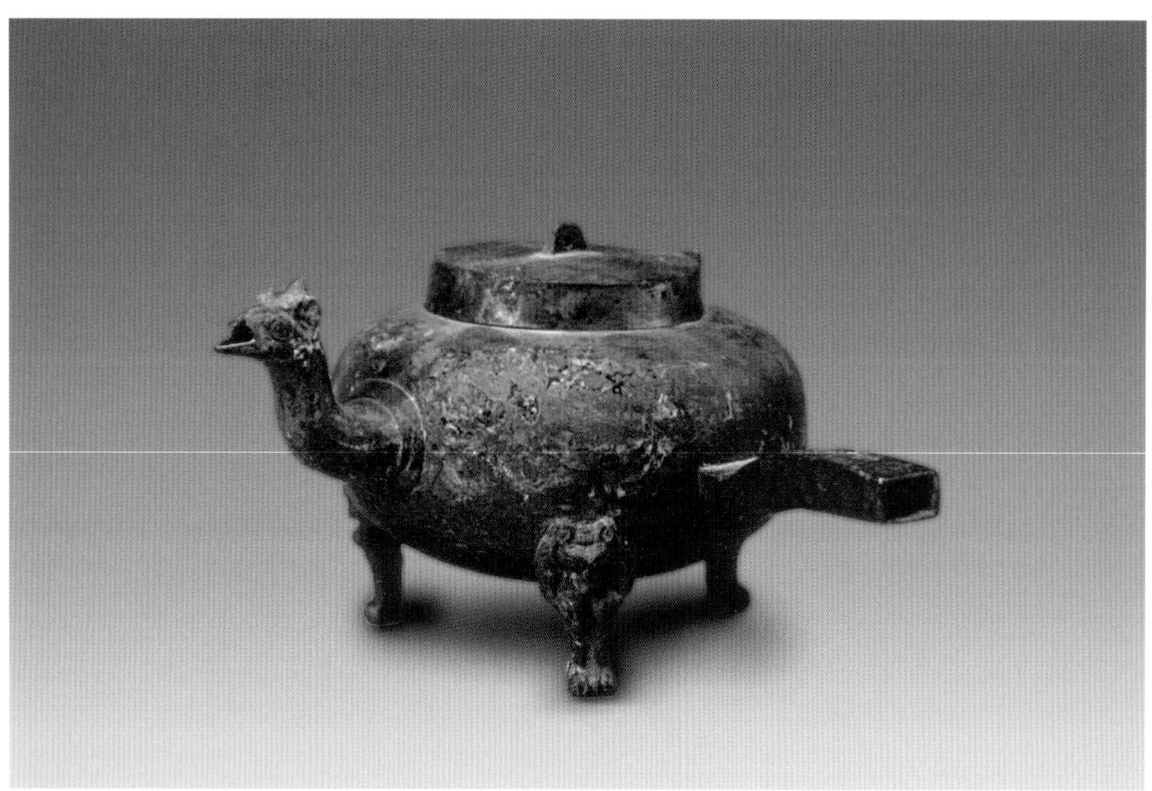

孙氏家鐎

汉

铜质

腹径 15 厘米，柄长 27 厘米，通高 12.7 厘米

Jiao of Sun Family

Han Dynasty

Copper

Belly Diameter 15 cm/ Handle Length 27 cm/ Total Height 12.7 cm

扁圆体，子母口，有盖，鼓腹，圆底，下承三熊形足。

山西博物院藏

The piece is oblate in shape with two matching mouths, a cover, a swelling belly, and three bear-shaped feet.

Preserved in Shanxi Museum

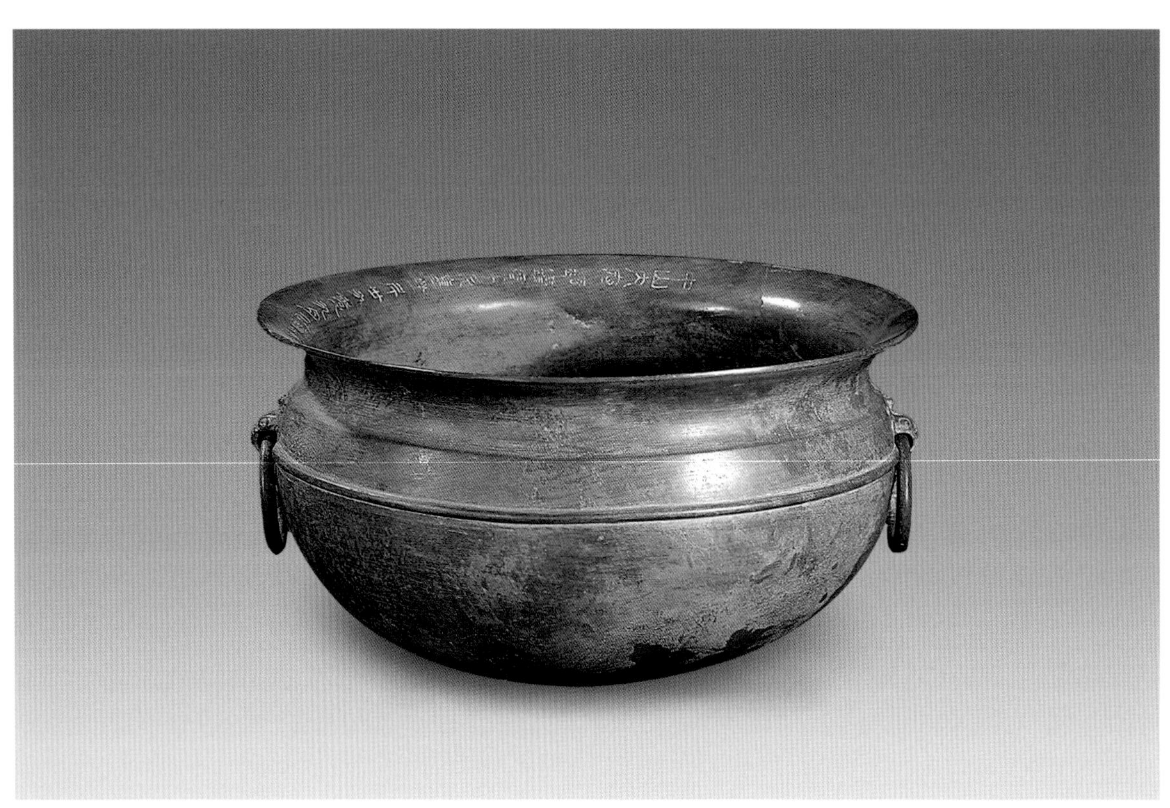

“中山内府”铜镬

西汉

铜质

口径 41 厘米，腹径 37.3 厘米，高 22.5 厘米，重 11200 克

Copper Wok with Characters “Zhong Shan Nei Fu”

Western Han Dynasty

Copper

Caliber 41 cm/ Belly Diameter 37.3 cm/ Height 22.5 cm/ Weight 11,200g

敞口，束颈，口沿外侈，腹微鼓，假圈足。腹部有蟾蜍形铺首衔环一对。上腹部饰凸弦纹一周。

河北博物院藏

The wok has an open mouth with its edge protruding outward, a tightened neck, a slightly swelling belly, and a fake circular foot. On each side of its belly are two rings with toad-shaped design. The upper belly is patterned with a circle of convex string.

Preserved in Hebei Museum

華

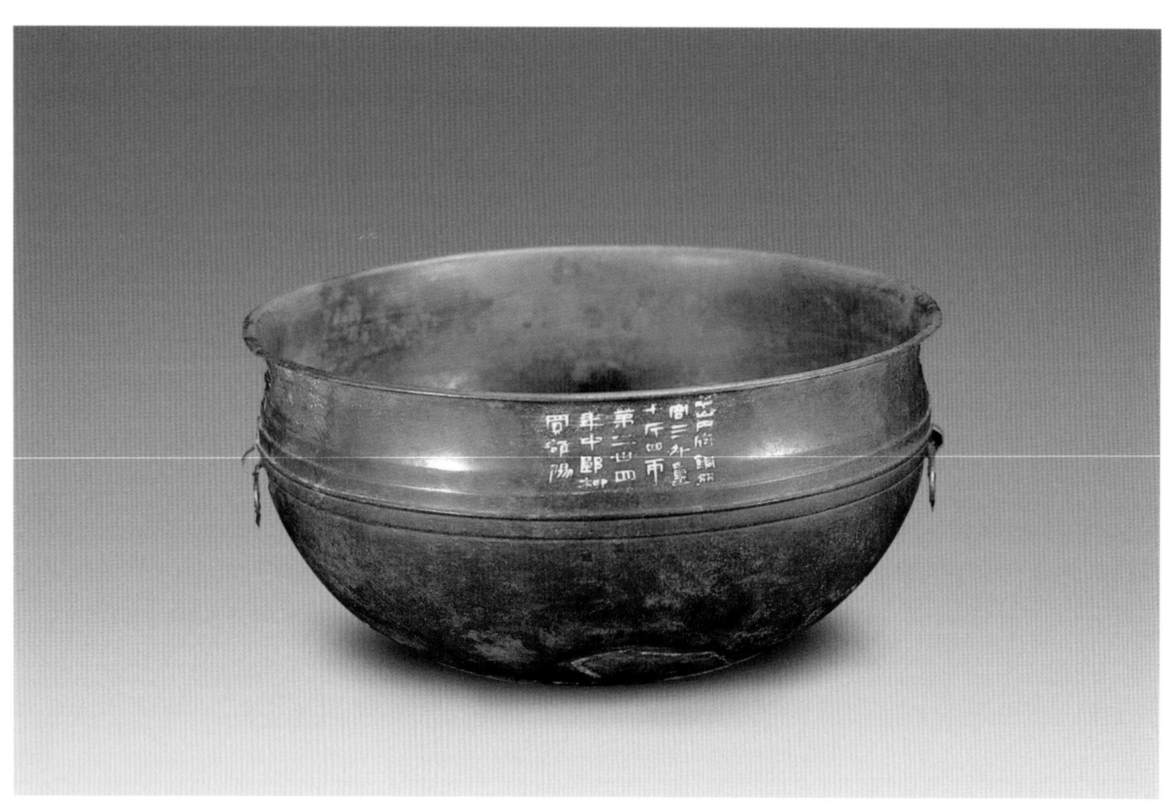

“中山内府”铜铜

西汉

铜质

高 12.5 厘米，重 1700 克

Copper Kettle with Characters “Zhong Shan Nei Fu”

Western Han Dynasty

Copper

Height 12.5 cm/ Weight 1,700g

敞口，沿微外卷，腹微鼓，矮圈足。腹部有一对铺首衔环，并饰宽带凸弦纹一周。

河北博物院藏

The kettle has an open mouth with its edge rolling outward slightly, a slightly swelling belly, and a short circular foot. One animal head applique holding rings is on each side of the belly. Meanwhile, the belly is patterned with a circle of wide convex belt.

Preserved in Hebei Museum

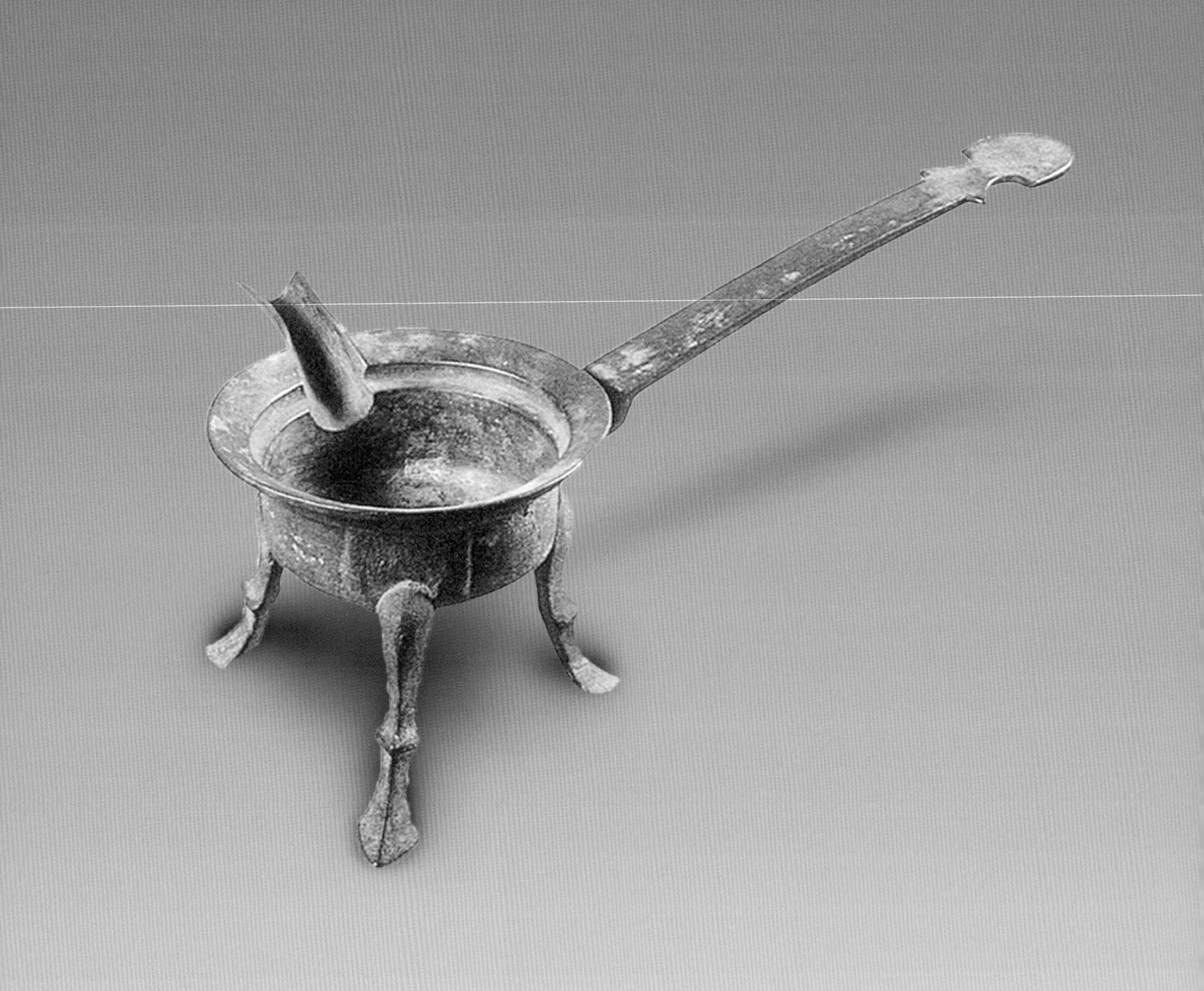

铜鐎斗

汉

铜质

口径 14.4 厘米，柄长 25.4 厘米，高 17.5 厘米

鐎斗是汉代新出现的一种炊器。文献中记载说“鐎，温器也，三足有柄”，与实物形状相合。器身为宽折沿的深腹盆，沿部一侧带有斜长的流，底部有三条外撇的两节兽蹄足。盘沿下部安有扁条形长柄以备握持。汉墓中屡有出土。

北京大学赛克勒考古与艺术博物馆藏

Copper Jiao Dou

Han Dynasty

Copper

Caliber 14.4 cm/Length of the Handle 25.4 cm/Height 17.5 cm

The piece was a new type of cooking utensil in the Han Dynasty. By literature, it was recorded as “Jiao, a warming utensil with a handle and three feet”. This is accordance with the real object. Its body is in the shape of a deep pot with a wide-folded edge. There is a long oblique spout on one side of the edge. The bottom is decorated with three horseshoe-shaped feet which are oblique outward. Below the plate edge, a long strip-shaped handle is made for convenience to take. Many utensils of this kind have been unearthed from tombs of the Han Dynasty.

Preserved in Arthur M. Sackler Museum of Art and Archaeology at Peking University

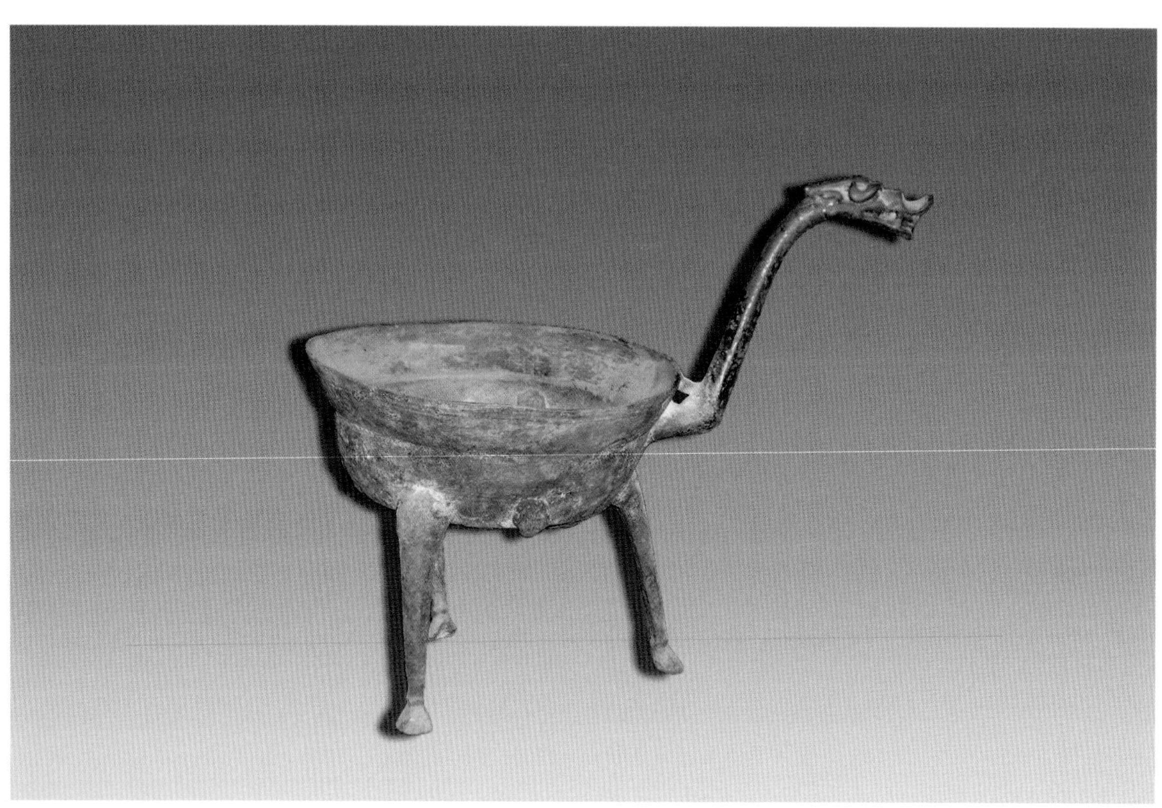

铜鐎锥斗

汉

铜质

口径 12.3 厘米，底径 9 厘米，足高 7.2 厘米，通高 15.8 厘米，重 750 克

Copper Jiao Dou

Han Dynasty

Copper

Caliber 12.3 cm/ Base Diameter 9 cm/ Height of the Feet 7.2 cm/ Height 15.8 cm/ Weight 750 g

盘口，直腹，平底，三兽足，腹中间连接一兽头把。炊器。完整无损。陕西省西安市征集。

陕西历史博物馆藏

The piece has a flat mouth, an upright belly, a flat base, and three animal-like feet. The middle part of the belly is connected to an animal head handle. This a cooking utensil is well preserved. It was collected from Xi’an, Shaanxi Province.

Preserved in Shaanxi Museum of Medical History

華

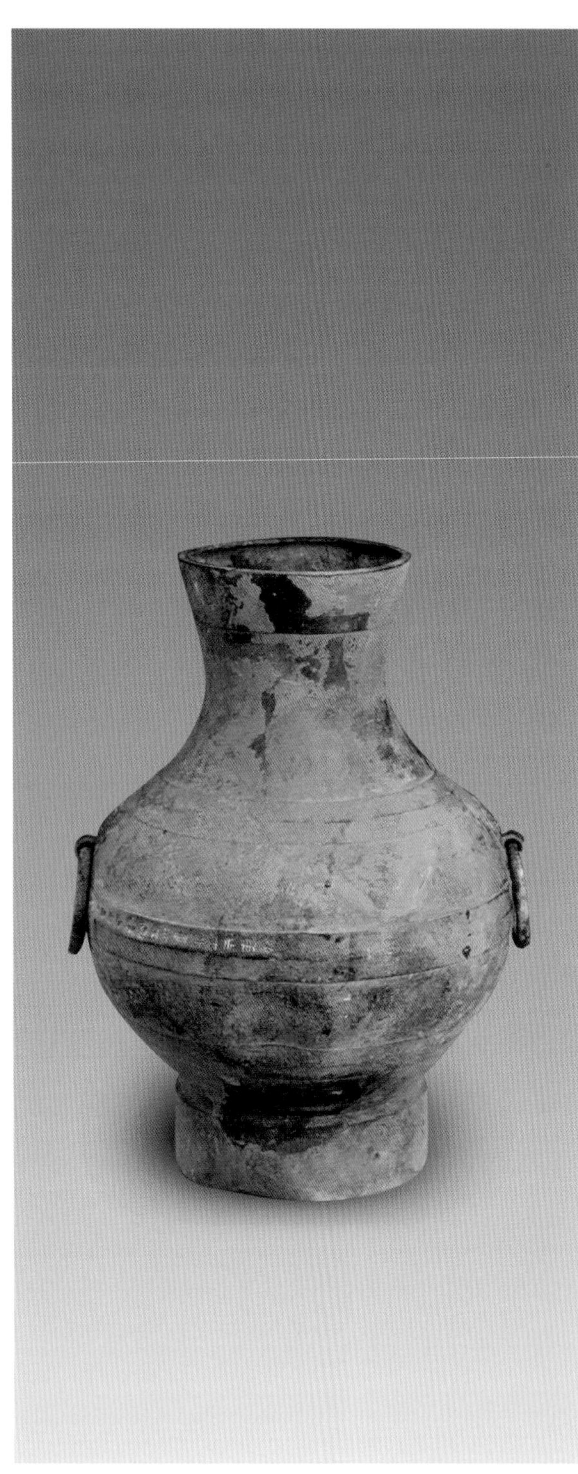

代食官糟锺

汉

铜质

口径 18 厘米，腹径 31.5 厘米，通高 46 厘米

"Dai Shi Guan" Dregs Vessel

Dai Shi Guan—ancient Chinese officer who eat the food to test if the food has been poisoned.

Han Dynasty

Copper

Mouth Diameter 18 cm/ Belly Diameter 31.5 cm/ Height 46 cm

敞口，短束颈，鼓腹下收，高圈足。腹侧置铺首衔环一对。口、腹部凸饰宽带纹四道。

山西博物院藏

The vessel has an open mouth, a short contracted neck, a swelling belly with a tapered lower end, and a tall circular foot. There is one animal head applique holding rings on each side of the belly. Meanwhile, four convex broad strip patterns are decorated on the mouth and the belly.

Preserved in Shanxi Museum

華

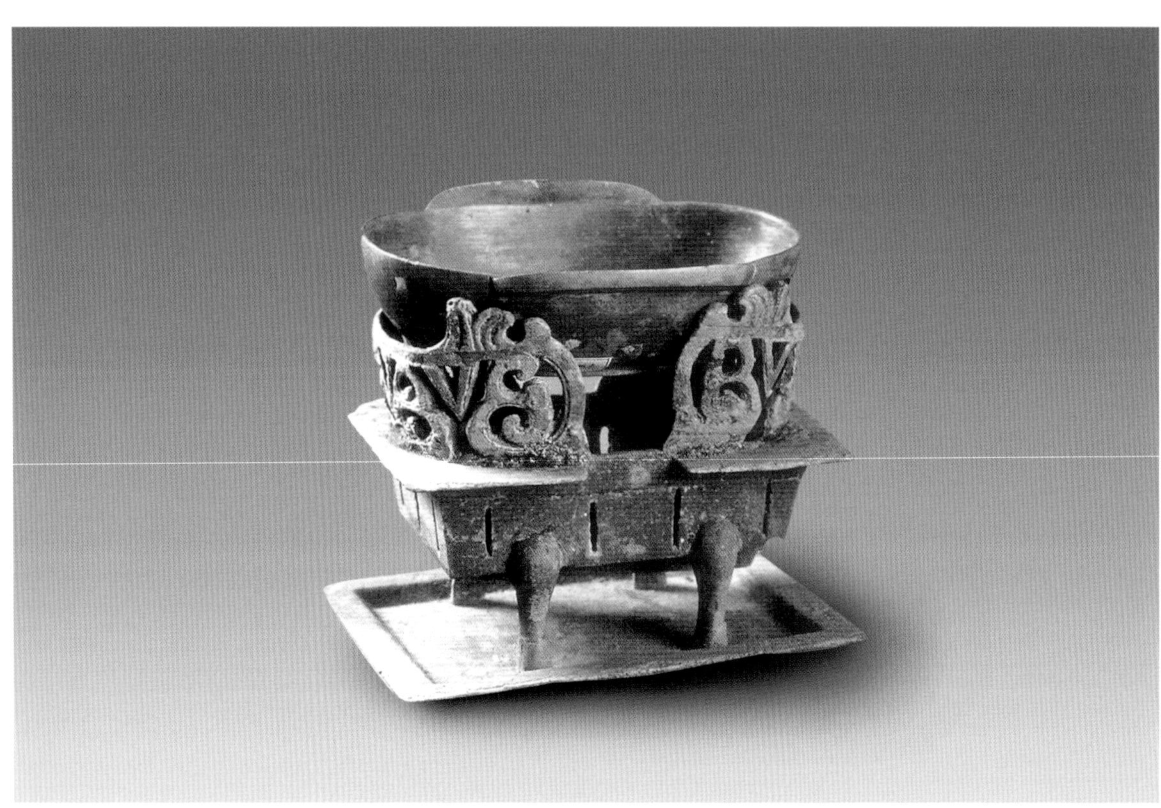

铜染炉

西汉

铜质

长 16.6 厘米，宽 12 厘米，通高 14.2 厘米

Copper Dying Stove

Western Han Dynasty

Copper

Length 16.6 cm/ Width 12 cm/ Height14.2 cm

染炉由承盘、炉和耳杯组成。炉身呈长方形，口大底小，斜直壁，平底镂空。炉身腰部有宽平方边的腰尚，腰沿上方为镂空博山式支边，悬空支撑着耳杯，腰沿下为炉膛。炉壁四周有十四道竖条状气孔十道，炉下为长方形宽平沿承盘。经考证其用途当为一套组合式烹饪炊具。1988 年在邗江区甘泉乡姚庄村出土。

扬州博物馆藏

The stove is made of a tray, a stove, and an ear cup. The stove is rectangular with a big mouth, a smaller base, and an oblique wall. The base is flat with hollow design. A flat square trestle on the waist works to support the cup. Above the waist is hollow out designed Boshan (a hill in China) trestle. Below the waist is the chamber of the stove. The stove wall is equipped with ten vertical air holes. Below the stove is a rectangular tray with flat edge. Textual research proves that this is a set of cooking utensils. This piece was unearthed in Yaozhuang Village, Ganquan Township, Hanjiang District, in 1988.

Preserved in Yangzhou Museum

華

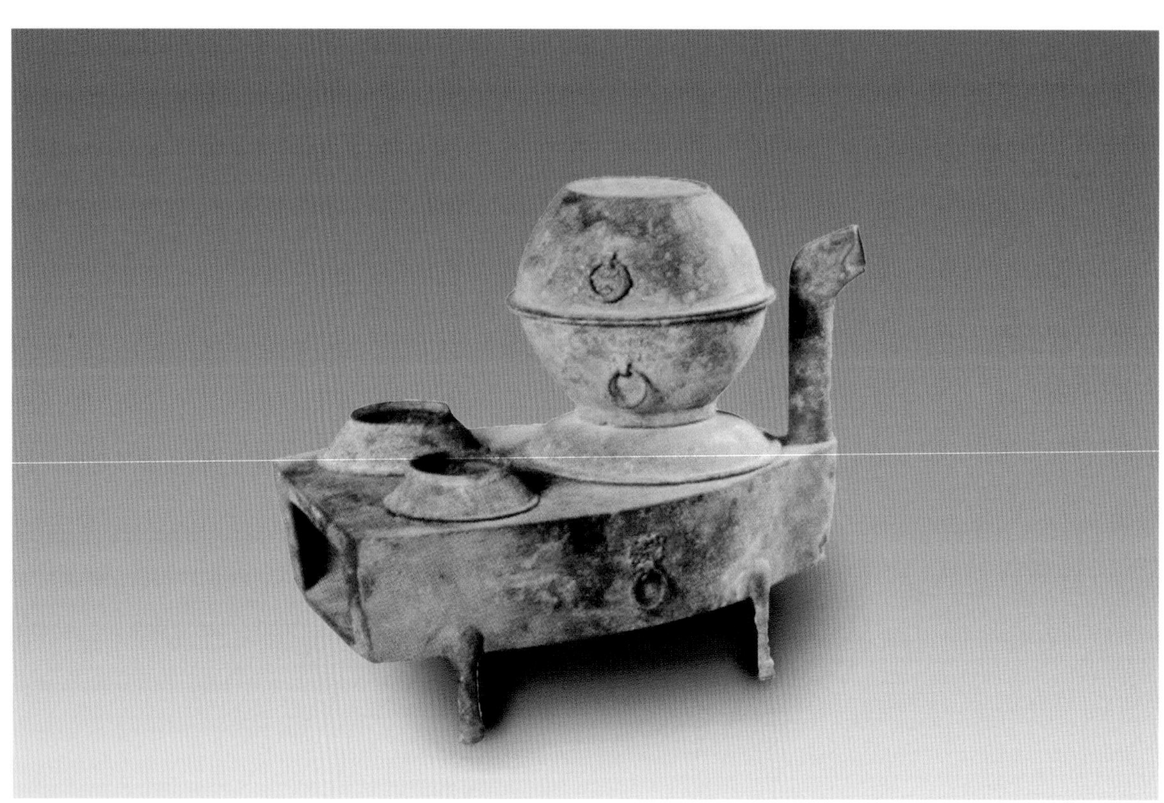

青铜灶

西汉

青铜质

通长 34.3 厘米

Bronze Kitchen Range

Han Dynasty

Bronze

Height 34.3 cm

平面近船形，圆头外突近尖，灶面上有一大二小三个火孔。小火孔内各安放一折腹敛口的釜，大火孔中放置由折腹釜、深腹甑和甑盖组成的甗，釜折腹处有一周平沿，防止其从火孔脱落，甑与盖外形相同，均深腹平沿，腹部有一对铺首衔环。灶一端是长方形火门通向灶膛，另一端上置直柱式烟囱，但烟囱的头部弯向一侧，而不是直接排烟向上。灶底为四条瘦削的蹄状足。此灶于山西省朔州市平朔露天煤矿出土。

山西省考古研究所藏

The shape of the stove resembles a ship. There is a circular protruding head and three fire holes, one big and two smaller on the surface. A cauldron with folded belly and a tightened mouth is placed inside of each smaller hole. Inside the big hole is placed a steamer composed of a folded belly cauldron, a deep belly vessel, and a cover. The circular flat edge on the belly of the cauldron can stop the cauldron from dropping into the fire. The steamer and its cover are in the same shape: a flat edge and a deep belly with a pair of animal head applique holding rings. At one end of the stove is a rectangular fire door to the chamber of the stove. At the other end is a cylindrical chimney standing upward. The head of the chimney is designed to bend to one side to avoid to discharge smoke directly. The bottom of the range are four thin horseshoe-shaped feet. This piece was unearthed from an opencast coal mine site of Pingshuo region in Shuozhou, Shanxi Province.

Preserved in Shanxi Provincial Institute of Archaeology

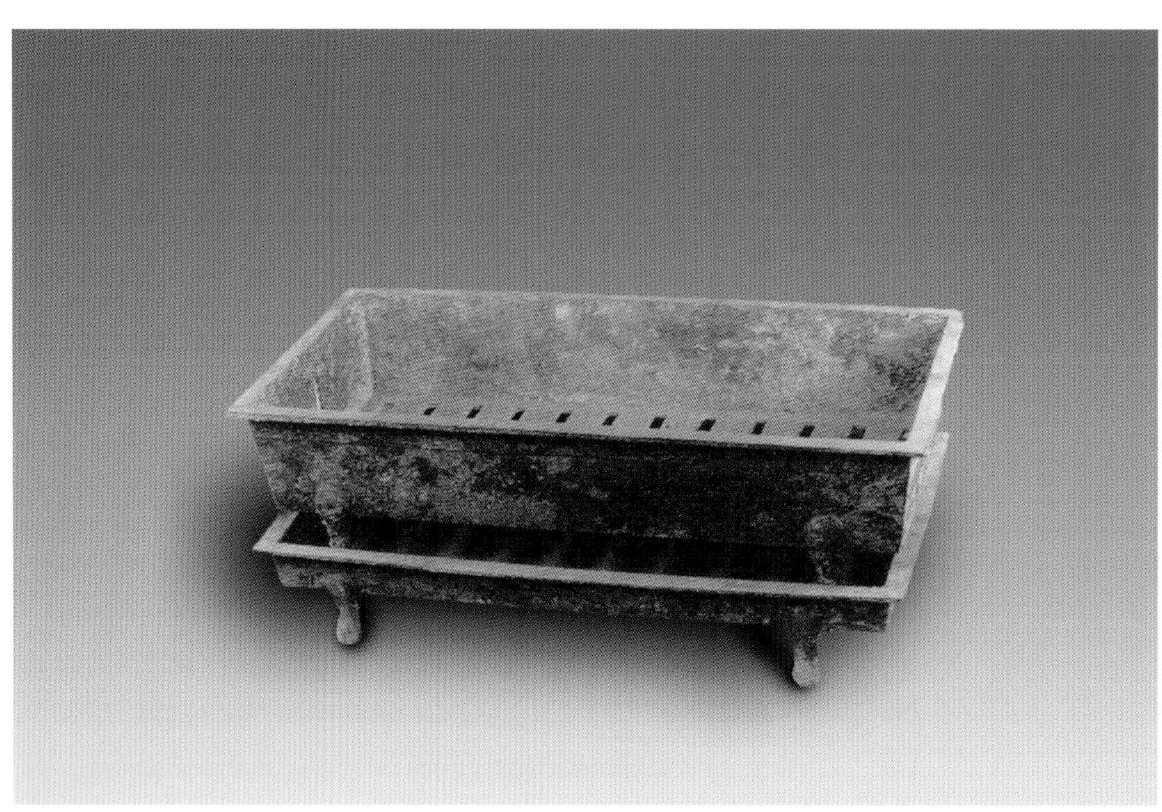

上林方炉

西汉

铜质

长 47 厘米，宽 23.25 厘米，通高 16 厘米

"Shanglin" Square Censer

Western Han Dynasty

Copper

Length 47 cm/ Width 23.25 cm/ Total Height 16 cm

分上下两层。上层是长槽形炉身，其底部有数条条形镂孔而形同箅子。下层为浅盘式四足底座，炉身亦有 4 条蹄足安放于承盘之上。上层炉身平沿有 42 字铭文。据此可知，此件铜方炉为弘农宫之物，初元三年 (前 46) 被征调至上林荣官使用。1969 年陕西省西安市延兴门村出土。

陕西省历史博物馆藏

The furnace is divided into two parts. The upper part is a long groove-shaped body with multiple bar-type hollowed holes in the shape of grate. The lower part is a four-foot pedestal in the shape of a shallow plate. The body also has four hoof-like feet placed upon the pedestal to uphold the upper part. There are forty-two characters inscribed on the rim of the upper body, which proves that this bronze censer was a collection of the Hongnong Palace and it was transferred and used by an official named Shang Lin Rong in 46 B.C. This piece was unearthed in Yan Xing Men Village, Xi'an City, Shaanxi Province in 1969.

Preserved in Shaanxi History Museum

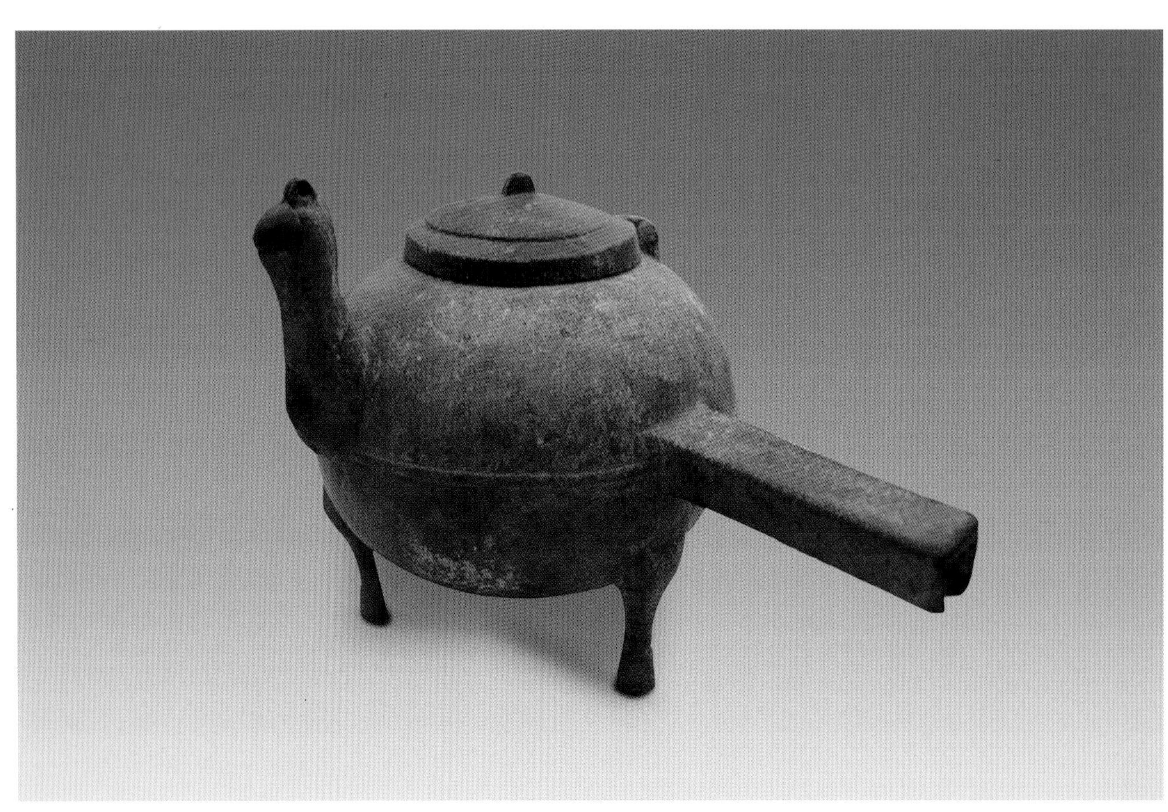

素面鐎壶

东汉早期

青铜

直径 26 厘米，手柄 20 厘米

Plain Jiao Pot

Early years in Eastern Han Dynasty

Bronze

Diameter 26 cm/ Handle 20 cm

直口，平唇，矮颈，扁腹饰粗弦纹，圈足。肩部置鸟首流，腹部装方管状执柄。该壶造型简朴，为生活中的实用器，多用于煎煮中药。

北京御生堂中医药博物馆藏

The pot has a vertical mouth, a flat lip, a short neck, ring feet and a flat and round belly which is carved with thick ring motifs and the square tube-shaped handle. The bird's head-shaped spout is welded onto the shoulder. The design of the pot was simple and was used in daily life, mainly for boiling medicine.

Preserved in Chinese Medicine Museum of Beijing Yu Sheng Tang Drugstore

華

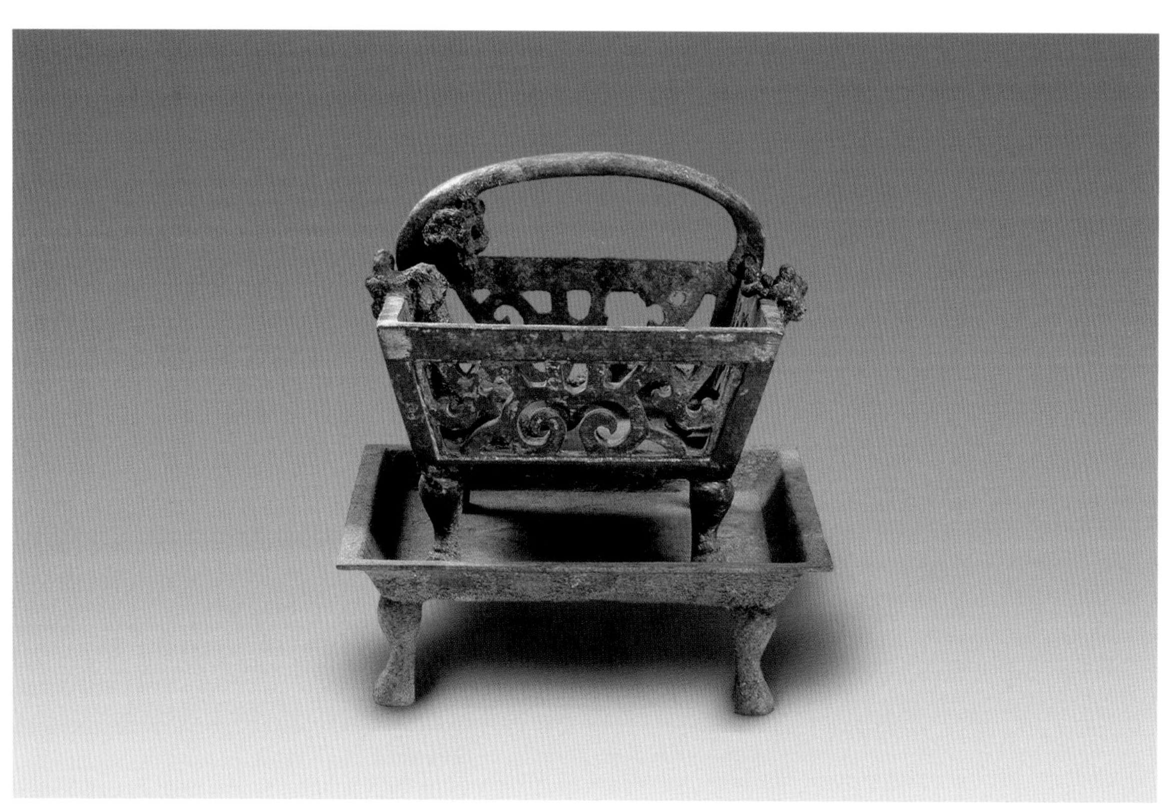

铜方炉

东汉

铜质

高 17 厘米，宽 22.7 厘米

Copper Square Censer

Astern Han Dynasty

Copper

Height 17 cm/ Width 22.7 cm

分上下两层，上层为方形炉体，斜壁，平底，蹄足，无盖，四壁镂孔形似卷草，口沿两边各有一钮，穿以铜提梁，炉底有四个对称的小方孔，便于净除灰烬。下层为方形承盘，用来承接灰烬。盘平底，斜壁，平沿，蹄足。该器用块模浇铸，再焊接成一体，造型古朴，器体厚重，是当时贵族才能拥有的生活用品。南京象山出土。

南京市博物馆藏

The censer is divided into two parts. The upper part is a square censer body with an oblique wall, a flat base, hoof-shaped feet, and no cover. The four walls are made in hollowed holes in the shape of scrolled grass. One both sides of the mouth rim, there is a knob through which a bronze handle goes. There are four small symmetrical square holes with the purpose of clearing ashes. The lower part is a square tray to hold the fallen ashes. The tray is made of a flat base, oblique walls, flat rims and hoof-shaped feet. The censer was weld with components which were first made with mold. The censer is of primitive simplicity with a solid body. It was only used by nobles at ancient time. This piece was unearthed in Xiangshan, Nanjing City.

Preserved in Nanjing Municipal Museum

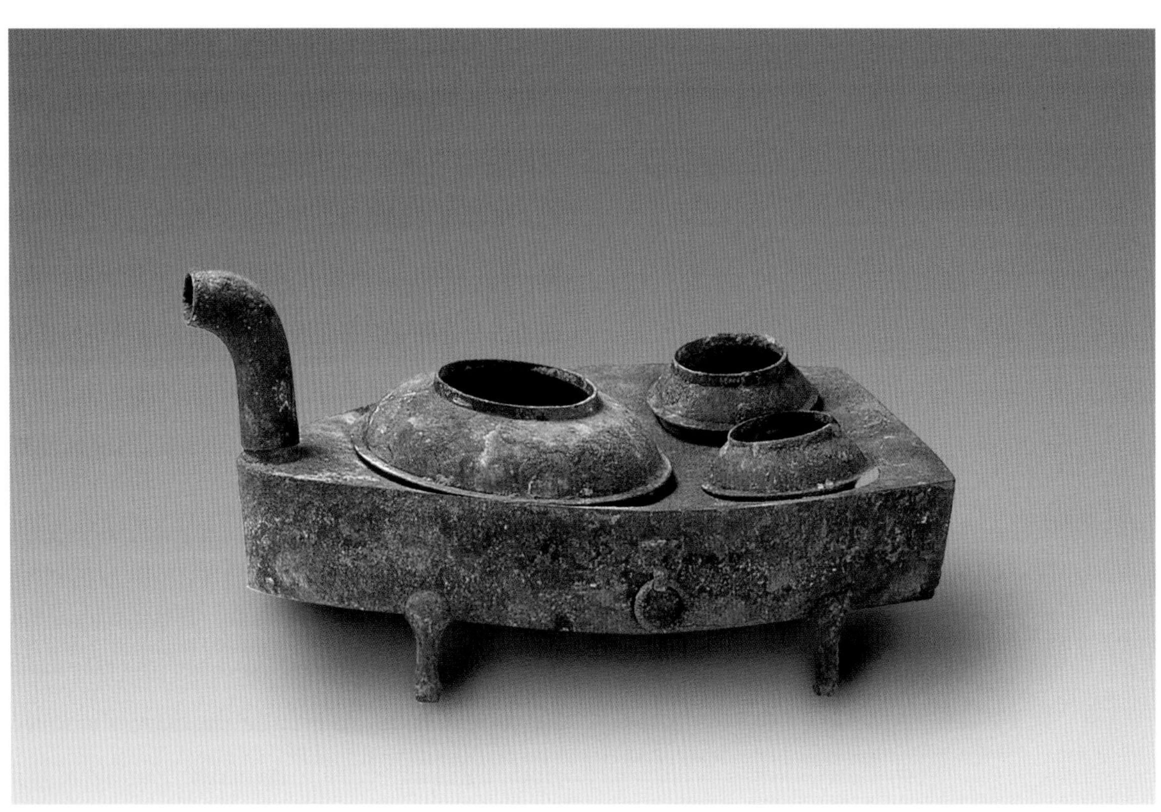

铜灶

汉

铜质

长 32 厘米，宽 19.5 厘米，高 17.2 厘米，重 1926 克

Copper Kitchen Range

Han Dynasty

Copper

Length 32 cm/ Width 19.5 cm/ Height 17.2 cm/ Weight 1,926 g

灶体平面略近舟形，两侧饰铺首衔环，下承四蹄足。灶面有三个火眼，其上分别置二釜一甑，并有铜勺一柄，灶尖端置一烟囱，顶部曲弯。六合区境内出土。

南京博物院藏

The stove is like a ship. It is decorated with animal head appliques holding rings on both sides of the body and is held by four hoof-shaped feet. There are three burners: one for steamer and the other two for boilers. The stove is equipped with a bronze spoon. A chimney with a curly roof is set up on the stove's pointed-end. This piece was unearthed in Liuhe District, Nanjing City, Jiangsu Province.

Preserved in Nanjing Museum

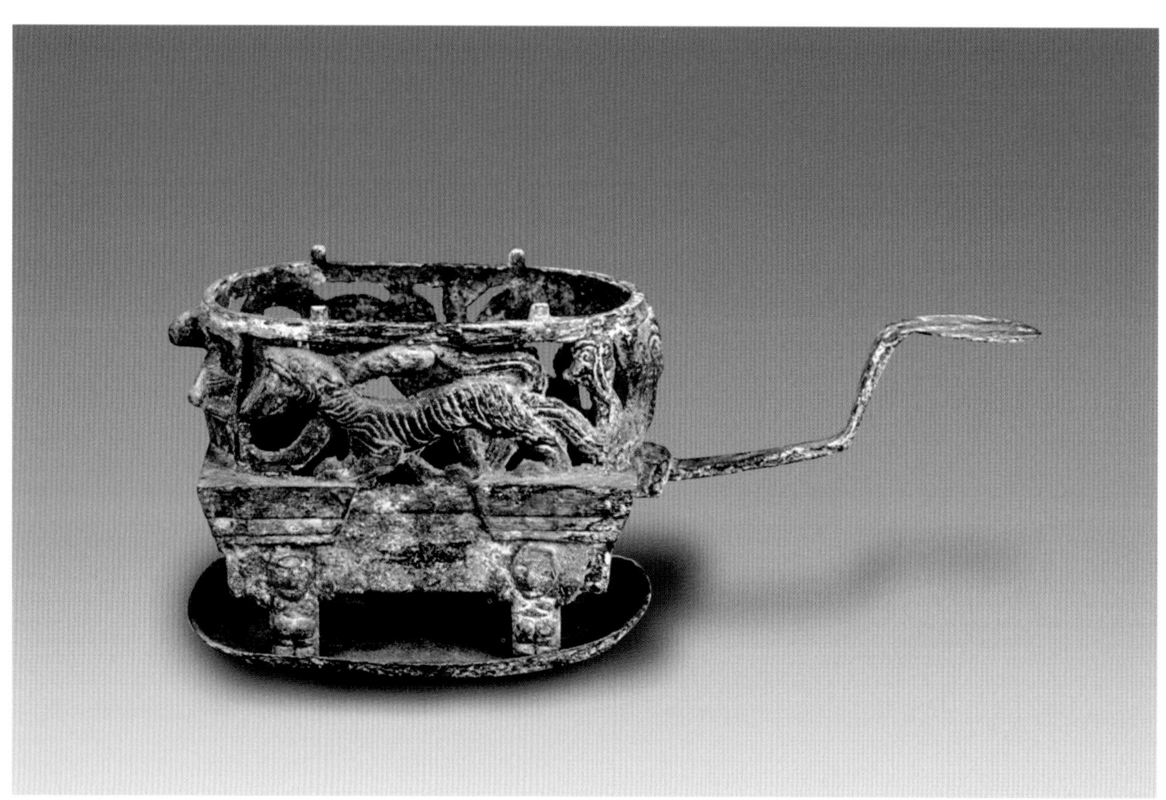

四神炉

汉

铜质

通长 24 厘米，宽 7.5 厘米，通高 11.5 厘米

Four Immortals Censer

Han Dynasty

Copper

Length 24 cm/ Width 7.5 cm/ Total Height 11.5 cm

圆口，大腹，圈足。上腹原有两个对称的环耳，其一已失。

首都博物馆藏

The kettle has a circular mouth, a large belly, and a circular foot. The upper belly was originally equipped with two symmetrical circular ears, but one of them is missing.

Preserved in the Capital Museum

華

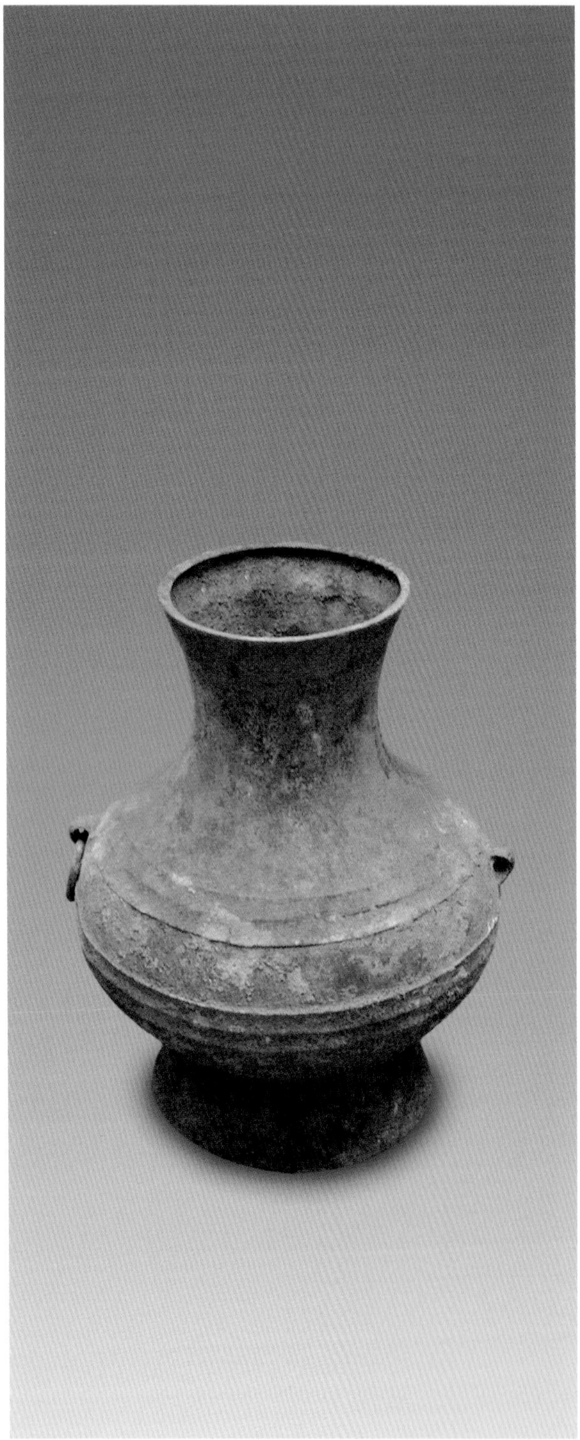

铜钟

汉

铜质

腹经 26 厘米，高 33 厘米

Copper Wine Vessel

Han Dynasty

Copper

Belly Diameter 26 cm/ Height 33 cm

口微侈，长颈，鼓腹，喇叭形圈足，腹中部及下部饰旋纹，有两个对称的环耳，耳上吊一圆环，器物表面泛铜绿色，保存完整，由民间征集。

成都中医药大学中医药传统文化博物馆藏

The utensil has a relatively wide mouth, a long neck, a swelling belly, and a trumpet-shaped circular foot. The middle and lower parts of the belly are decorated with a paisley pattern. It is installed with two symmetrical circular ears linked with two rings. Its surface bears a copper green color and it has been preserved well. The relic was collected in the folk.

Preserved in Museum of Traditional Chinese Medicine Culture, Chengdu University of Traditional Chinese Medicine

華

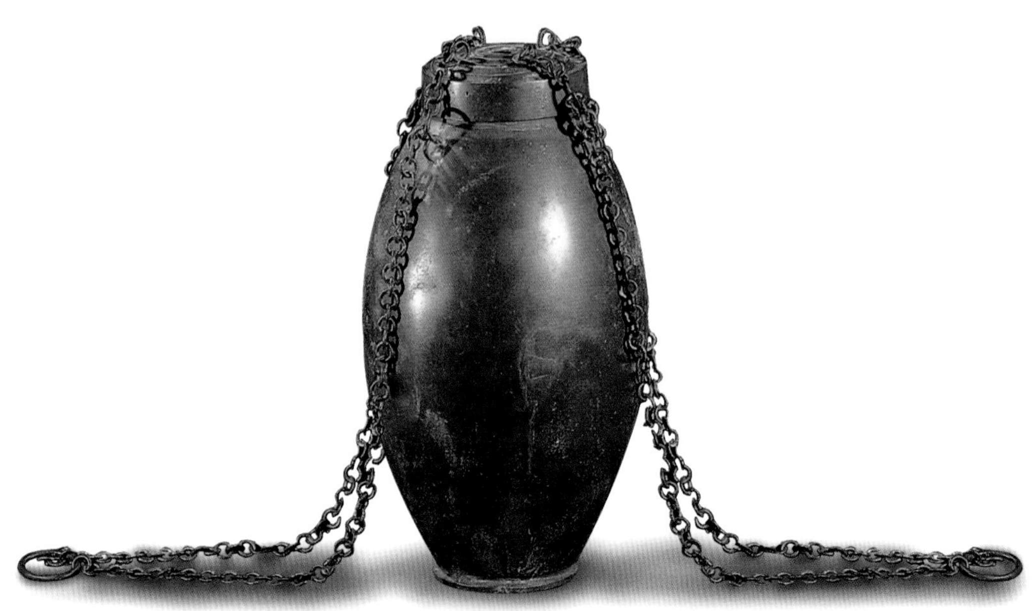

橄榄形铜链壶

西汉

铜质

口径 9.4 厘米，圈足径 8.5 厘米，通高 30.6 厘米

Olive-Shaped Copper Kettle with Chains

Western Han Dynasty

Copper

Caliber 9.4 cm/ Foot Diameter 8.5 cm/ Total Height 30.6 cm

壶身作橄榄形，小直口，长鼓腹，小平底，矮圈足。盖作覆钵形，盖面饰凸弦纹四圈，并作对称等距的四个小环钮，钮上各系短链。壶身肩部也有相应的四小环钮，钮上各系长链。每条长链分别穿过短链末端的环，再两两相连，形成两条长背链。开启或合盖时，须将穿于短链中之长链松开或拉紧，利用链环间卡阻作用，使盖不能自行启开。

河北博物院藏

The olive-shaped kettle has a small straight mouth, a tall swelling belly, a small flattened base, and a short circular foot. The cover appears in bowl shape. Its top is adorned with four circles of convex string patterns. Meanwhile four small symmetrical circular knobs are equidistantly set on the top of the cover. The knobs are tied with short chains. The utensil shoulder has another four small circular knobs tied with long chains. Every long chain is linked with the circular at the end-point of every short chain. The long chains and short ones intertwine with each other to form two long chains on the utensil back. The opening and closing of the cover are controlled respectively by loosening and straining the intertwined long chains. The chain jamming prevents the cover from opening by itself.

Preserved in Hebei Museum

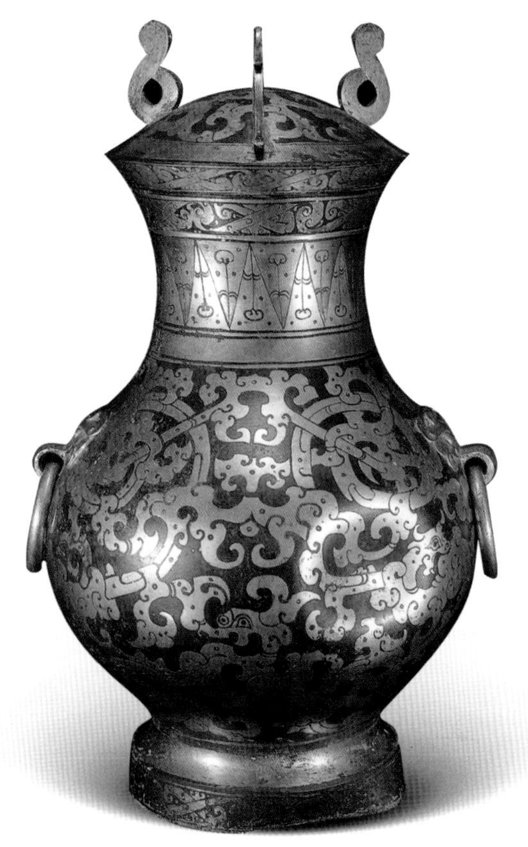

乳钉纹铜壶

西汉

鎏金铜质

圈足径 17.9 厘米，通高 45 厘米

Copper Kettle with Nipple-Nail Pattern

Western Han Dynasty

Gilded copper

Foot Diameter 17.9 cm/ Total Height 45 cm

壶口微敞，束颈，鼓腹，高圈足，腹部有一对铺首衔环。盖上有三云形钮。盖缘饰鎏金宽带纹，盖面上作方格纹、乳钉，填嵌绿琉璃。颈和腹部的宽带纹间作鎏金斜方格纹，方格纹的交叉点上镶嵌鎏银乳钉。方格纹中填嵌绿琉璃，琉璃上划出小方格圆点纹。色彩缤纷，绚丽异常。

河北博物院藏

The kettle has a relatively wide open mouth, a tightened neck, a swelling belly, and a tall circular foot. The belly is decorated with a pair of animal head applique holding rings. The cover is decorated with three cloud-like knobs. The cover rim is adorned with gilding broad strip patterns and the cover surface is decorated with grid shaped pattern and nipple-nail design which is filled with green decorative glass. Between each broad strip design on the utensil neck and belly are decorated oblique gilded grid patterns. The crossing points in the grid design are inlaid with silver nipple nails. The smaller boxes in the grid design are inlaid with green decorative glass on which faillette patterns are outlined. The relic appears rather colorful and florid.

Preserved in Hebei Museum

華

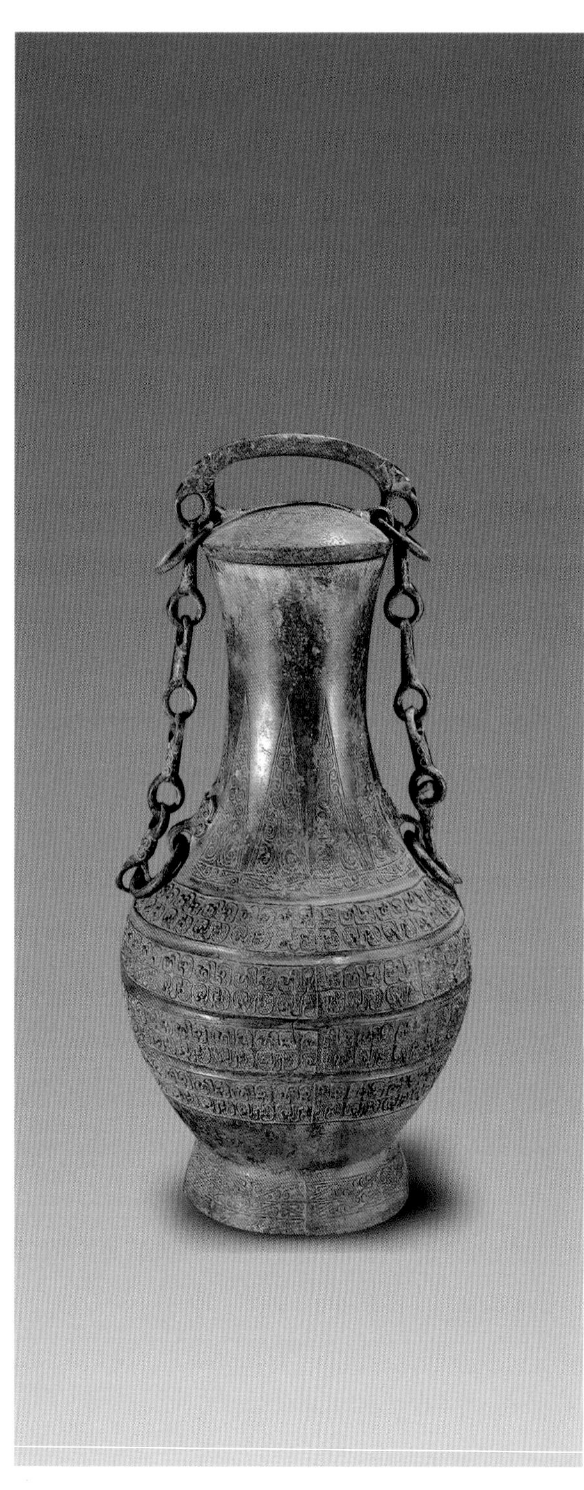

蟠螭蕉叶纹提梁铜壶

西汉

铜质

圈足径 10.3 厘米，通高 29.8 厘米

Copper Kettle with “Pan Chi”-Banana Leaf Patterns and Chain-Handles

Western Han Dynasty

Copper

Foot Diameter 10.3 cm/ Height 29.8 cm

长颈，鼓腹，平底，高圈足。壶带盖，两则各有一兽鼻衔环。壶肩两侧各有一铺首衔环，每侧环上系链索四节，向上穿过器盖两侧的环，与弓形兽首提梁连接。壶颈肩部饰蕉叶纹，蕉叶内填卷云纹。腹部以凹弦纹为界，分为四条蟠螭纹带。圈足饰斜角卷云纹两周。花纹细密繁缛。

河北博物院藏

The kettle has a long neck, a swelling belly, a flat base, and a tall circular foot. It has a cover with each side ornamented with animal nose appliqué holding rings. So does the body. The holding rings on the body is tied with a four-knob chain link which is connected to go through the cover circles and further connected with the bow-shaped animal head handles. The neck and shoulders are adorned with banana leaf design with scrolled cloud patterns inside. The belly is adorned with four intaglio-cut Pan-chi dragon designs. The circular foot is decorated with two circles of oblique-cornered scrolled cloud patterns. The decorative design is compact and elaborate.

Preserved in Hebei Museum

華

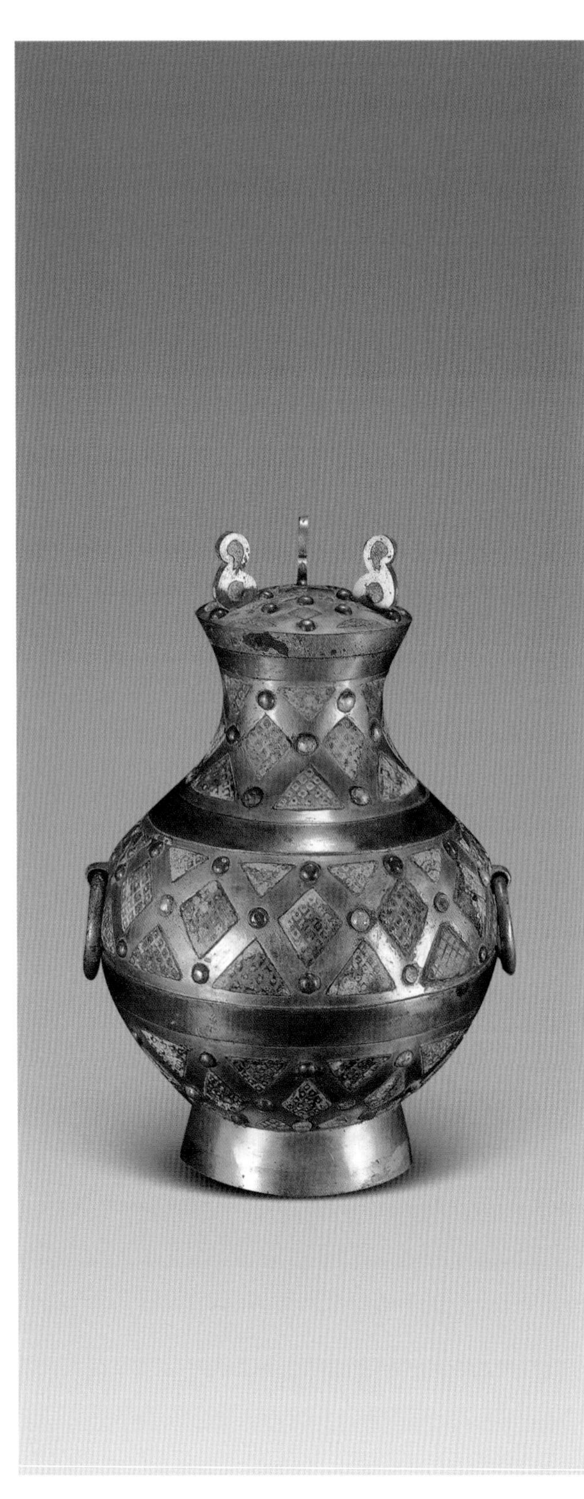

鎏金银蟠龙纹铜壶

西汉

鎏金鎏银铜质

通高 59.5 厘米，腹径 37 厘米，重 16250 克

Gilded Copper Kettle with Yin-Pan Dragon Patterns

Western Han Dynasty

Gold and silver-plated copper

Total Height 59.5 cm/ Belly Diameter 37 cm/ Weight 16,250g

壶通体用鎏金、鎏银工艺装饰。口部和圈足饰鎏银卷云纹带，颈部饰金银相间的三角纹带，腹部饰四条独首双身的金龙相互翻卷蟠绕，并缀以金色卷云纹。铺首鎏金。盖面饰鎏金夔凤，盖缘饰鎏银卷云纹，卷云钮鎏银。纹饰金银相映，富丽堂皇。壶内壁髹朱漆一层。

河北博物院藏

The whole kettle is gilded by gold and silver. Scrolled cloud pattern gilded with silver is applied to the utensil mouth and the circular foot. The neck is decorated with triangle-shaped strips which are interphase with gold and silver. The belly is ornamented with four gold dragons, each of which has one head and two bodies. The dragons intertwine with each other and are dotted with gold scrolled cloud patterns and gilded animal head applique holding rings. The cover surface is decorated with Kui dragon and phoenix design gilded with gold. The cover rim is adorned with silver-gilded scrolled cloud patterns and knobs. The kettle's splendid decoration shines with gold and silver. The inner wall is varnished with a layer of red paint.

Preserved in Hebei Museum

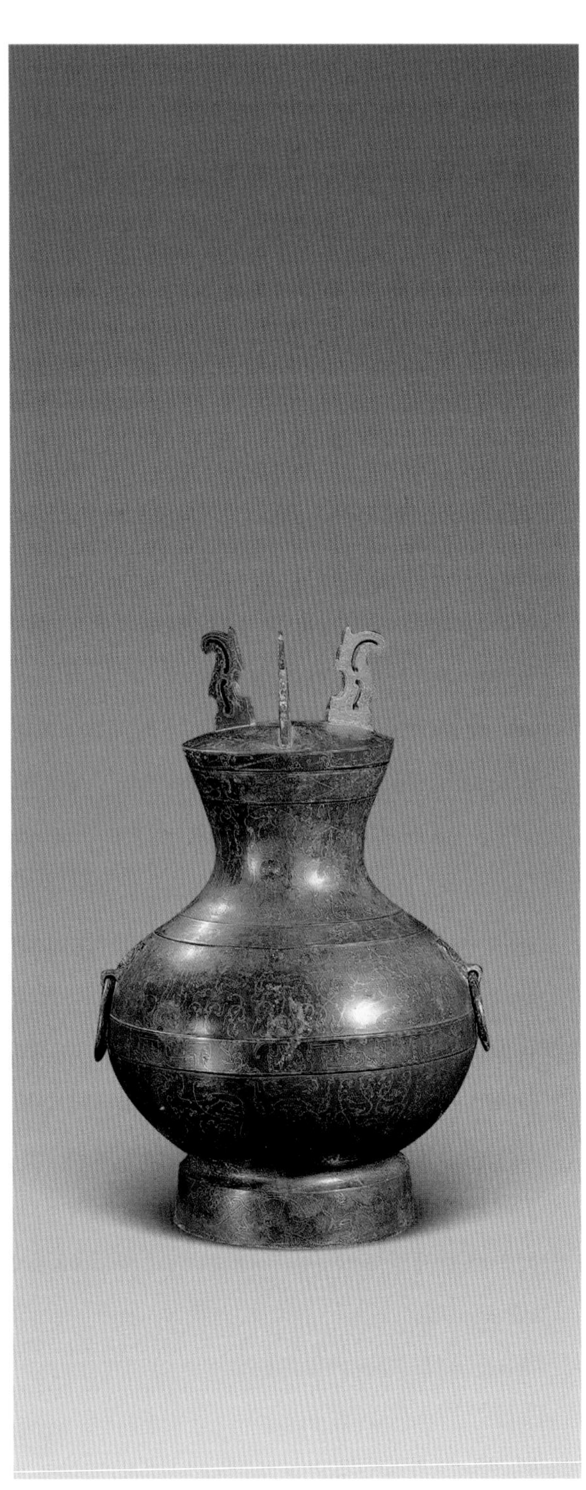

错金银鸟篆文铜壶

西汉

错金银铜质

腹径 28.5 厘米，通高 44.2 厘米

Copper Kettle Bird Seal Script Inlaid with Silver and Gold

Western Han Dynasty

Gold and silver-inlaid copper

Belly Diameter 28.5 cm/ Height 44.2 cm

子口盖，环钮。壶口略外侈，鼓腹，高圈足。双铺首衔环。器通体饰鸟篆文吉祥语和动物纹带，文字和图案均用纤细的金银丝双勾错出。下腹有铭文“口味。充润血肤，延寿却病，万年有余”。

河北博物院藏

The kettle has a swelling belly and a tall circular foot. The cover with a circular knob is designed with seam allowance to fit into the utensil body. The mouth is slightly outstretched. The body also has a pair of animal head applique holding rings. The whole kettle is decorated with auspicious seal scripts in bird shape as well as animal patterns. Both the seal scripts and patterns are outlined with fine gold and silver threads. The lower belly is inscribed with fourteen inscriptions which means that "The kettle adds flavor to drinks. The drink can flourish and nourish blood and skin and build up lifespan for a long time as well as prevent diseases."

Preserved in Hebei Museum

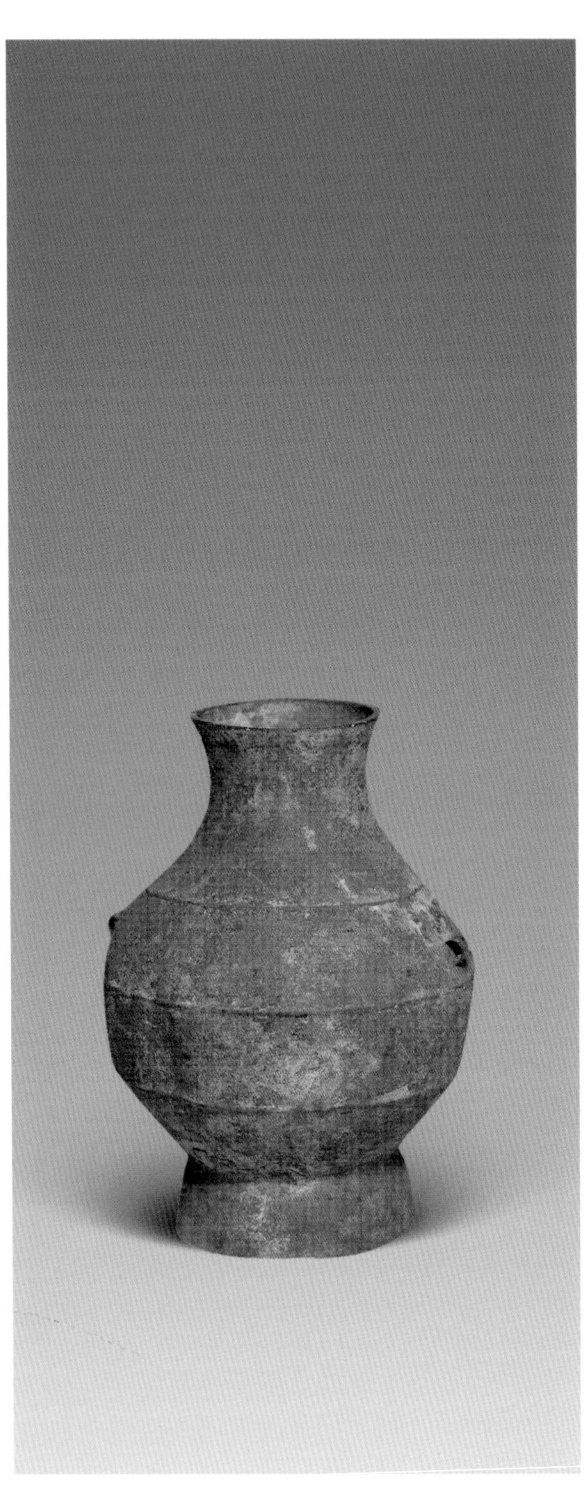

圆铜壶

汉

铜质

口径 10.2 厘米，腹围 27 厘米，底径 13 厘米，高 28 厘米

Circular Copper Kettle

Han Dynasty

Copper

Caliber 10.2 cm/ Belly Diameter 27 cm/ Base Diameter 13 cm/ Height 28 cm

侈口，圈足。上腹有两对称系环，腹身圈内有三道凸弦纹。也称为“钟”，系酒器和盛水器。

北京中医药大学中医药博物馆藏

The kettle has a wide mouth and a circular foot. The upper belly is equipped with two symmetrical knobs for handling. The utensil's body is adorned with three convex string patterns. The relic is also called “Zhong”, used as a wine or water vessel.

Preserved in the Museum of Chinese Medicine, Beijing University of Chinese Medicine

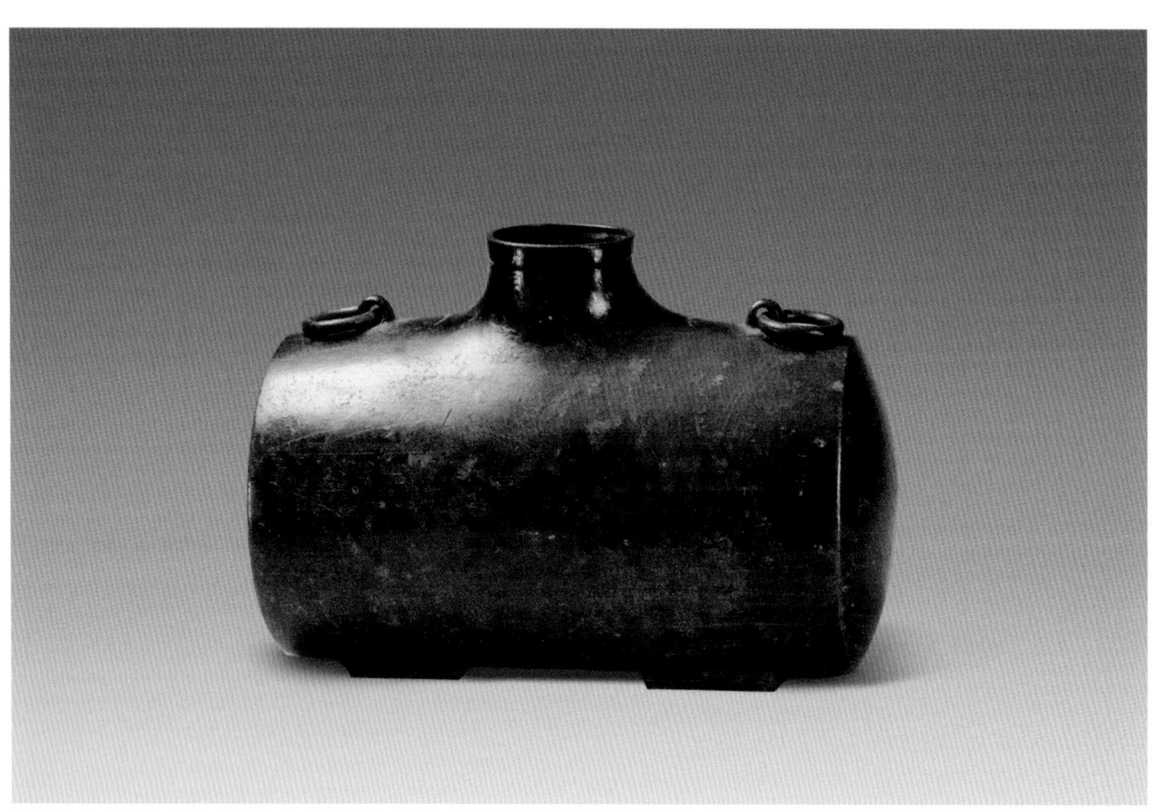

杨氏容二斗壶

汉

铜质

口径 6.6 厘米，横长 29.5 厘米，端径 14.5 厘米，高 19 厘米

Two Dou Kettle of Yang Family

Dou (an ancient Chinese volume unit)

Han Dynasty

Copper

Caliber 6.6 cm/ Transverse Length 29.5 cm/ End Diameter 14.5 cm/ Height 19 cm

圆口，矮颈，为横圆筒形，下附2方足，口两边有活环。形体似蚕形壶，造型奇特。底一侧铸阴文1行5字“杨氏容二斗”，刻阴文1行4字“重十四斤”。

山东省博物馆藏

The kettle has a circular mouth and a short neck. It appears in a transverse cylinder shape, equipped with two rectangle feet. A mobilizable ring is attached to each side of the mouth. The body is in an uncommon shape of silkworm. On one side of the base are engraved five characters as “Yang Shi Rong En Dou” (Yang Family Tow Dou Kettle) in one line in intaglio and four Chinese characters as “Zhong Shi Si Jin” (Weighing Shi Si Jin) in one line in intaglio. (Shi Si means fourteen in English.)

Preserved in Shandong Museum

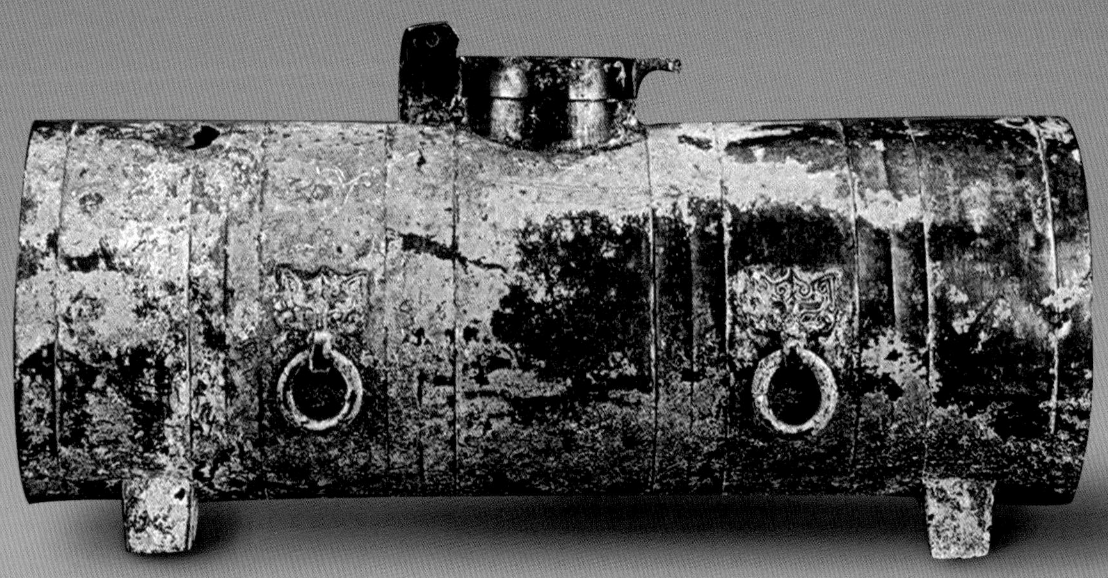

筒形器

汉

铜质

直径 17 厘米，长 47 厘米，高 22 厘米

器为横置圆筒形，下承两长方支足，筒中央置圆形直口。口一侧出一小鋬，一侧置长方轴槽，原有可开启的盖，盖失。腹两侧饰铺首衔环两对。筒身有六道凸起圈带。依其形制当为榼。

山西博物院藏

Barrel-Shaped Vessel

Han Dynasty

Copper

Diameter 17 cm/ Length 47 cm/ Height 22 cm

The vessel is in a transverse cylinder shape supported by two long and square feet. A circular straight mouth is positioned on the top of the central body. A handles attached to one side of the mouth. On the other of the mouth is a rectangular axial groove which was originally matched with a movable cap but the cap was lost. A pair of animal head appliqué holding rings is decorated on each side of the belly. The belly is also circulated with six convex string patterns. It should be an ancient wine vessel by its shape.

Preserved in Shanxi Museum

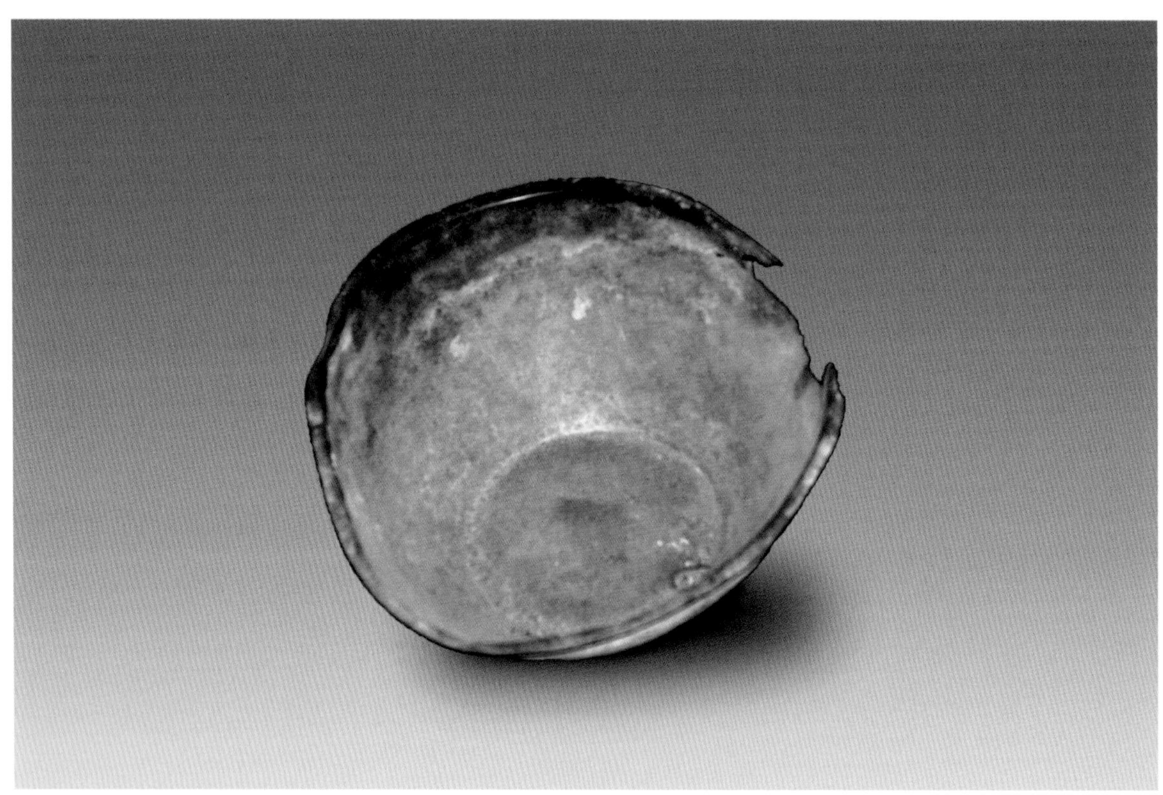

铜盆

汉

铜质

口径 32 厘米，底径 14.5 厘米，通高 12 厘米，重 950 克

Copper Basin

Han Dynasty

Copper

Caliber 32 cm/ Base Diameter 14.5 cm/ Height 12 cm/ Weight 950 g

圆唇，斜腹，平底，上腹有一道凸棱。盛贮器。口沿残。陕西省渭南市征集。

陕西医史博物馆藏

The basin has a circular lip, an oblique belly and a flattened base. The upper belly is adorned with a ridge. The basin was used as a reservoir. The mouth rim is not complete. The relic was collected in Weinan City, Shaanxi Province.

Preserved in Shaanxi Museum of Medical History

華

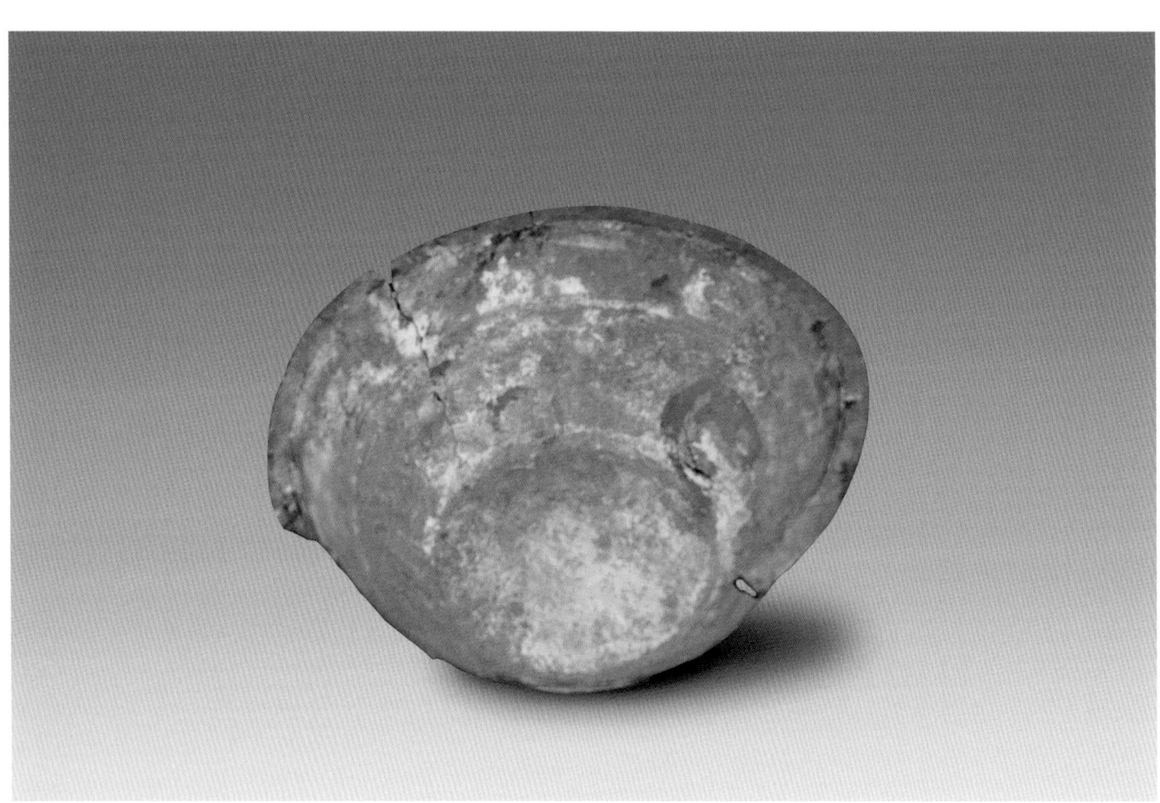

铜盆

汉

铜质

口径 31 厘米，底径 15 厘米，通高 11 厘米，重 1000 克

Copper Basin

Han Dynasty

Copper

Caliber 31 cm/ Base Diameter 15 cm/ Height 11 cm/ Weight 1,000 g

平口，斜腹，平底，口沿三分之二残。盛贮器。口沿有残。陕西省渭南市征集。

陕西医史博物馆藏

The basin has a flat mouth, an oblique belly, and a flat base. Two thirds of the mouth rim is missing. The basin was used as a reservoir. It was collected from Weinan City, Shaanxi Province.

Preserved in Shaanxi Museum of Medical History

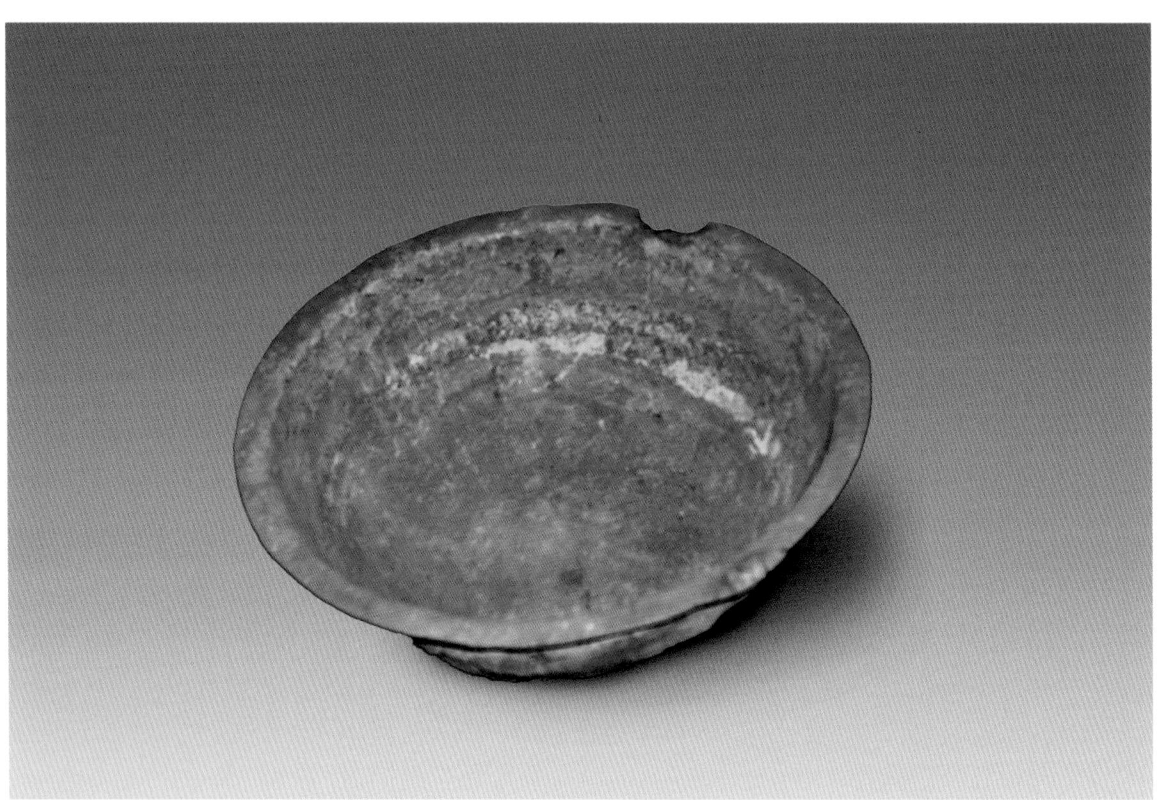

铜盆

汉

铜质

口径 32.5 厘米，底径 16 厘米，通高 10.7 厘米，重 1500 克

Copper Basin

Han Dynasty

Copper

Caliber 32.5 cm/ Base Diameter 16 cm/ Height 10.7 cm/ Weight 1,500 g

平口沿，斜腹，平底。盛贮器。口沿有残。陕西省咸阳市征集。

陕西医史博物馆藏

The basin has a flat mouth rim, an oblique belly, and a flat base. The basin was used as a reservoir. The mouth rim is not intact. The relic was collected from Weinan City, Shaanxi Province.

Preserved in Shaanxi Museum of Medical History

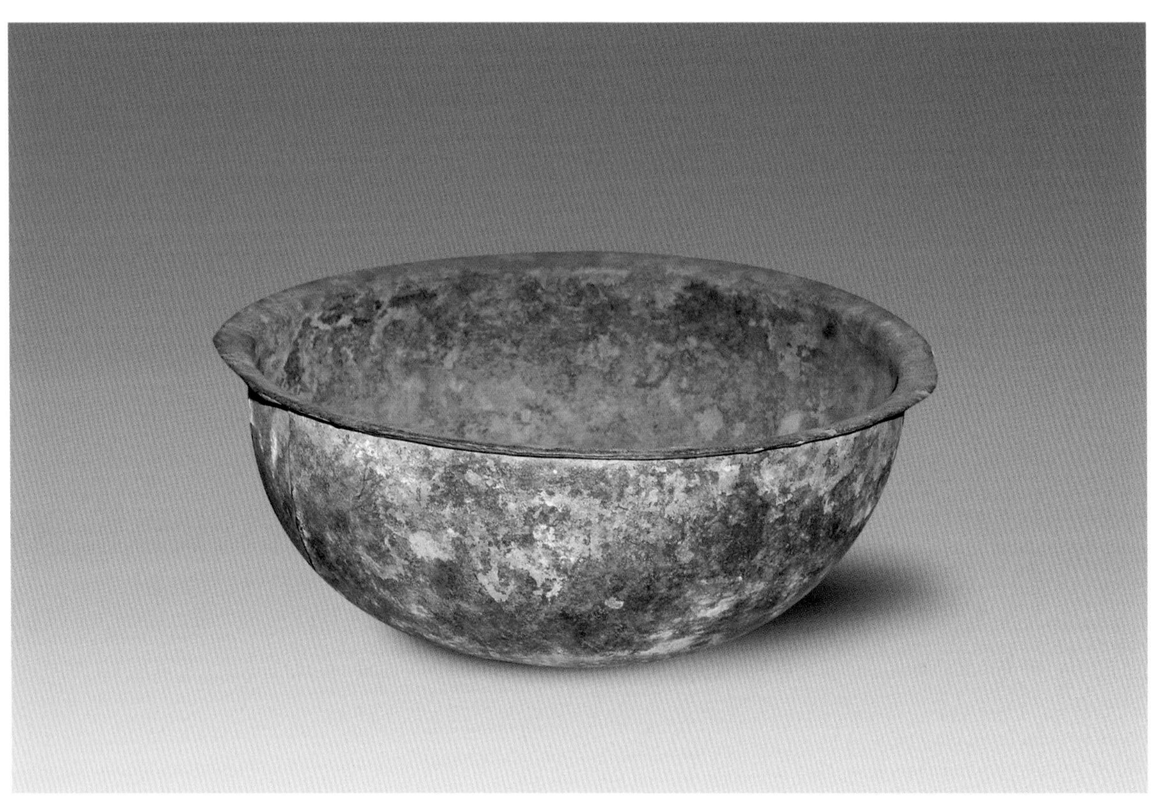

铜盆

汉

铜质

口径 30 厘米，通高 12 厘米，重 2300 克

Copper Basin

Han Dynasty

Copper

Caliber 30 cm/ Total Height 12 cm/ Weight 2,300 g

平口沿，圆腹，圜底，底内有一巴钉。生活用器。有残。陕西省白水县狄家河征集。

陕西医史博物馆藏

The basin has a flat mouth rim, a round belly, and a circular base with a nail. The basin is an article of daily use. It is not intact. The relic was collected from Dijiahe, Baishui County, Shaanxi Province.

Preserved in Shaanxi Museum of Medical History

華

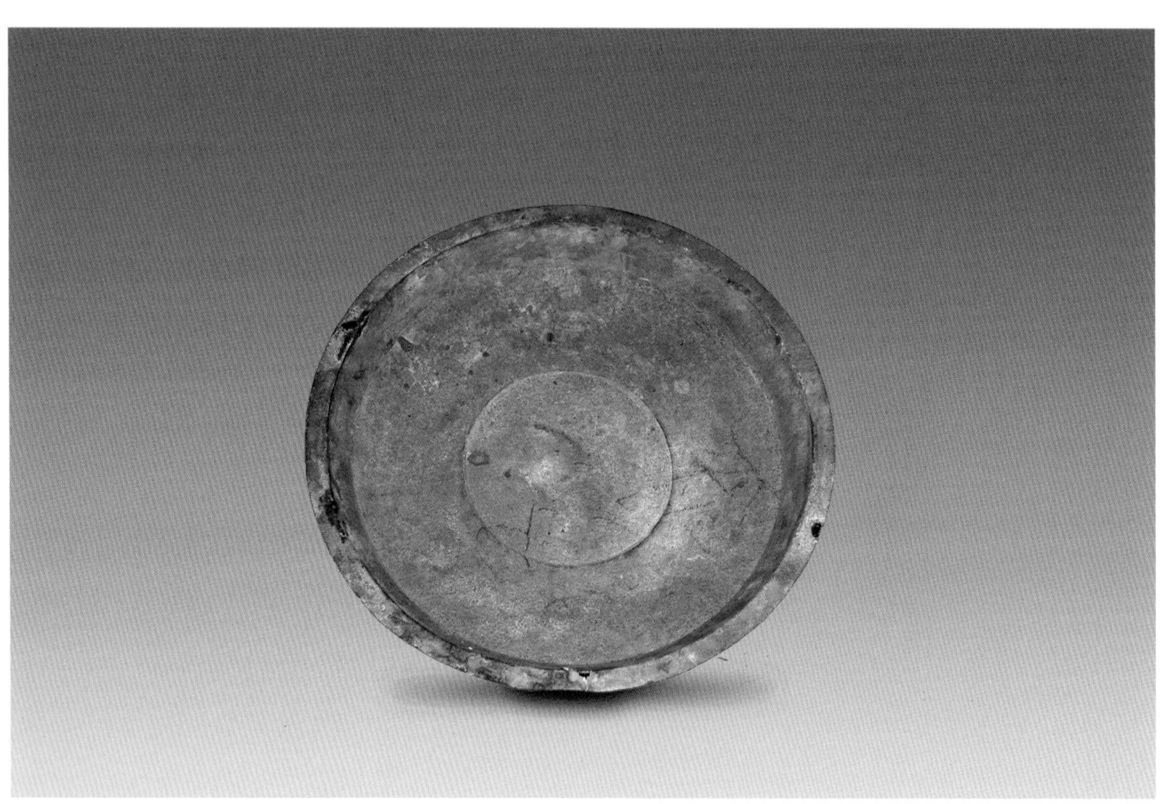

铜盘

汉

铜质

口径 37.3 厘米，底径 15.5 厘米，通高 4.5 厘米，重 1150 克

Bronze Plate

Han Dynasty

Copper

Caliber 37.3 cm/ Base Diameter 15.5 cm/ Height 4.5 cm/ Weight 1,150 g

敞口，平腹，平底。生活用器物。有残。陕西省西安市鄠邑区征集。

陕西医史博物馆藏

The plate has a wide mouth, a flat belly, and a flat base. It was an article of daily use. It is not intact. The relic was collected from Huyi District, Xi'an City, Shaanxi Province.

Preserved in Shaanxi Museum of Medical History

華

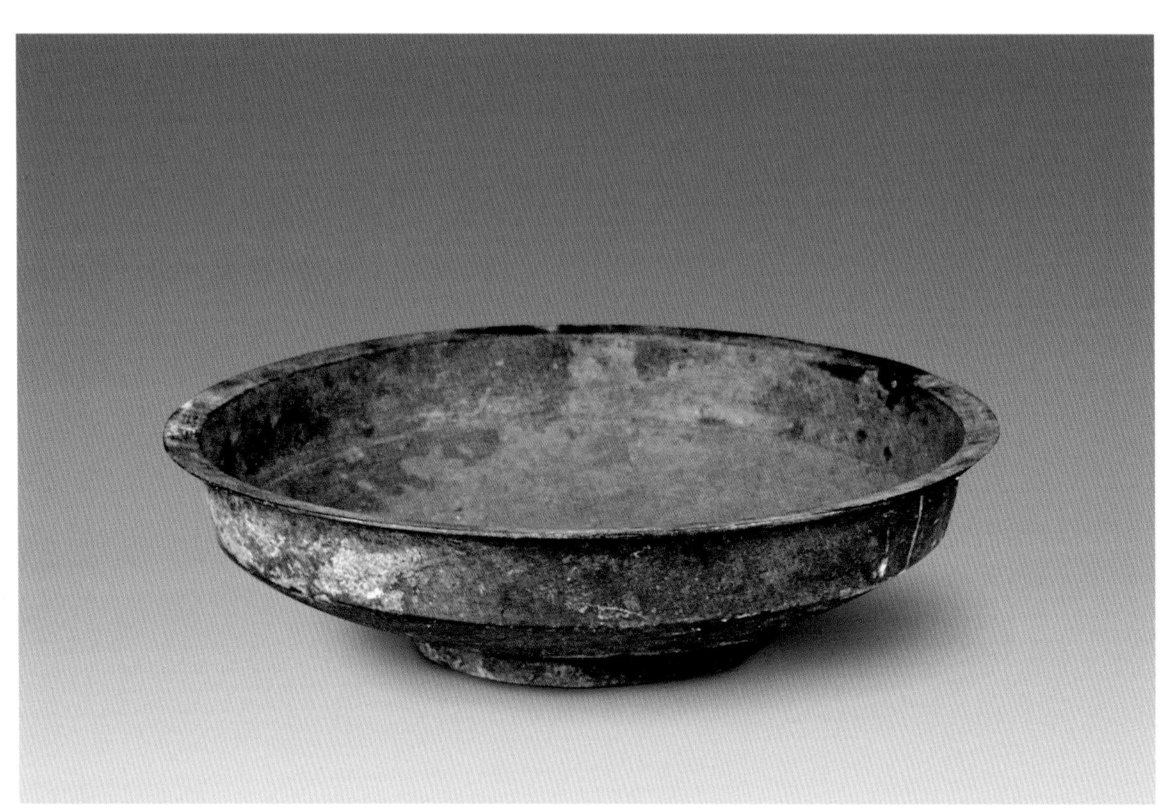

上郡小府盘

汉

口径 23 厘米，通高 25 厘米

敞口，平唇，折肩，圈足，通体光素无纹。

山西博物院藏

"Shang Jun Xiao Fu" Plate

Han Dynasty

Mouth diameter 23 cm/ Height 25 cm

The Plate has a wide mouth, a flat lip, a folded shoulder, and a circular foot. The whole plate is simple and unpatterned.

Preserved in Shanxi Museum

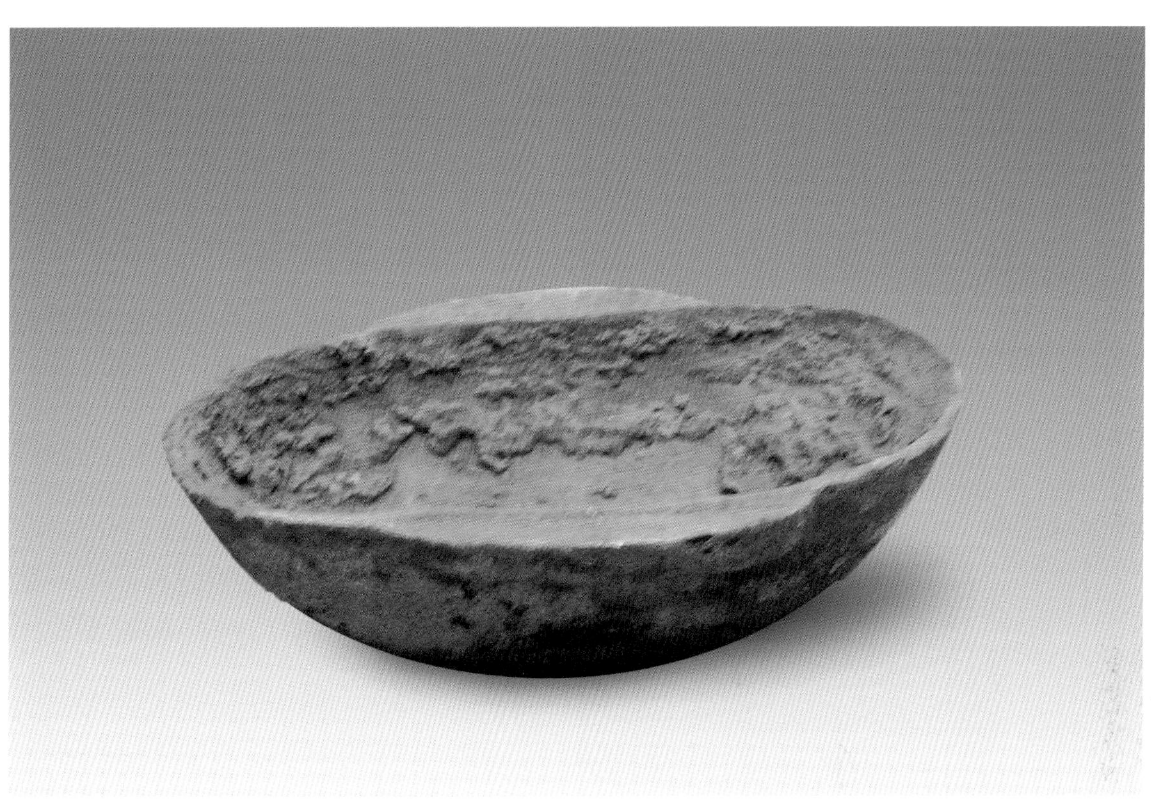

耳杯

汉

铜质

口径 7.5 厘米，高 12 厘米

器身泛铜绿色，保存完整，是饮酒用具，由成都市博物馆调拨。

成都中医药大学中医药传统文化博物馆藏

Ear Cup

Han Dynasty

Copper

Caliber 7.5 cm/ Height 12 cm

The cup body bears the color of copper green. The cup is well preserved and it was used as a drinking vessel. The relic was allocated by Chengdu City Museum.

Preserved in Museum of Traditional Chinese Medicine Culture, Chengdu University of Traditional Chinese Medicine

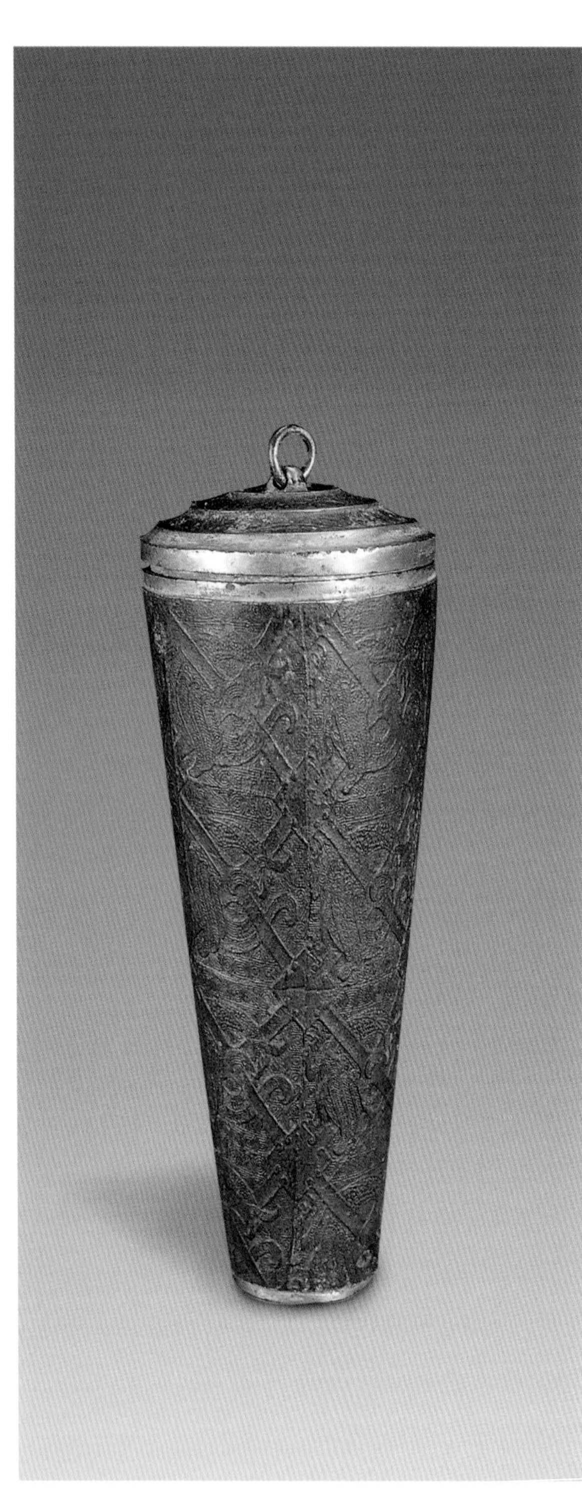

桶形盖杯

西汉

鎏金铜质

口径 5.5 厘米，圈足径 2.9 厘米，通高 14.5 厘米

Barrel-Shaped Cup with Cover

Western Han Dynasty

Gilded copper

Caliber 5.5 cm/ Foot Diameter 2.9 cm/ Height 14.5 cm

杯为直桶形，口大底小，矮圈足。盖作弧面、子口，盖顶有环钮，盖面饰三圈凸弦纹，以形象化的鸟纹为主题。器身通体饰方格图案花纹，以凤鸟为主题。器的口沿、圈足、盖缘、环钮和凸弦纹均鎏金。

河北博物院藏

The cup is like a straight barrel with a large mouth, a small base, and a short circular foot. The cover, with a knob on its top, has an arc surface and seam allowance. The cover surface is adorned with three circular convex string patterns whose theme is of picturesque bird patterns. The whole body is decorated with grid-like patterns which are primarily in the theme of phoenix. The mouth rim, the circular foot, the cover rim, the circular knob, and the convex string patterns are all gilded.

Preserved in Hebei Museum

華

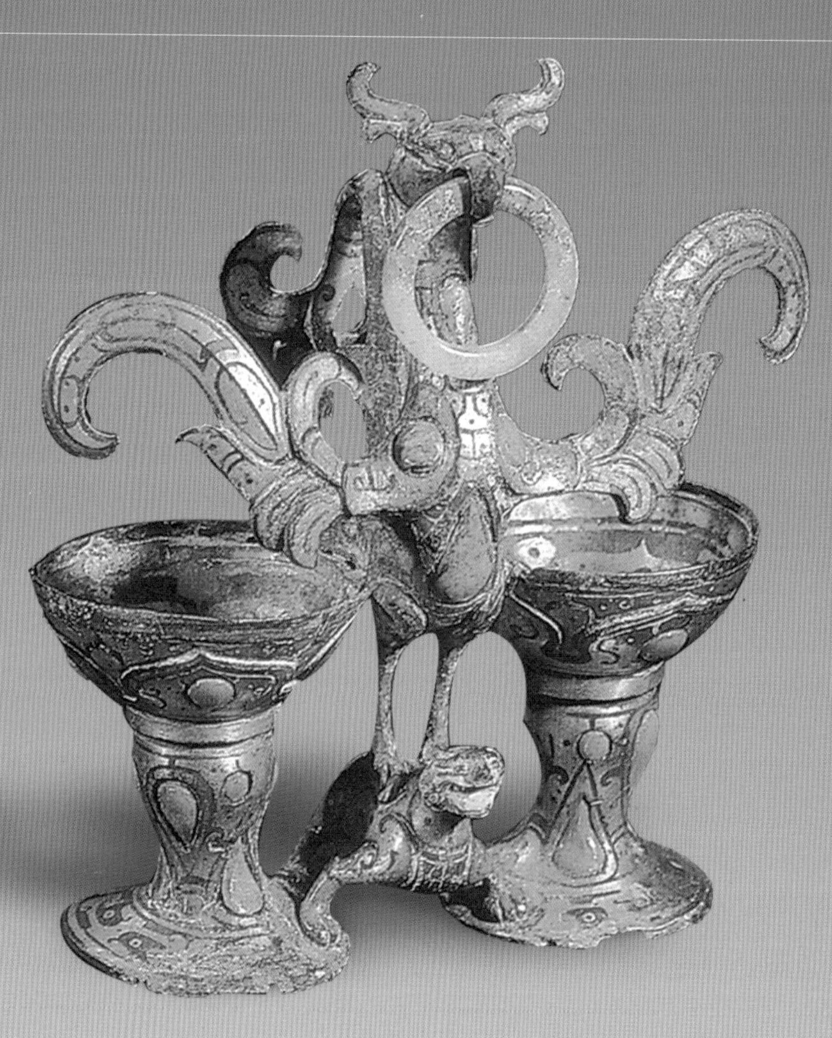

朱雀衔环杯

西汉

铜质

宽 9.5 厘米，通高 11.2 厘米

朱雀衔环矗立于两高足杯之间的兽背上，通体错金。朱雀展翅翘尾，神采飞扬，喙部衔一能自由转动的白玉环。兽匍匐，四足分踏在两高足杯底座上。朱雀的颈、腹与两杯的表面嵌有圆形和心形绿松石十三颗，色彩斑斓。出土时两杯内尚存朱红色痕迹，推测为化妆品。1980 年河北满城汉墓出土。

河北博物院藏

Rosefinch Biting Ring Cup

Western Han Dynasty

Copper

Width 9.5 cm/ Height 11.2 cm

The rosefinch biting rings stands at the animal back between the two stem cups. The whole cup is gilded. The rosefinch stretches its wings and upholds its tail in high spirit with its beak biting a mobilizable white jade ring. The bird is in a creeping position while its four feet are standing on the pedestal of the two stem cups. The rosefinch's neck, belly, as well as the cup surface are inlaid with thirteen gorgeous calaites in circular and heart shape. A trace of vermilion which was supposed to be cosmetics was found when this piece was unearthed. It was unearthed from a tomb of Han in Man County of Hebei Province in 1980.

Preserved in Hebei Museum

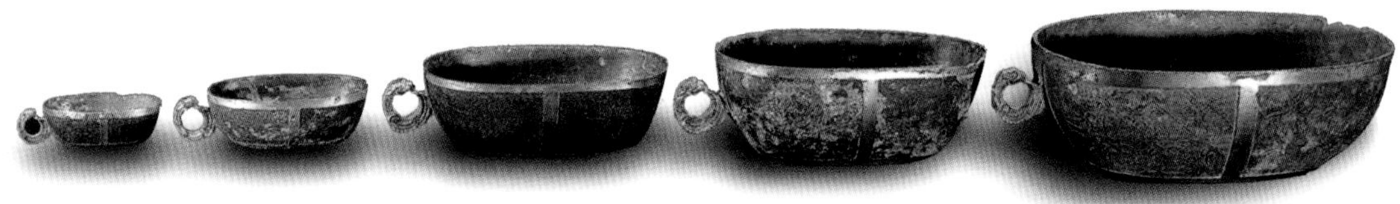

椭圆形铜套杯

西汉

鎏金铜质

口径 5.2~25.9 厘米，高 2.8~9 厘米，容量 65~1800 毫升

A Set of Oval Copper Cups

Western Han Dynasty

Gilded copper

Caliber 5.2–25.9 cm/ Height 2.8-9 cm/ Volume 65-1,800 mL

五件，形状相同，大小逐渐递增，属于一套。器身椭圆，敞口，弧腹，平底。一端附鎏金凤鸟环耳，凤回首衔住凤尾形成环状。口沿和底边鎏金，四道鎏金竖带将器身分为四格，器身和底部饰方格图案，以纤细的云雷纹为地，两带对角勾连，以形象化的鸟纹蟠绕于上。

河北博物院藏

As a set, the five cups bear the same shape but different size in an ascending order. The oval cup body has a wide mouth, an arc-like belly, and a flat base. A gilded bird ear adorns one side of the cup's body. A gilded circular phoenix ear is attached to the cup body. Meanwhile, the bird is turning around to bite its tail. The mouth rim and the base are gilded. Four gilded vertical strips divided the cup body into four parts. The cup body and base are ornamented with checkerboard pattern shaded by fine cloud-thunder pattern. The two strips are colluded with each other in opposite angles and coiled with vivid bird design.

Preserved in Hebei Museum

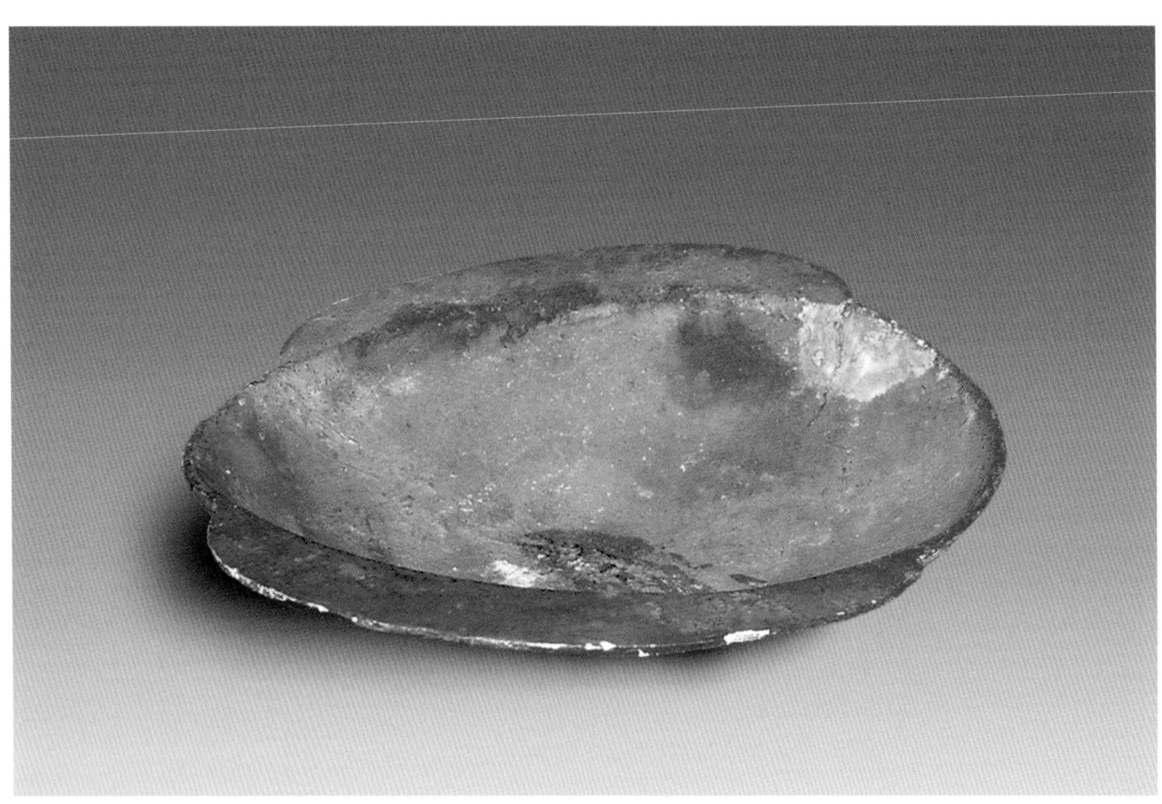

铜耳杯

汉

铜质

口径 9.5 厘米，底径 4 厘米，通高 2 厘米，重 50 克

Copper Ear Cup

Han Dynasty

Copper

Caliber 9.5 cm/ Base Diameter 4 cm/ Height 2 cm/ Weight 50 g

椭圆形口，两平耳，半圆底。酒器。有残。陕西省西安市边家村出土。

陕西医史博物馆藏

The cup has an oval mouth, two flat ears, and a semicircular base. It is a wine vessel but not intact. This piece was unearthed in Bianjia Village, Xi'an City, Shaanxi Province.

Preserved in Shaanxi Museum of Medical History

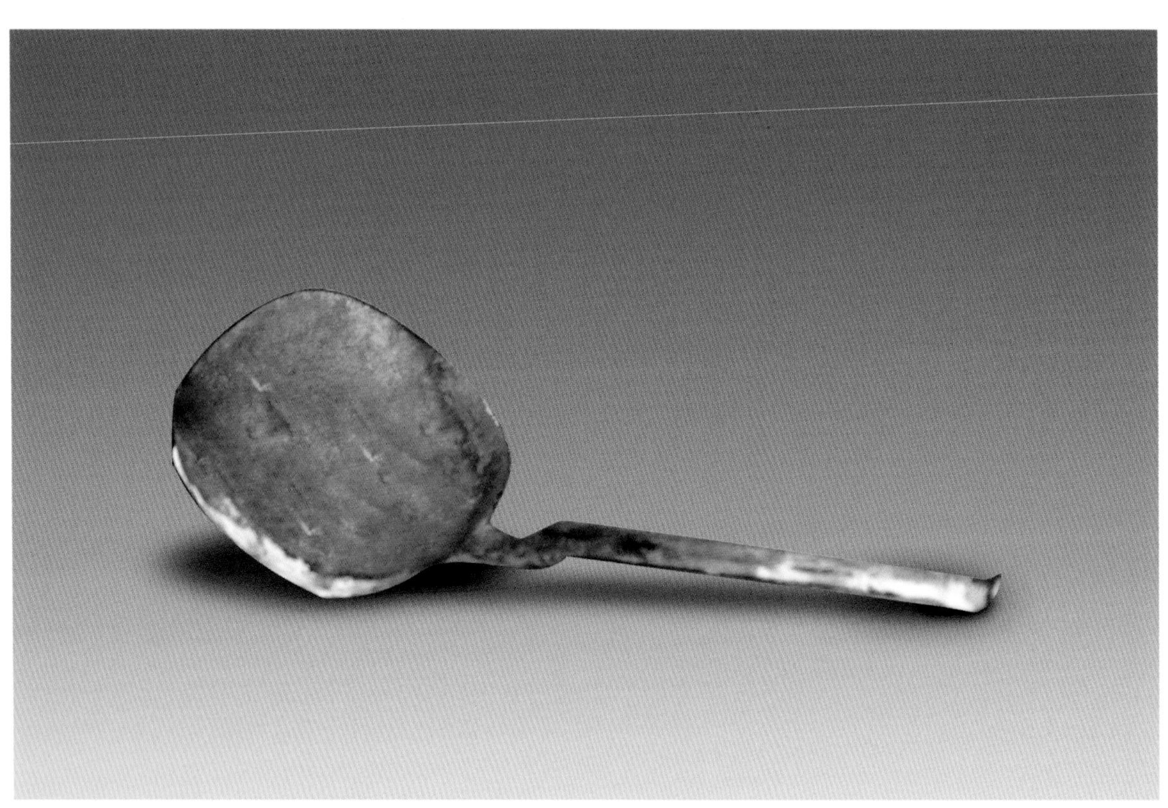

铜勺

汉

铜质

宽 10 厘米，重 150 克

Copper Spoon

Han Dynasty

Copper

Width 10 cm/ Weight 150 g

勺状，勺柄呈长条状，勺头浅椭圆形。生活器具。完整无损。陕西省西安市二府街征集。

陕西医史博物馆藏

The relic is in spoon shape with a long and slim handle. The spoon head appears shallow oval shape. It was an article for daily use. The relic is intact. It was collected in Erfu Street, Xi'an City, Shaanxi Province.

Preserved in Shaanxi Museum of Medical History

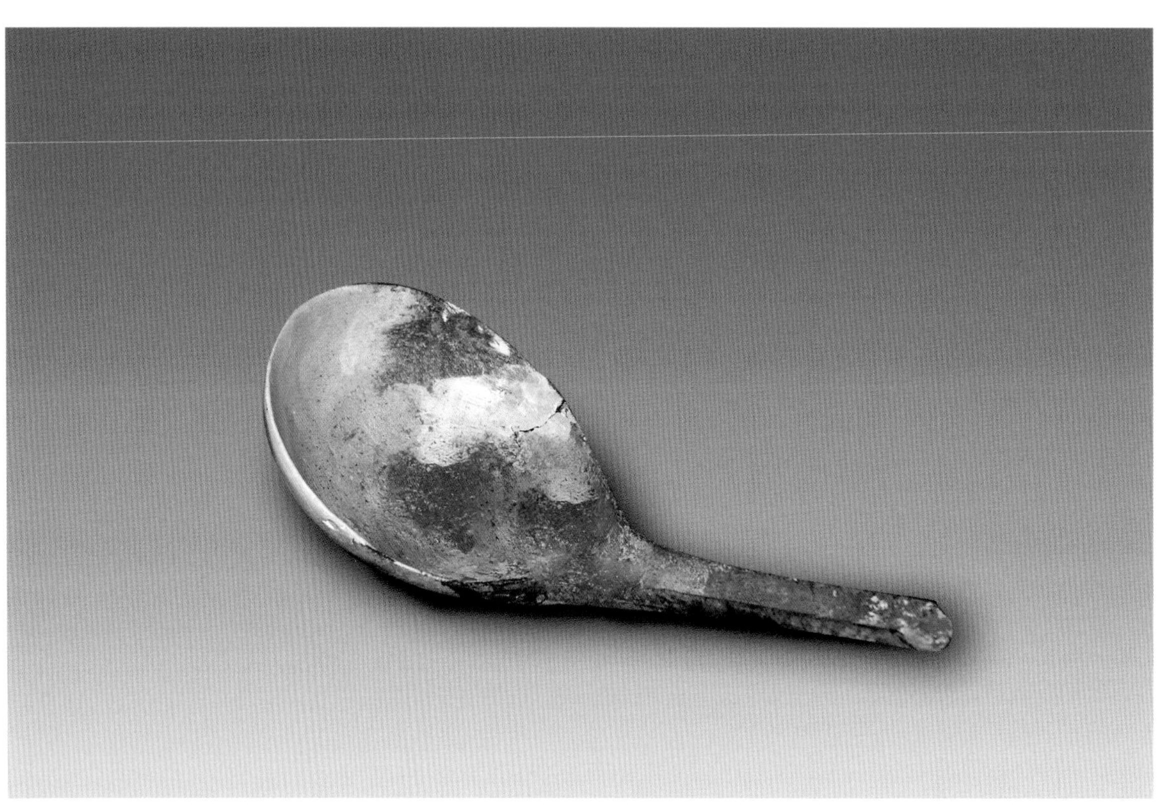

铜勺

汉

铜质

长 23.5 厘米，宽 11 厘米，重 150 克

Copper Spoon

Han Dynasty

Copper

Length 23.5 cm/ Width 11 cm/ Weight 150 g

勺状，勺柄呈渠状，勺头大而深。生活器具。有修补。陕西省西安市边家村征集。

陕西医史博物馆藏

The relic has a trench-like handle and is in spoon shape. The spoon head is large and deep. The spoon was an article of daily use. The spoon has a trace of repair. It was collected from Bianjia Village, Xi'an City, Shaanxi Province.

Preserved in Shaanxi Museum of Medical History

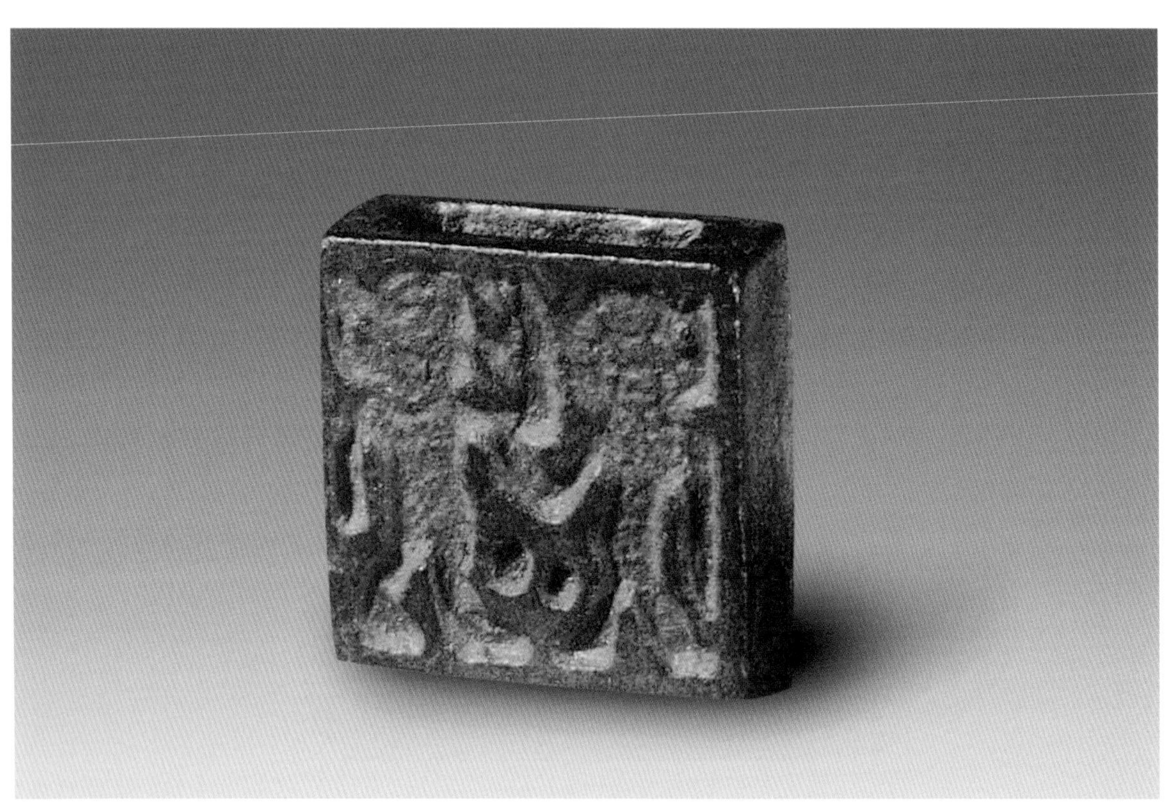

蹴鞠纹肖形印

汉

铜质

边长1. 4 厘米

Cu Ju Pictorial Seal (Cu Ju- Ancient Chinese Football)

Han Dynasty

Copper

Side Length 1.4 cm

印为铜质，印面为正方形。图中两头后束发髻的蹴鞠者，正做出欲踢的样子。两人之间有二鞠已被踢起。此当为古代蹴鞠"白打"形式中较早的一种。

故宫博物院藏

The seal surface is square. With their hair tied up with a bus, the two Cu Ju players appear to be kicking the balls. Two balls have been kicked up between the players. This represents an early form of "unarmed fighting" in Cu-ju games dating back to ancient times.

Preserved in the Palace Museum

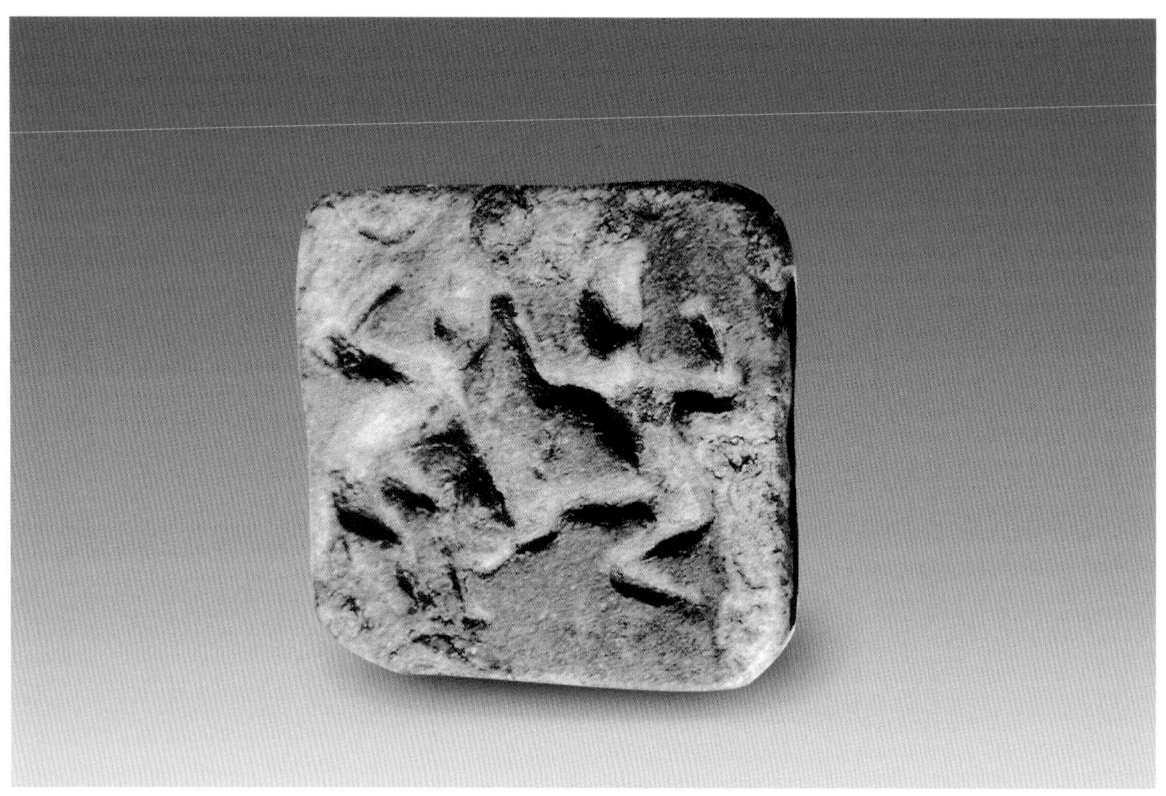

角抵纹肖形印

汉

钢质

边长 1.1~1.4 厘米

Ancient Wrestling Pattern Pictorial Seal

Han Dynasty

Steel

Side Length 1.1-1.4 cm

印为钢质，印面近于正方形。印纹中两摔跤力士正斗得难分难解，一方以右手撼对方左脚，一方在奋力挣脱，场面显得殊为紧张。

故宫博物院藏

The seal is made of steel. Its surface is approximately in square shape. Two wrestlers are fighting fiercely in the seal pattern. One of then is trying to shake his rival's left foot by his right hand while the other side is shielding hard. The scene is rather tense.

Preserved in the Palace Museum

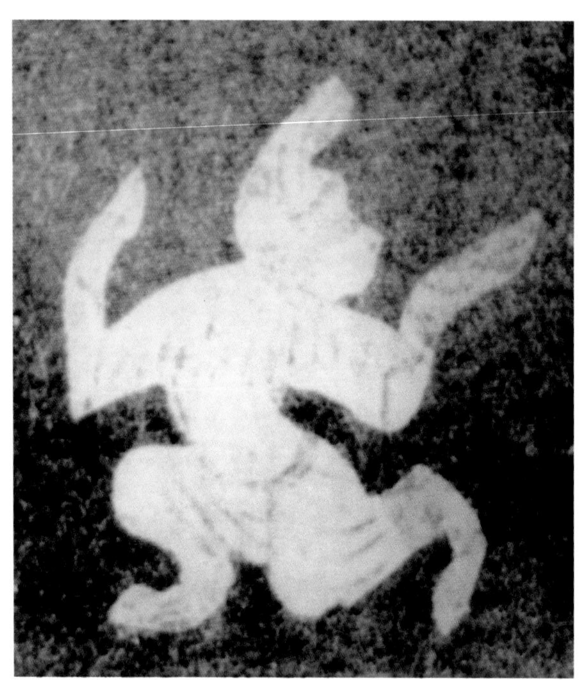

漆盒武术纹贴花片

西汉

金质

Lacquer Box Decal with Wushu Pattern

Western Han Dynasty

Gold

贴花片为金箔制成，为一漆盒上面的贴花装饰。这一武术纹贴花片的习武者头梳高髻，戴猴形面具，呈蹲步，双肘上扬，正做出拳术中猴拳的姿势。1978 年湖南省长沙市杨家山 304 号西汉墓出土。

湖南省博物馆藏

The decal made of gold foil is a decoration on the lacquer box surface. The martial art player in the pattern has his hair pulled up high in a bun. Wearing a monkey-shaped mask, he appears monkey boxing gestures by crouching and raising both elbows upward. It was unearthed in No. 304 Western Han Tomb in Yangjiashan, Changsha City, Hunan Province in 1978.

Preserved in Hunan Provincial Museum

華

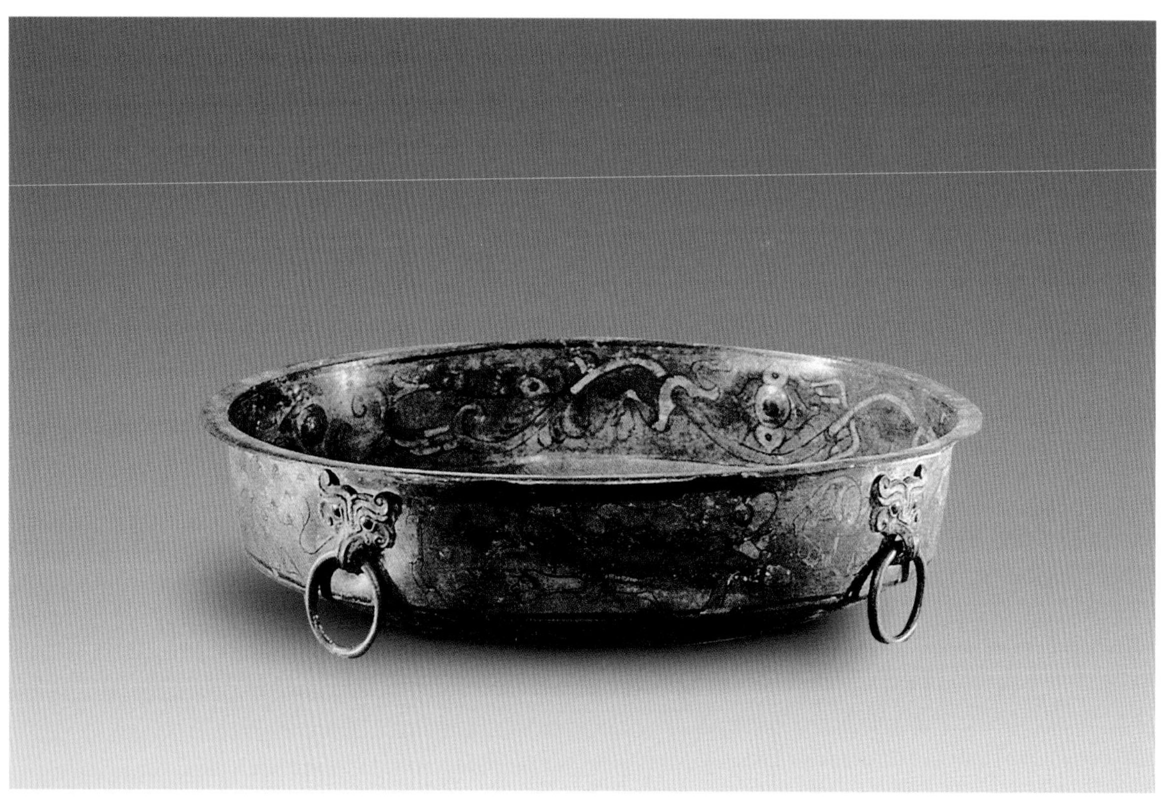

技击图漆画铜鉴

西汉

铜质

口径 50 厘米，高 13.5 厘米

Copper Mirror with Wushu Lacquer Painting

Western Han Dynasty

Copper

Caliber 50 cm/ Height 13.5 cm

鉴为平口，宽唇沿外折，浅直腹，腹侧有一对铺首衔环。漆画主要见于其口沿和腹壁内外。其中腹外壁所饰是以技击为主要内容的漆画，包括徒手对打、持器械相击等形式，再现了当时武艺活动的精彩场景。1976 年广西壮族自治区贵县罗泊湾 1 号西汉墓出土。

广西壮族自治区博物馆藏

The mirror has a flat mouth, a broad and outstretched lip rim, and a shallow and straight belly. On one side of the belly is decorated with two animal head holding rings. The lacquer painting is seen on the mouth rim and both sides of the belly wall. The outer belly wall is primarily lacquer painting about attack and defense in wushu such as armed or unarmed fighting. The painting represents the highlights of ancient wushu activities. It was unearthed in NO.1 Western Han Tomb, Luopowan, Gui County, Guangxi Zhuang Autonomous Region, in 1976.

Preserved in the Museum of Guangxi Zhuang Autonomous Region

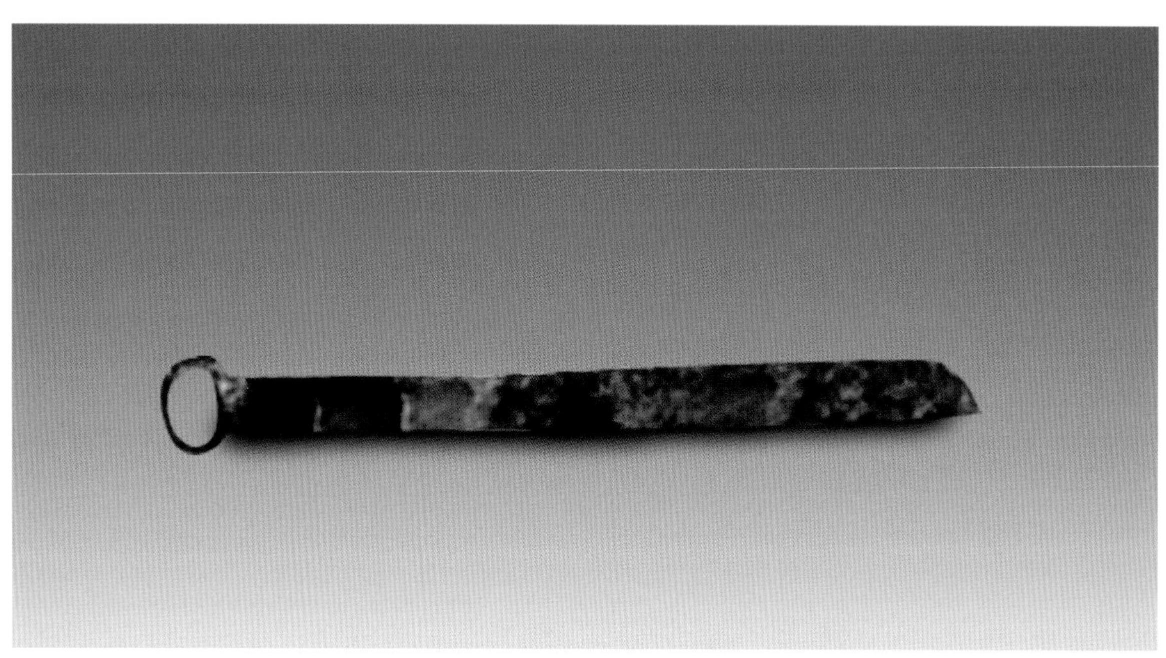

铜削刀

汉

铜质

长 15.2 厘米

条形，刀一端呈尖状，另一端半圆形，可用于削、切。

广东中医药博物馆藏

Copper Sharpener

Han Dynasty

Copper

Length 15.2 cm

The knife is in the shape of bar with one pointed end and one semicircular end. It was used for sharpening and cutting.

Preserved in Guangdong Chinese Medicine Museum

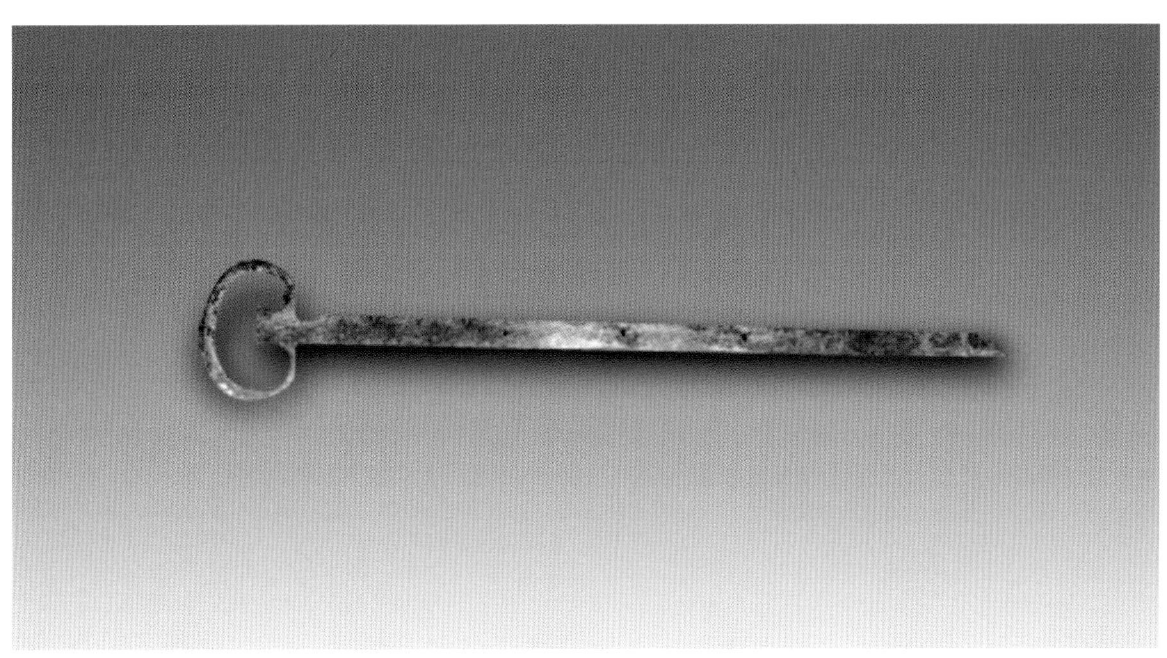

铜削刀

汉

铜质

长 22.5 厘米

条形，刀一端呈尖状，另一端半圆形，可用于削、切。

广东中医药博物馆藏

Copper Sharpener

Han Dynasty

Copper

Length 22.5 cm

The knife is in the shape of bar with one pointed end and one semicircular end. It was used for sharpening and cutting.

Preserved in Guangdong Chinese Medicine Museum

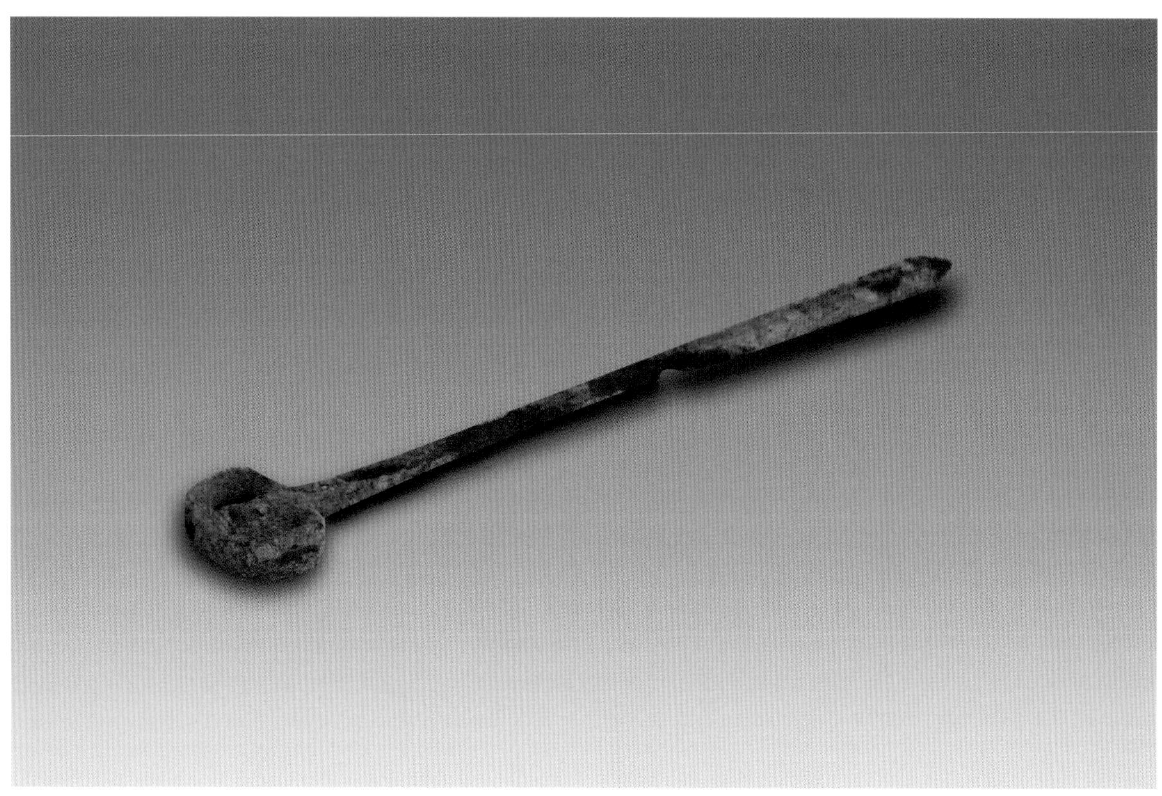

铁刀

秦

铁质

大：长 27 厘米

中：长 20 厘米

小：长 5 厘米

重：300 克

Iron Knife

Qin Dynasty

Iron

The large one: Length: 27 cm

The middle one: Length 20 cm

The small one: Length: 5 cm

Weight 300g

一套三件，圆把全锈。生活器具，有残，陕西省长安区征集。

陕西医史博物馆藏

There are three knives in one set. The circular handle of the knife is completely rusty. It is an article of daily use with some parts missing. It was collected from Chang'an District, Shaanxi Province.

Preserved in Shaanxi Museum of Medical History

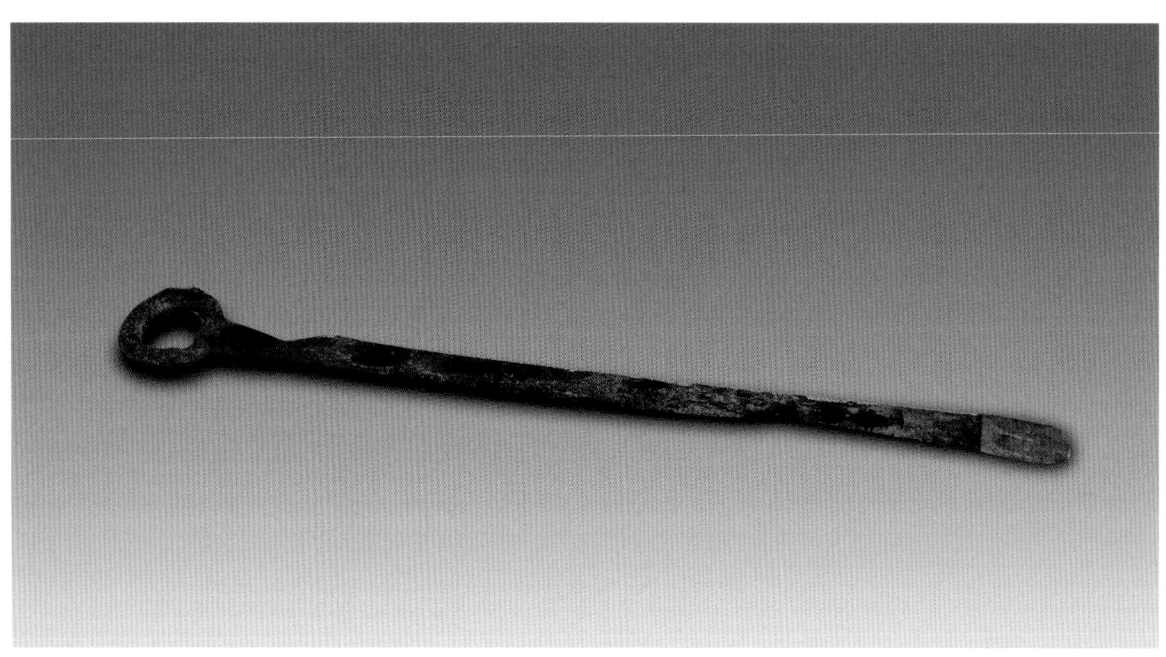

铁刀

秦

铁质

长 33 厘米，宽 1.5 厘米，重 200 克

Iron Knife

Qin Dynasty

Iron

Length 33 cm/ Width 1.5 cm/ Weight 200 g

手把为圆形环，尖带有银套，中间全锈。兵器，生活器具，有残，陕西省西安市长安区征集。

陕西医史博物馆藏

The handgrip of the knife is in the shape a ring. The end of the knife is covered with a silver sheath. The middle of the knife is completely rusty. It was a weapon or an article of daily use. It was collected from Chang’an District in xi’an, Shaanxi Province.

Preserved in Shaanxi Museum of Medical History

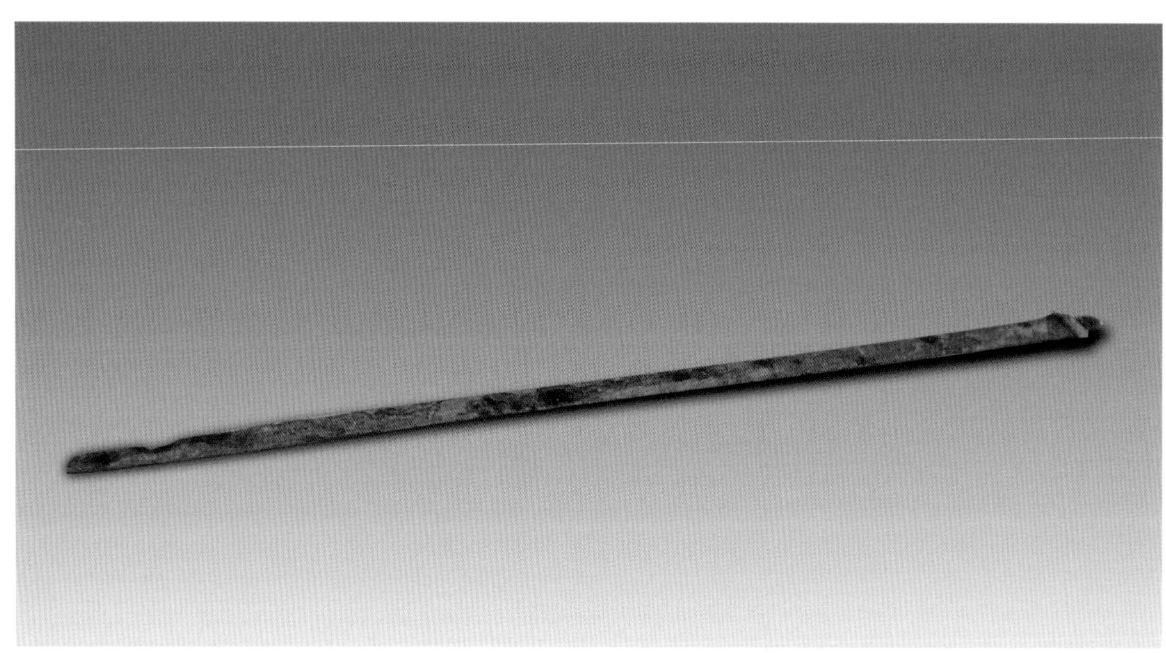

铁剑

秦

铁质

长 72 厘米，宽 3 厘米，重 500 克

Iron Sword

Qin Dynasty

Iron

Length 72 cm/ Width 3 cm/ Weight 500 g

无把，无尖，全锈。兵器，保健器具，有残。陕西省西安市长安区征集。

陕西医史博物馆藏

The sword has no handle or tip. It is completely rusty. It was a weapon or a health care appliance with some parts missing. It was collected from Chang'an District in Xi'an, Shaanxi Province.

Preserved in Shaanxi Museum of Medical History

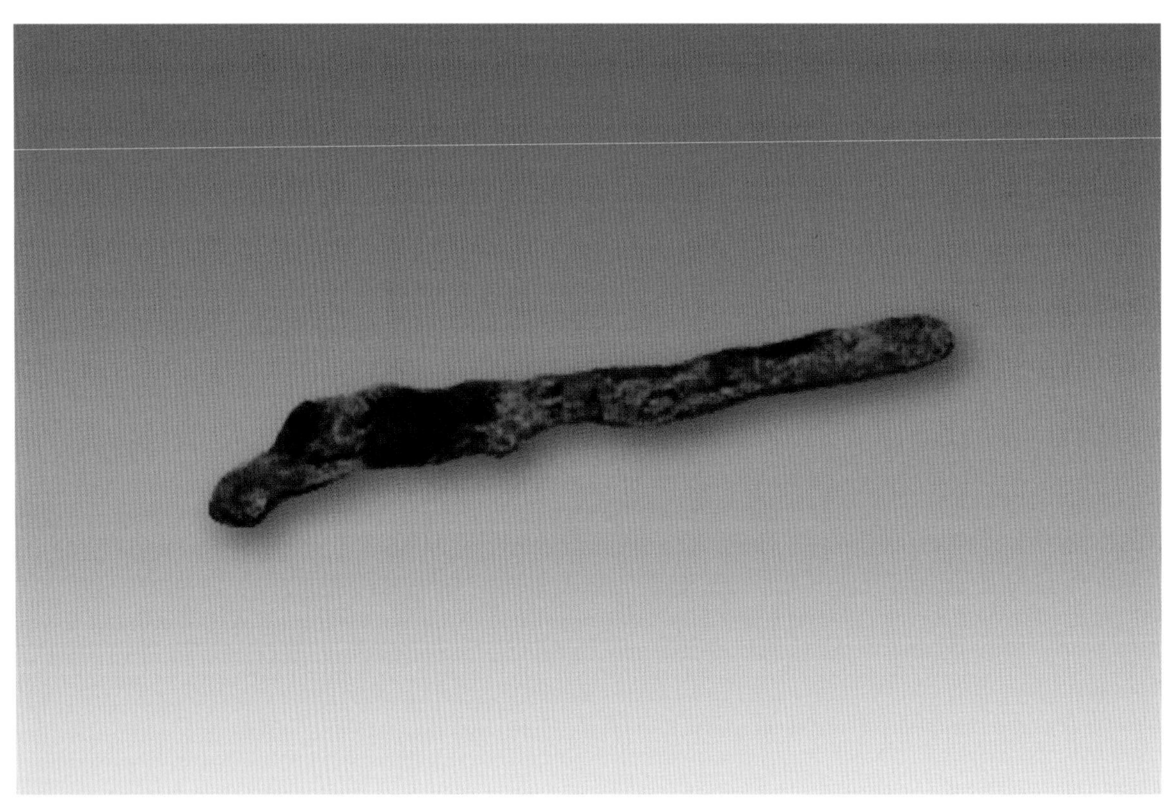

铁凿器

秦

铁质

长 12.5 厘米，重 150 克

Iron Chisel

Qin Dynasty

Iron

Length 12.5 cm/ Weight 150 g

长条形，中间有孔，全锈。生活、生产工具，有残，陕西省长安区征集。

陕西医史博物馆收藏

This chisel, all rusted and damaged, is a long strip with a hole in the middle. It has been used as a living and producing tool. It was collected from Chang'an district of Shaanxi Province.

Preserved in Shaanxi Museum of Medical History

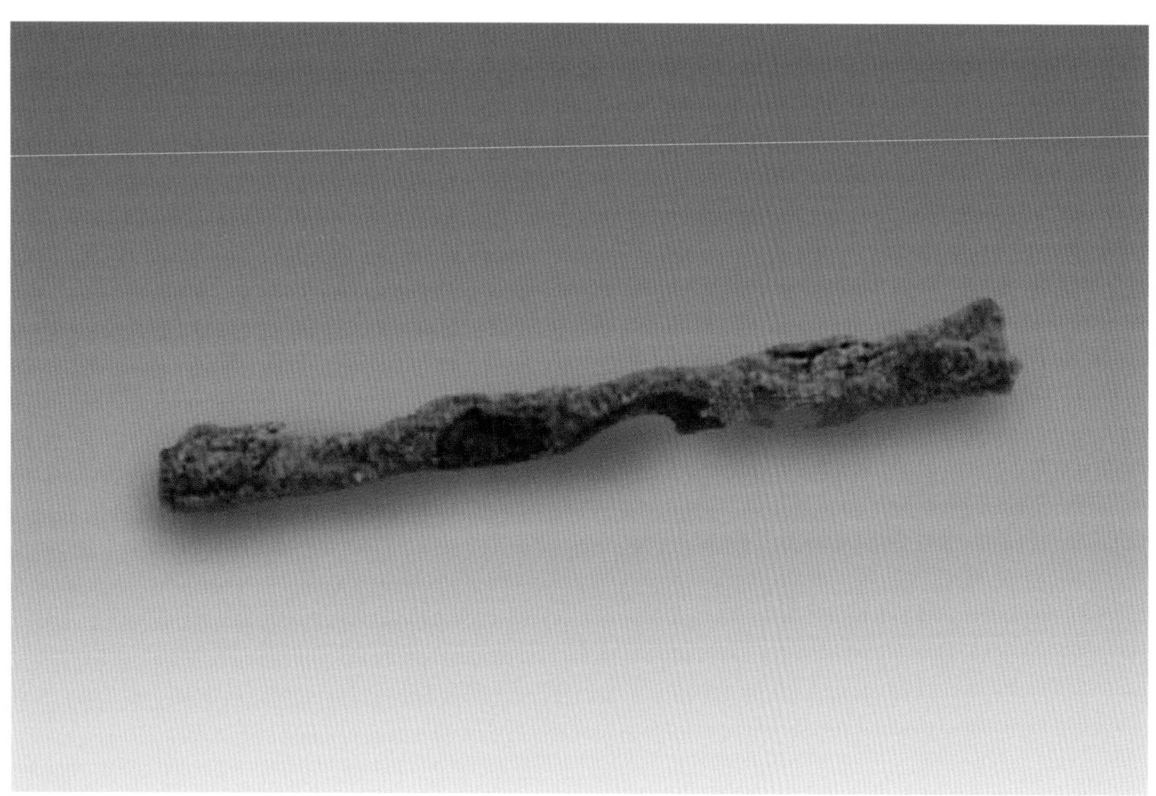

铁凿器

秦代

铁质

长 13 厘米，重 150 克

Iron Chisel

Qin Dynasty

Iron

Length 13 cm/ Weight 150 g

长勺状，全锈。生活、生产工具有残，陕西省长安区征集。

陕西医史博物馆收藏

This chisel, all rusted and damaged, is in the shape of a spoon. It has been used as a living and producing tool. It was collected from Chang'an District of Shaanxi Province.

Preserved in Shaanxi Museum of Medical History

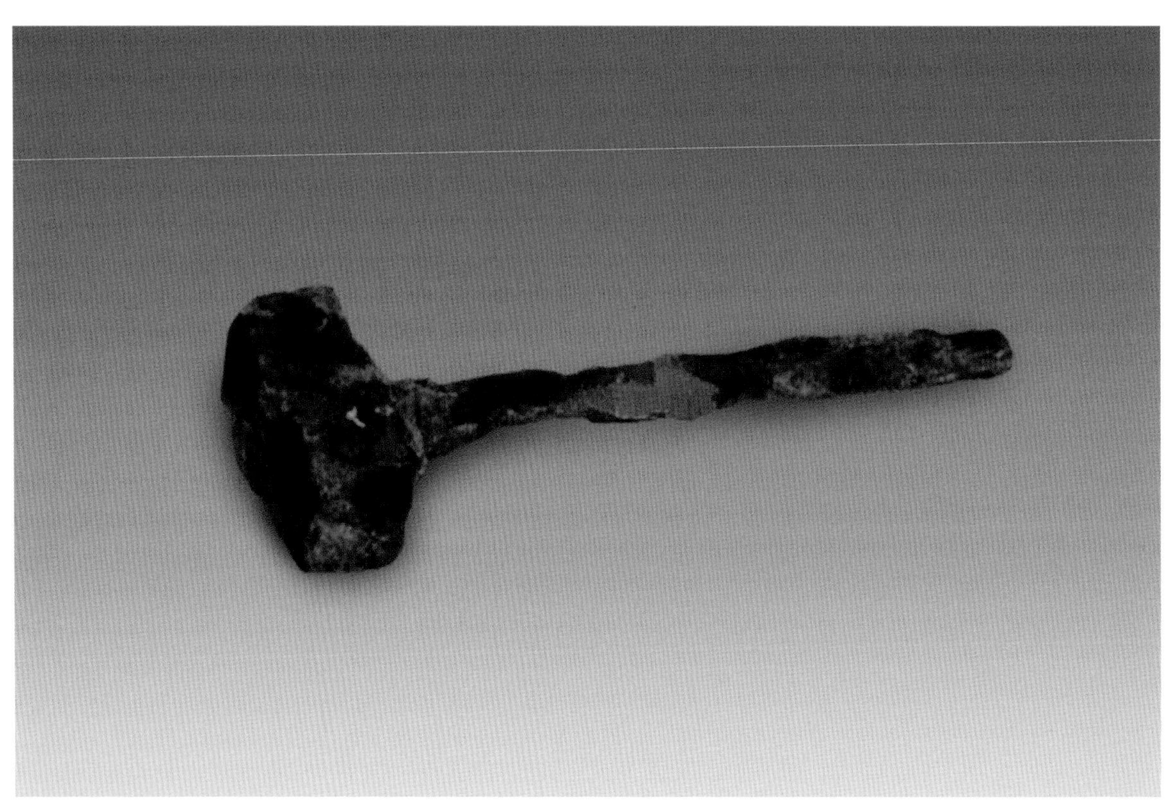

铁锤

秦代

铁质

长 13 厘米，宽 5 厘米，重 150 克

Iron Hammer

Qin Dynasty

Iron

Length 13 cm/ Width 5 cm/ Weight 150 g

头为长方形，一圆把。生活用具，有残，陕西省长安区征集。

陕西医史博物馆收藏

The hammer has a rectangular top and a round handle. It has been used as a living and production tool. It was collected from Chang'an District of Shaanxi Province.

Preserved in Shaanxi Museum of Medical History

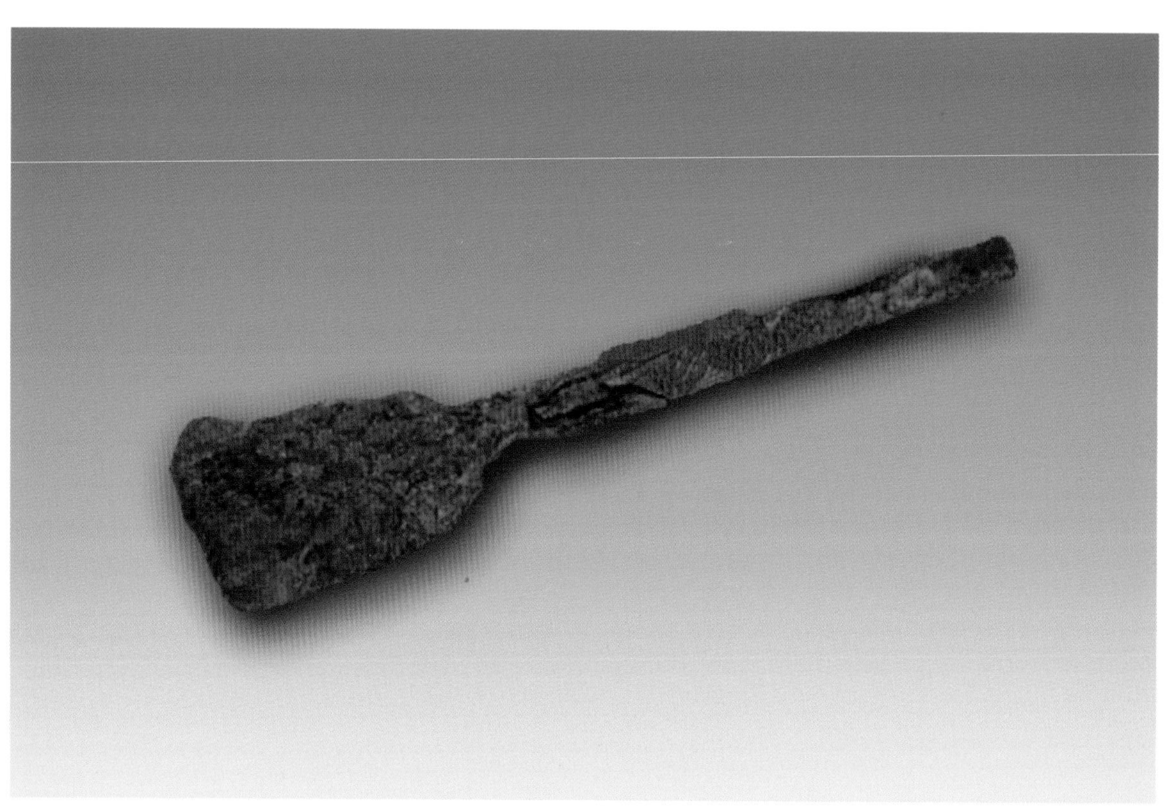

铁铲

秦

铁质

长 16 厘米，宽 4.5 厘米，重 50 克

Iron Shovel

Qin Dynasty

Iron

Length 16 cm/ Width 4.5 cm/ Weight 50 g

铲状，头为铲，一圆把。生产工具，有残，陕西省长安区征集。

陕西医史博物馆收藏

The tool, in the shape of shovel, has a round handle. It has been used as a labor tool. It is damaged. It was collected from Chang'an District of Shaanxi Province.

Preserved in Shaanxi Museum of Medical History

華

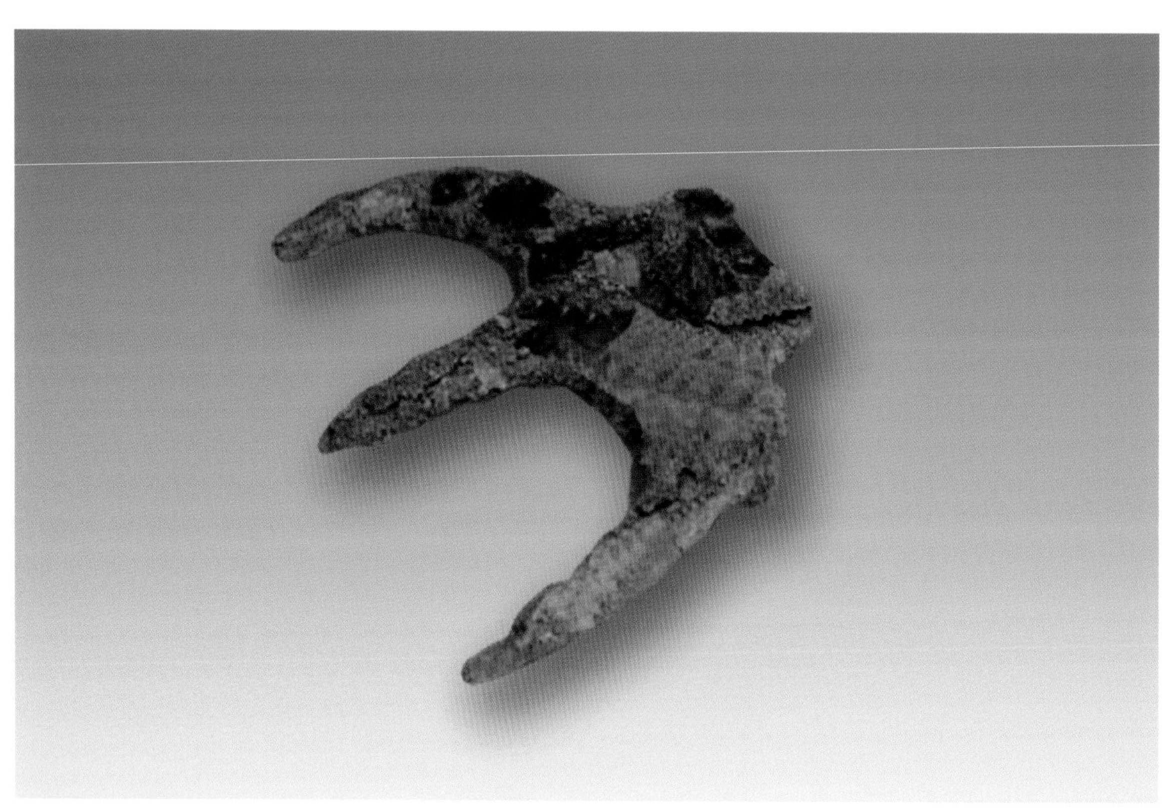

铁钯

秦

铁质

长 12 厘米，宽 16 厘米，重 500 克

耙状三齿，齿上有一方孔。生产工具，有残，陕西省长安区征集。

陕西医史博物馆收藏

Iron Rake

Qin Dynasty

Iron

Length 12 cm/ Width 16 cm/ Weight 500 g

The tool, damaged, is in the shape of a rake with three forks in which there is a square hole. It has been used as a labor tool. It was collected from Chang'an District of Shaanxi Province.

Preserved in Shaanxi Museum of Medical History

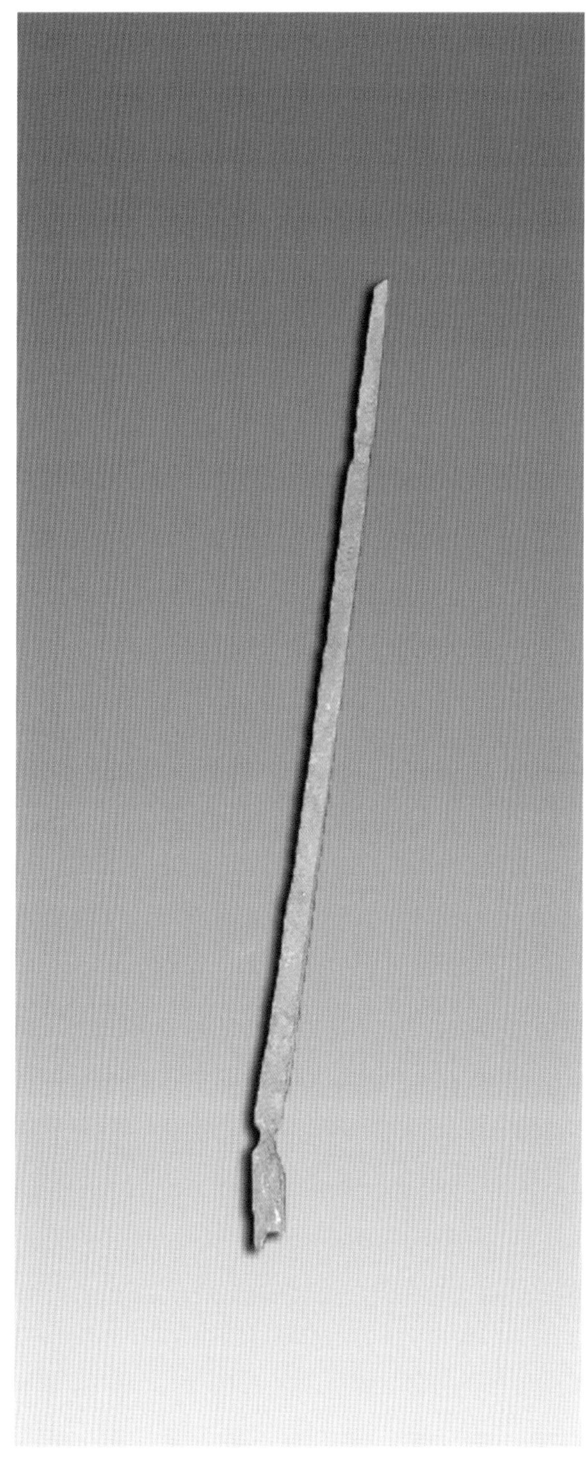

铁剑

汉

铁质

长 76.5 厘米，宽 2.6 厘米

击刺短器械。剑身扁平细长，单刃，柄部上翘。此为汉代北方游牧民族常用的武术器械。

内蒙古博物院藏

Iron Sword

Han Dynasty

Length 76.5 cm/ Width 2.6 cm

The sword is a short weapon used for fencing or stabbing. With an upturned hilt, the sword body has a single-edged blade, flat and slender. It is a martial arts weapon commonly used by northern nomadic people in the Han Dynasty.

Preserved in Inner Mongolia Museum

華

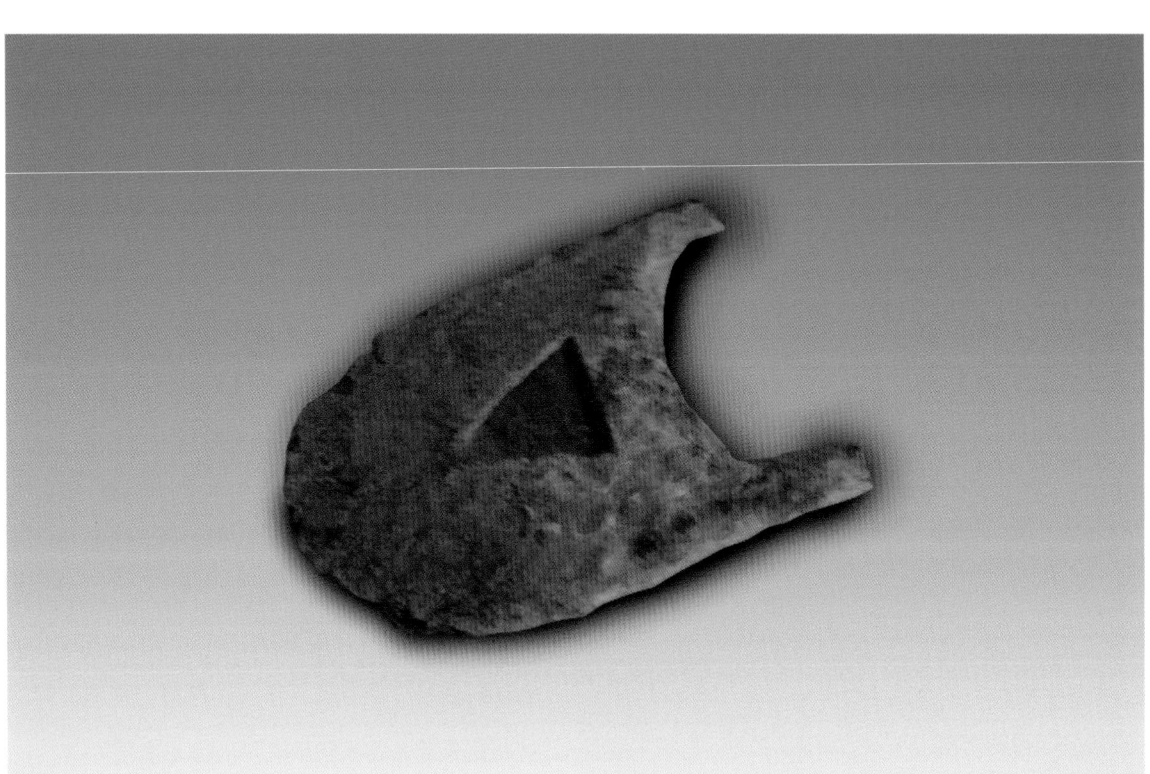

铁铧

汉

铁质

长口径 34 厘米，宽 23 厘米，重 3900 克

Iron Plowshare

Han Dynasty

Iron

Length 34 cm/ Width 23 cm/ Weight 3,900 g

铧状。生产工具，完整无损，陕西省澄城县征集。

陕西医史博物馆收藏

The tool is in the shape of a plowshare. It has been used as a labor tool. It is intact and undamaged. It was collected from Chengcheng of Shaanxi Province.

Preserved in Shaanxi Museum of Medical History

华

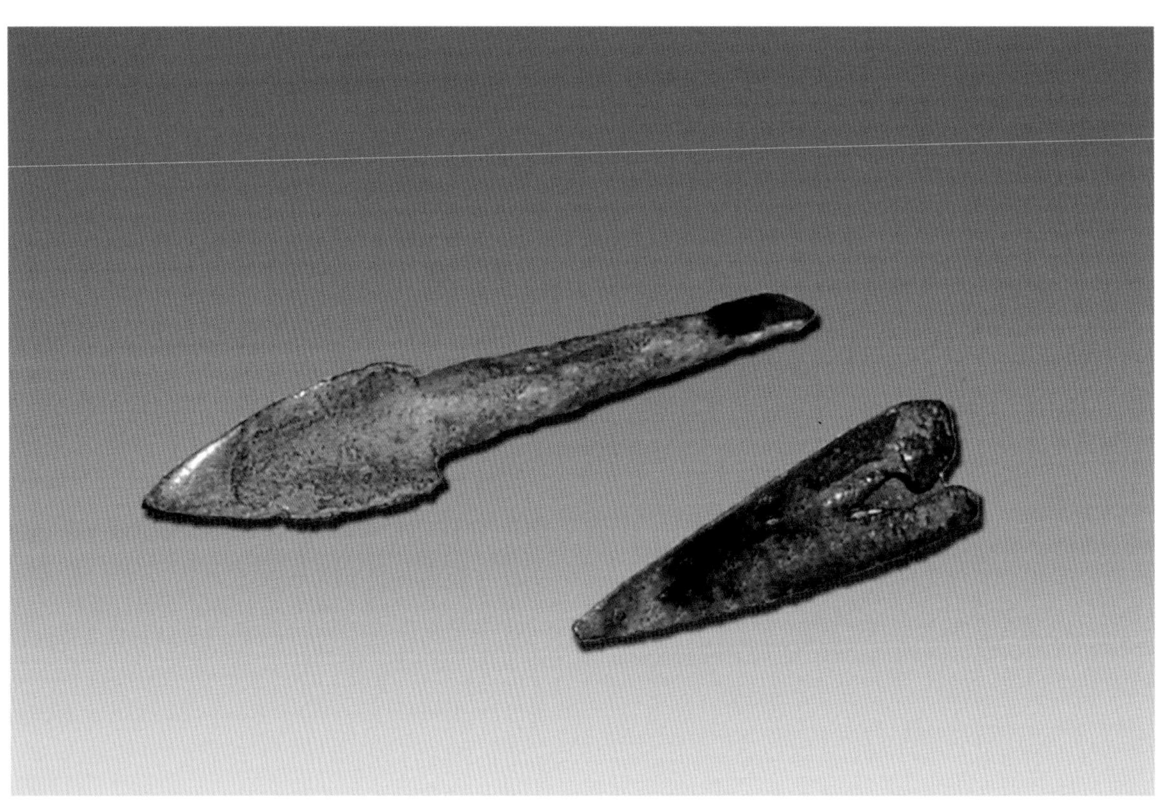

铜箭镞

汉

铜质

长 5.5 厘米，宽 3.2 厘米，重 30 克

Copper Arrowheads

Han Dynasty

Copper

Length 5.5 cm/ Width 3.2 cm/ Weight 30 g

一个带把，镞头呈三棱形；一个无把，镞头有三个小孔。兵器。完整无损。内蒙古自治区成陵废品站征集。

陕西医史博物馆藏

One arrowhead has a handle with its tip in triangular prism while the other one does not have but the tip has three small holes. The arrowheads, which remain intact, were collected from Cheng Ling Waste Station in the Inner Mongolia Autonomous Region.

Preserved in Shaanxi Museum of Medical History

華

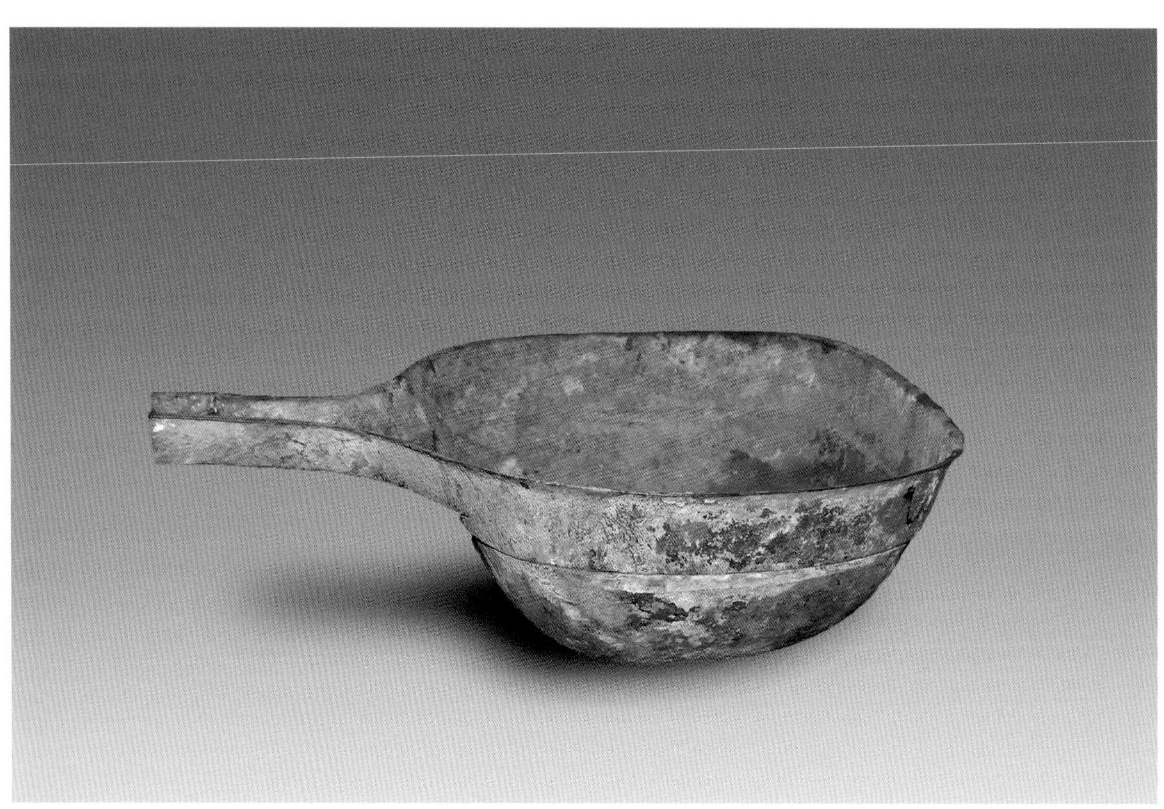

铜匜

汉

铜质

长 37.4 厘米，宽 29.6 厘米，高 10.8 厘米

Copper Yi

(Yi-ancient water vessel)

Han Dynasty

Copper

Length 37.4 cm/ Width 29.6 cm/ Height 10.8 cm

方口，斜腹，假圈足，口处有一流。生活器具。稍残。陕西省咸阳市博物馆调拨。

陕西医史博物馆藏

The vessel has a square mouth, an oblique belly, a fake circular foot, and a spout on the mouth. It is an article of daily use with some parts missing. It was allotted by the Xianyang Museum, Shaanxi Province.

Preserved in Shaanxi Museum of Medical History

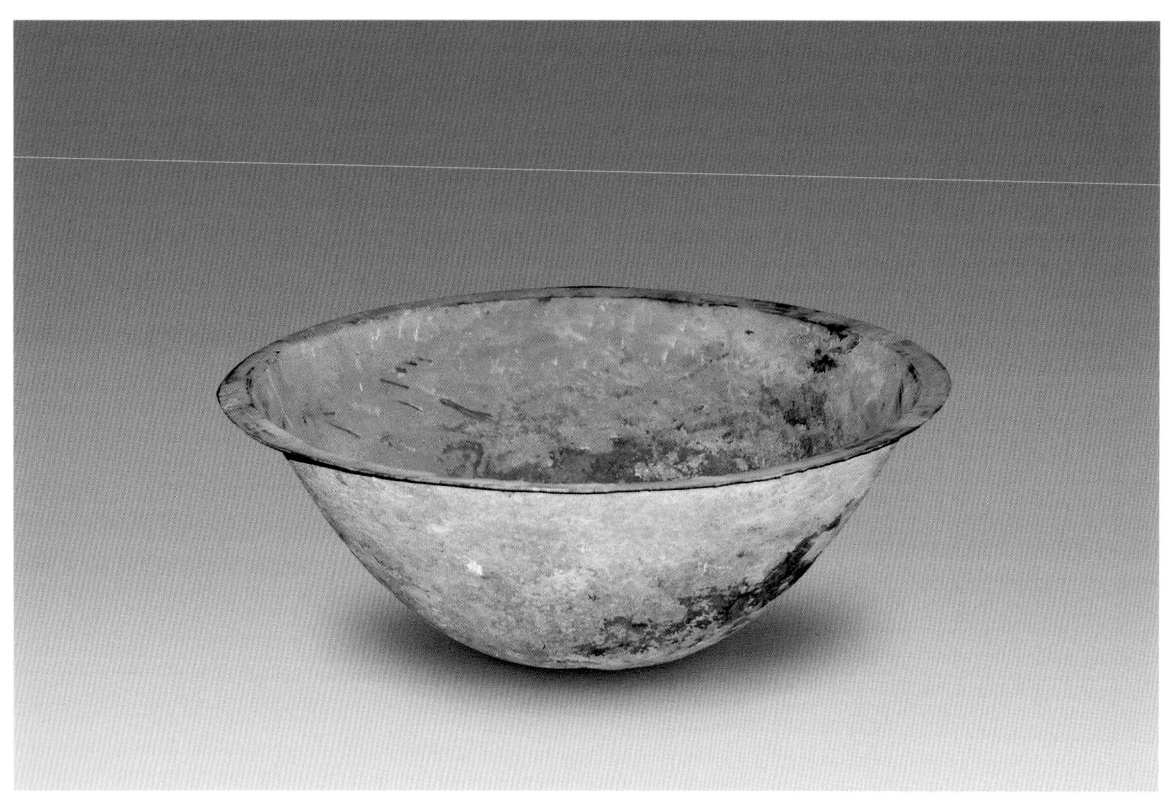

铜洗

汉

铜质

口径 12.3 厘米，底径 14.8 厘米，通高 10.5 厘米

Copper Basin

Han Dynasty

Copper

Caliber 12.3 cm/ Base Diameter 14.8 cm/ Height 10.5 cm

平口沿，侈口，斜腹，平底。生活器具。稍残。陕西省咸阳市博物馆调拨。

陕西医史博物馆藏

The basin has a flat edge, a wide flared mouth, an oblique belly, and a flat base. It is an article of daily use with some parts missing. It was allotted by the Xianyang Museum, Shaanxi Province.

Preserved in Shaanxi Museum of Medical History

華

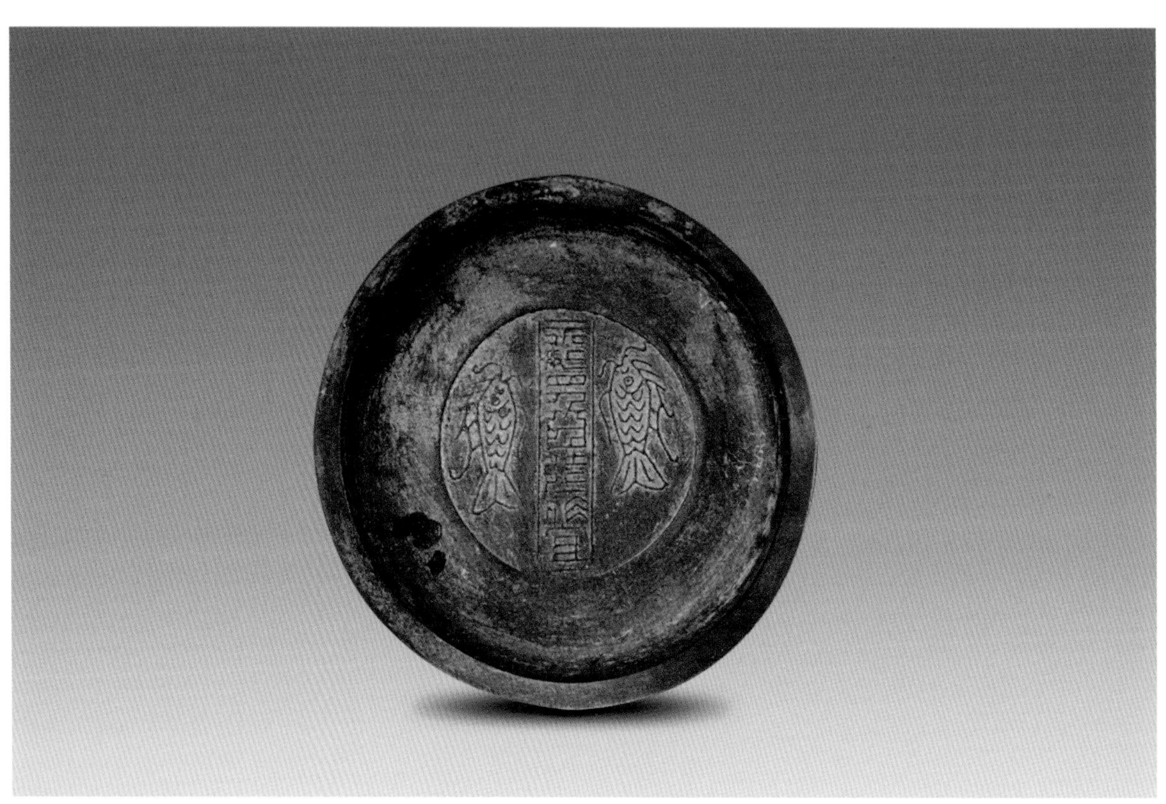

双鱼纹洗

汉

青铜质

口径 32.8 厘米，高 7.5 厘米

Double-Fish Pattern Basin

Han Dynasty

Bronze

Caliber 32.8 cm/ Height 7.5 cm

洗呈圆形，直口，斜折宽沿，浅腹平底。内底一圆，内篆铭一行："永和四年造作宜"7字。两侧饰双鱼纹。

山西博物院藏

The circular basin has a straight mouth, an oblique folded broad rim, a shallow belly, and a flat foot. There is a circle inside the base. A line of seven Chinese characters "Yong He Si Nian Zao Zuo Yi" is inscribed within the circle. A fish pattern is decorated on each side of the inscriptions.

Preserved in Shanxi Museum

華

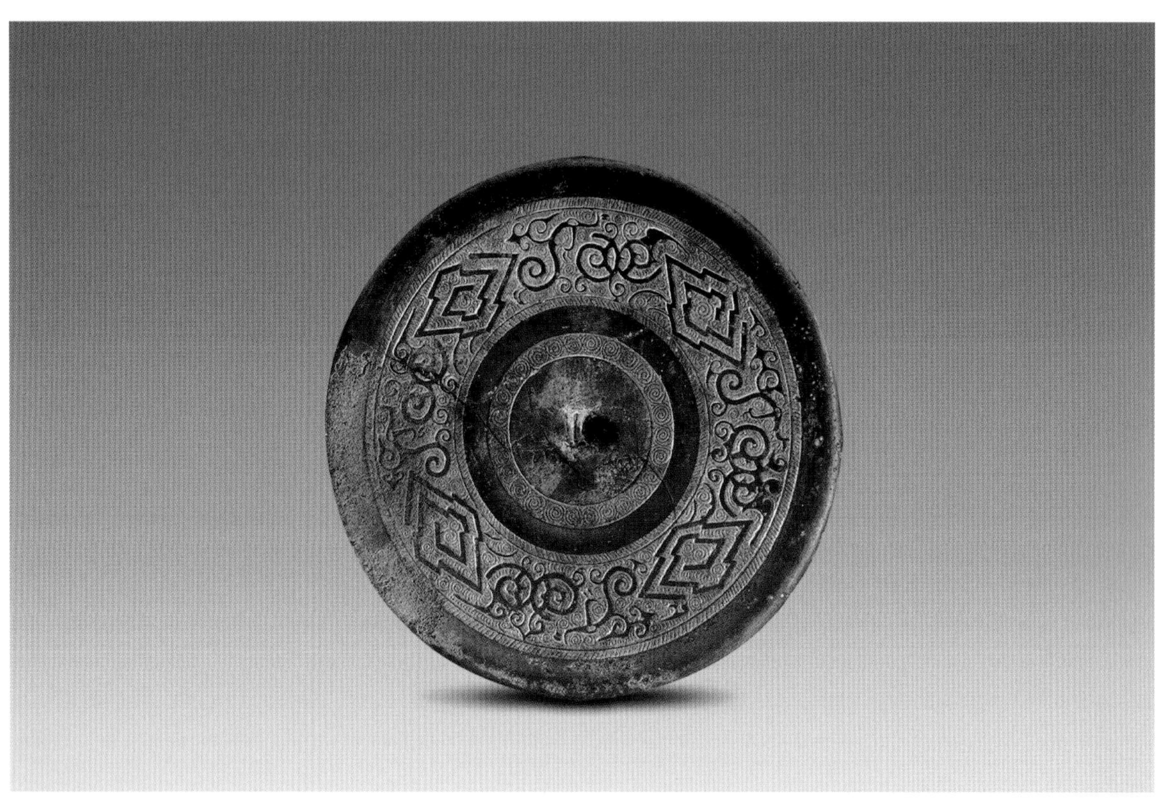

夔纹铜镜

秦

青铜质

直径 22.8 厘米

Copper Mirror with Kui Dragon Pattern

Qin Dynasty

Bronze

Diameter 22.8 cm

铜镜为古代梳妆照面用具。圆形，正面：磨砺光洁，背面：夔纹，有钮，可以宗系。1980 年咸阳淳化县秦河秦墓出土。

陕西省淳化县文化馆藏

The piece is round with a button through which a thread can go through. The obverse side is bright and clean polished and the reverse side is patterned with Kui (one-legged monster) lines (for good wishes). The copper mirror was a tool for girls to dress and make up. It was unearthed from a Qin tomb in Qinhe Village of Chunhua County, Xianyang, in 1980.

Preserved in Chunhua Cultural Center of Shaanxi Province

华

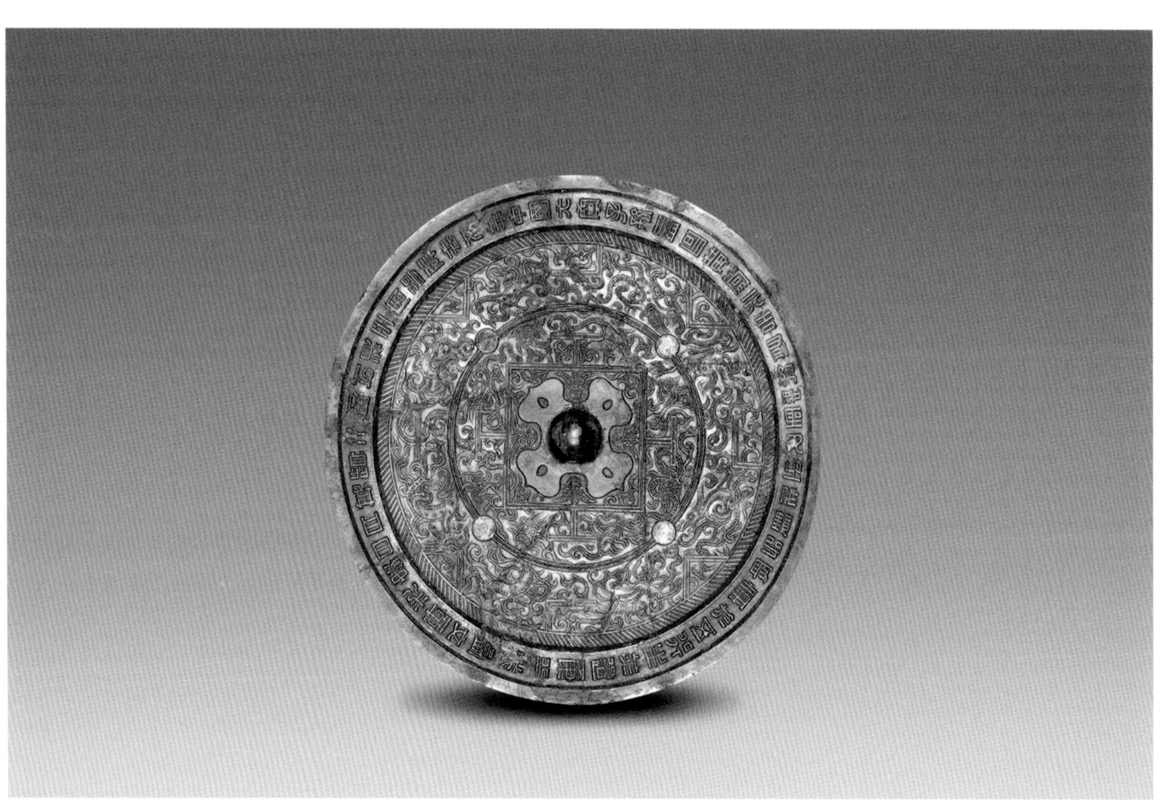

鎏金中国大宁博局纹镜

西汉

鎏金铜质

直径 18.6 厘米

Gilded Mirror with China Da Ning Bo Ju Pattern

Western Han Dynasty

Gilded Copper

Diameter 18.6 cm

圆钮，柿蒂纹钮座。柿蒂纹间各有一兽头，外围双线方栏。方栏外饰博局纹，间饰神人、鸟兽纹。周边有铭文一周。此镜表面鎏金，铭文工整。1952 年湖南长沙出土。

中国国家博物馆藏

The mirror surface is gilded. In the middle of the mirror is a circular knob with a calyx kaki pattern base beneath. There are four animal heads among the calyx kaki pattern. Outside the calyx kaki pattern is a square fence with double lines. Bo Ju pattern decorates the exterior of the square fence. God-human and bird-beast patterns alternate with the Bo Ju pattern. There is a circle of inscriptions on the circum. The inscriptions are carefully and neatly done. This piece was unearthed from Changsha City, Henan Province, in 1952.

Preserved in National Museum of China

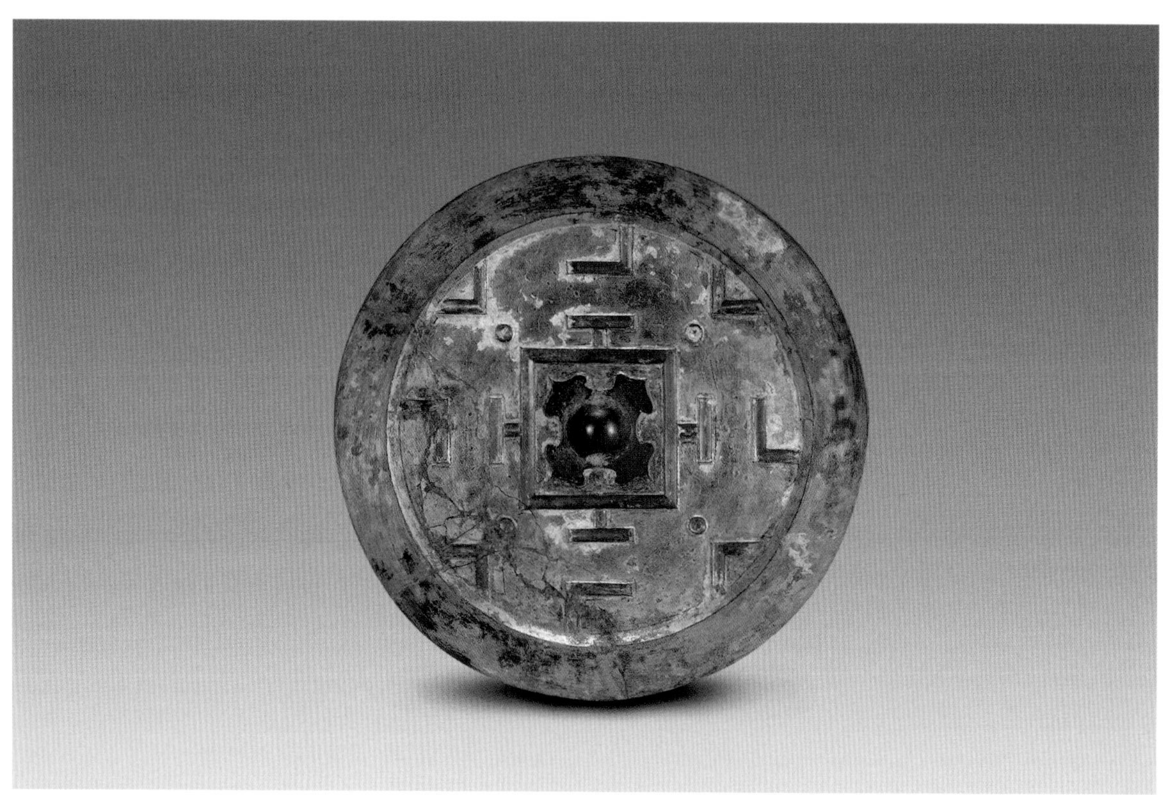

鎏金博局纹镜

西汉

鎏金铜质

直径 13.8 厘米

Gilded Mirror with Bo Ju Pattern

Western Han Dynasty

Gilded Copper

Diameter 13.8 cm

圆钮，柿蒂纹钮座。通体鎏金，主题纹饰为博局纹，素宽缘。1978 年湖南长沙杨家山 304 号墓出土。

湖南省博物馆藏

The whole body of the mirror is gilded. In the middle of the mirror is a circular knob with a calyx kaki pattern base beneath. The topical subject of the pattern is Ju Bo pattern with a simple broad edge. This piece was unearthed from No. 304 tomb in Yangjiashan Mountain, Changsha City, Hunan Province, in 1978.

Preserved in Hunan Provincial Museum

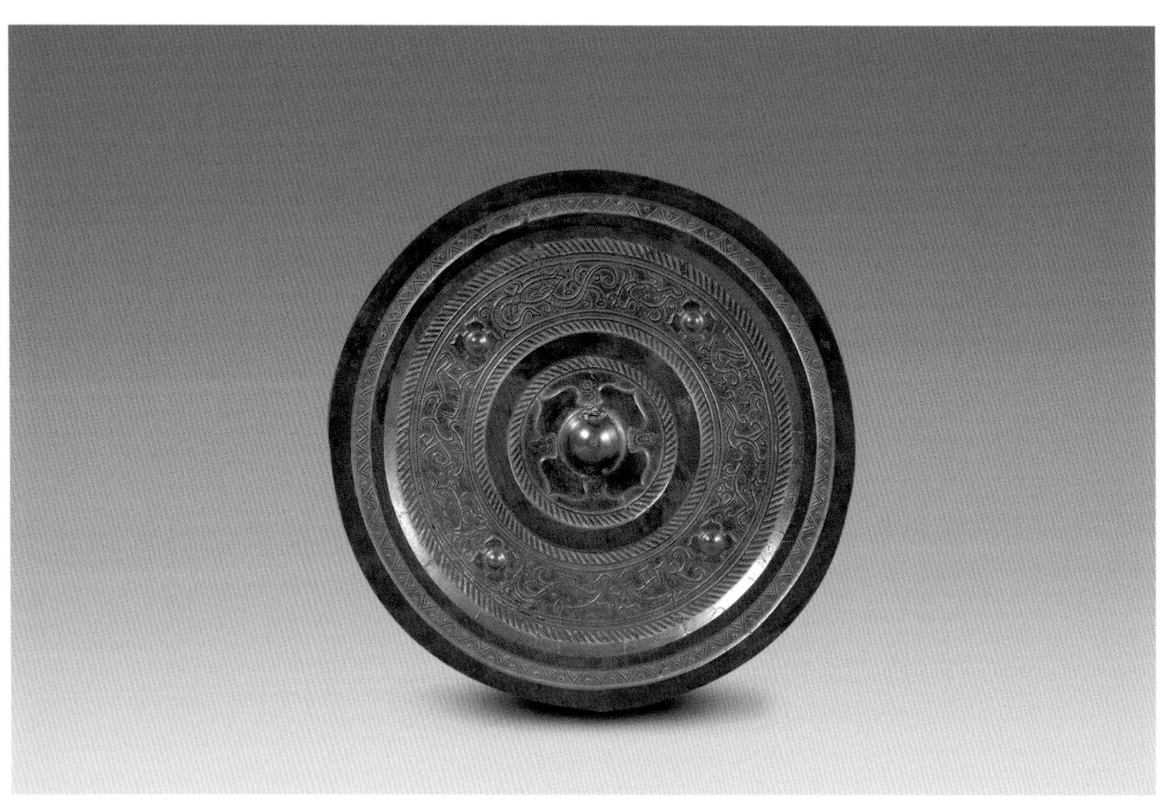

长宜子孙四神纹镜

西汉

青铜质

直径 17.7 厘米

“Chang Yi Zi Sun” Mirror with Four-God Pattern

Western Han Dynasty

Bronze

Diameter 17.7 cm

圆钮，柿蒂纹钮座。蒂叶间篆书铭文“长宜子孙”。座外饰射线纹、平素凸弦纹。主纹带为青龙、白虎、玄武、朱雀及天禄、辟邪、奔鹿等。四个柿蒂座乳钉纹将主纹均分为四组，环主纹带两边饰射线纹。镜边环饰双勾波折纹、点状纹。窄平素边。1975 年 7 月安徽天长汉墓出土。

天长博物馆藏

In the middle of the mirror is a circular knob with a calyx kaki pattern base beneath. There are four inscriptions “Chang Yi Zi”, “Sun” among the calyx kaki pattern. Radial patterns and normal raised-string patterns are ornamented around the base. The main pattern includes “Qing Long” (God in the East), “Bai Hu” (God in the West), “Zhu Que” (God in the South), and “Xuan Wu” (God in the North), as well as “Tian Lu”(Chinese mythical creature), “Bi Xie” (Chinese mythical creature), and “Ben Lu” (Chinese mythical creature) and so on. The main pattern is divided into four groups by four nipple nail patterns with calyx kaki base. Radial patterns are positioned on the two sides of the main pattern. Around the edge of the mirror are twists-turns patterns with a double hook and punctiform patterns. The narrow flat edge is undecorated. This piece was unearthed from Tianchang Han Dynasty tomb in Anhui Province in July, 1975.

Preserved in Tianchang Museum

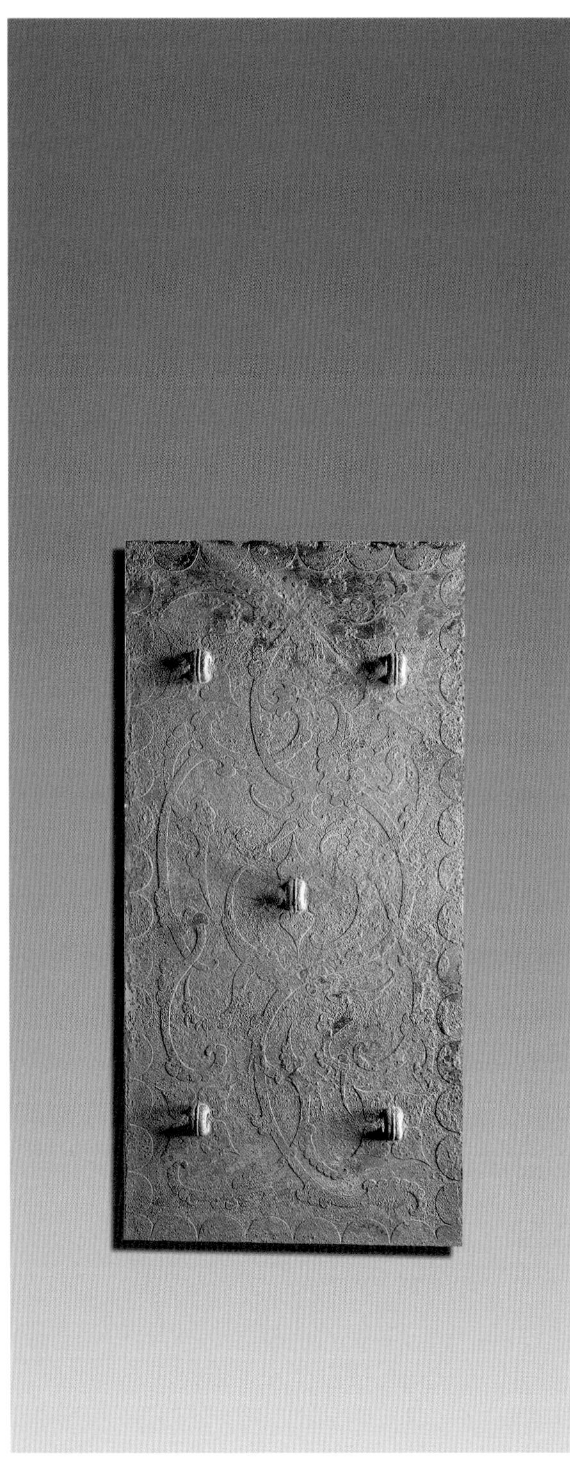

龙纹五钮长方镜

西汉

青铜质

长 115.1 厘米，宽 57.7 厘米

钮长 5 厘米，宽 3.5 厘米

Rectangular Mirror with Dragon Pattern and Five Knobs

Western Han Dynasty

Bronze

Length 115.1 cm/ Width 57.7 cm

The knob: Length 5 cm/ Width 3.5 cm

镜为长方形，镜面至今光亮可鉴。镜背边缘为连弧纹，四角及中心各一拱形弦纹钮。柿蒂纹钮座。主题纹饰为龙纹，龙首高昂，张口吐舌，龙身弯曲，舒展自如，形象生动，制作精良。1979 年山东淄博窝托村出土。

山东省淄博市博物馆藏

The mirror is rectangular and the surface is still bright for looking into today. The edge of the back is decorated with concatenated-arc pattern. There are five arch string patterned knobs in each corner and the middle of the mirror's back. There is a calyx kaki pattern on the base of the knob. The topical pattern is a dragon with its mouth open and its tongue sticking out. The body of the dragon bends naturally as if it could stretch out by itself. The pattern is vivid and perfect in workmanship. This piece was unearthed from Wotuo Village, Zibo City, Shandong Province in 1979.

Preserved in Zibo Museum of Shandong Province

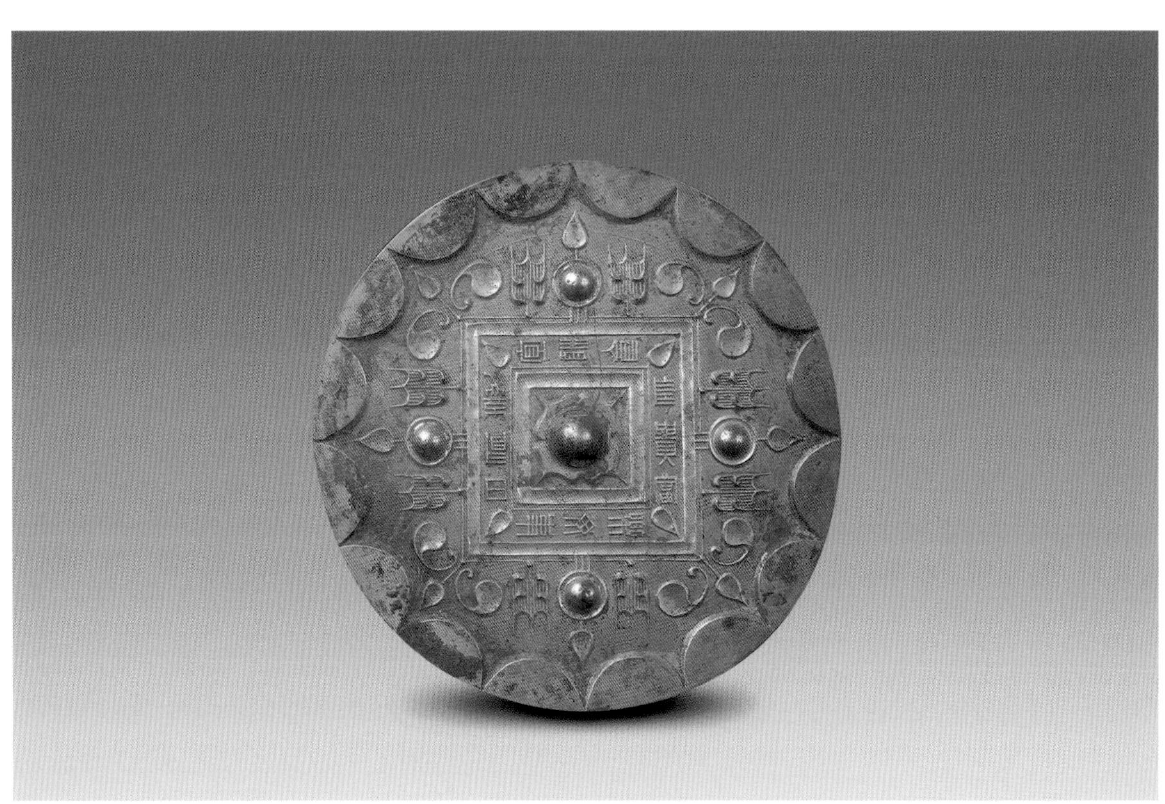

长贵富连弧纹镜

西汉

青铜质

直径 18 厘米

"Chang Gui Fu" Mirror with Connected-Arc Pattern

Western Han Dynasty

Bronze

Diameter 18 cm

圆钮，柿蒂纹钮座。其外方格内刻铭文：“日有喜，宜酒食，长贵富，乐毋事。”外区饰乳钉和叶纹。边缘饰连弧纹一周。1952年陕西咸阳出土。

陕西历史博物馆藏

In the middle of the mirror is a circular knob with a calyx kaki pattern base beneath. Within the outer square are inscriptions “Happy day when drinking is appropriate. It leads to a long rich life without any trouble.” Outside the outer square are decorated nipple nail and leaf patterns with a circle of concatenated-arch patterns on the edge. This piece was unearthed from Xianyang, Shaanxi Province in 1952.

Preserved in Shaanxi History Museum

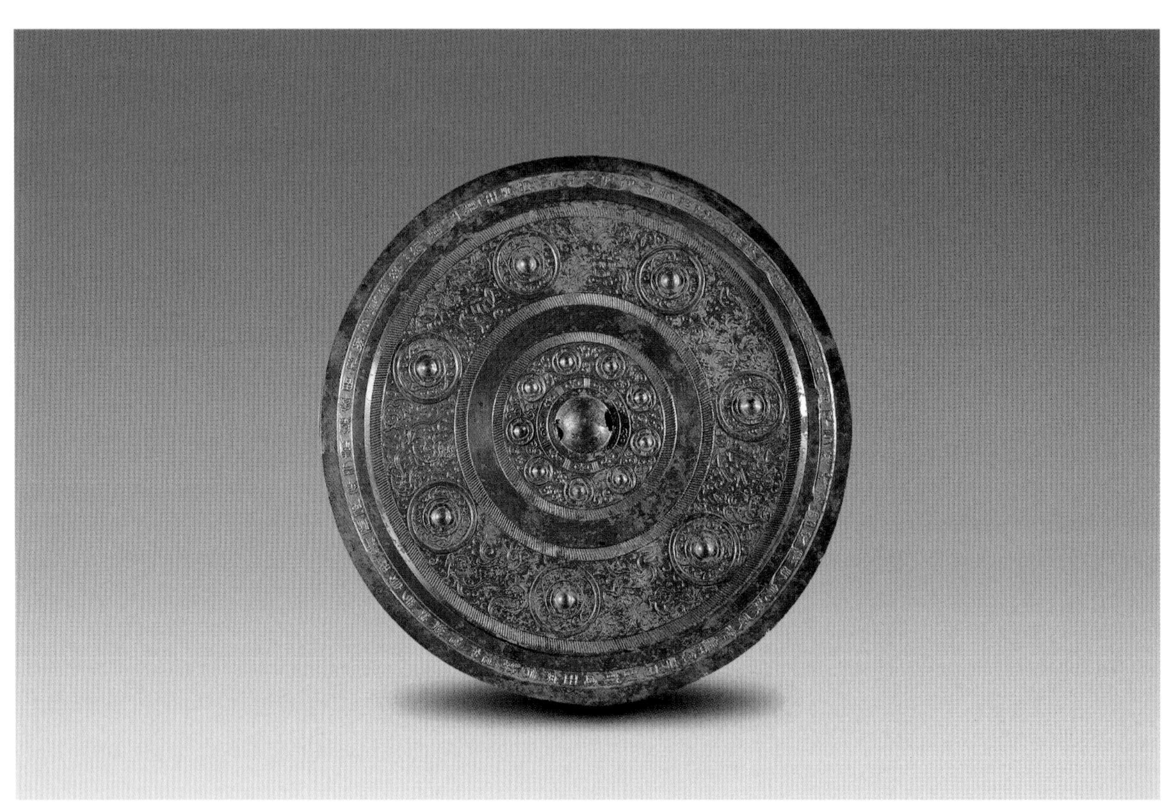

传子孙四神镜

西汉

青铜质

直径 25.4 厘米

Four-God Mirror Handing down to Offspring

Western Han Dynasty

Bronze

Diameter 25.4 cm

圆钮，圆钮座饰九乳钉纹，外绕宽带，主题纹饰为七乳钉纹，间饰四神及羽人、禽兽等形象。边缘有铭文七十四字。1964年陕西西安南郊出土。

西安市文物保护考古所藏

There is a circular knob with nipple nails pattern beneath the base of the knob. A broad strip circles the base. The topical theme of the pattern is one of seven nipple nails. Between the nails are four Gods, feather folks, birds, and beasts and so on. There are 74 inscriptions on the edge. This piece was unearthed from the southern suburbs in Xi'an, Shaanxi Province in 1964.

Preserved in Xi'an Municipal Institute of Archaeology and Cultural Relics Protection

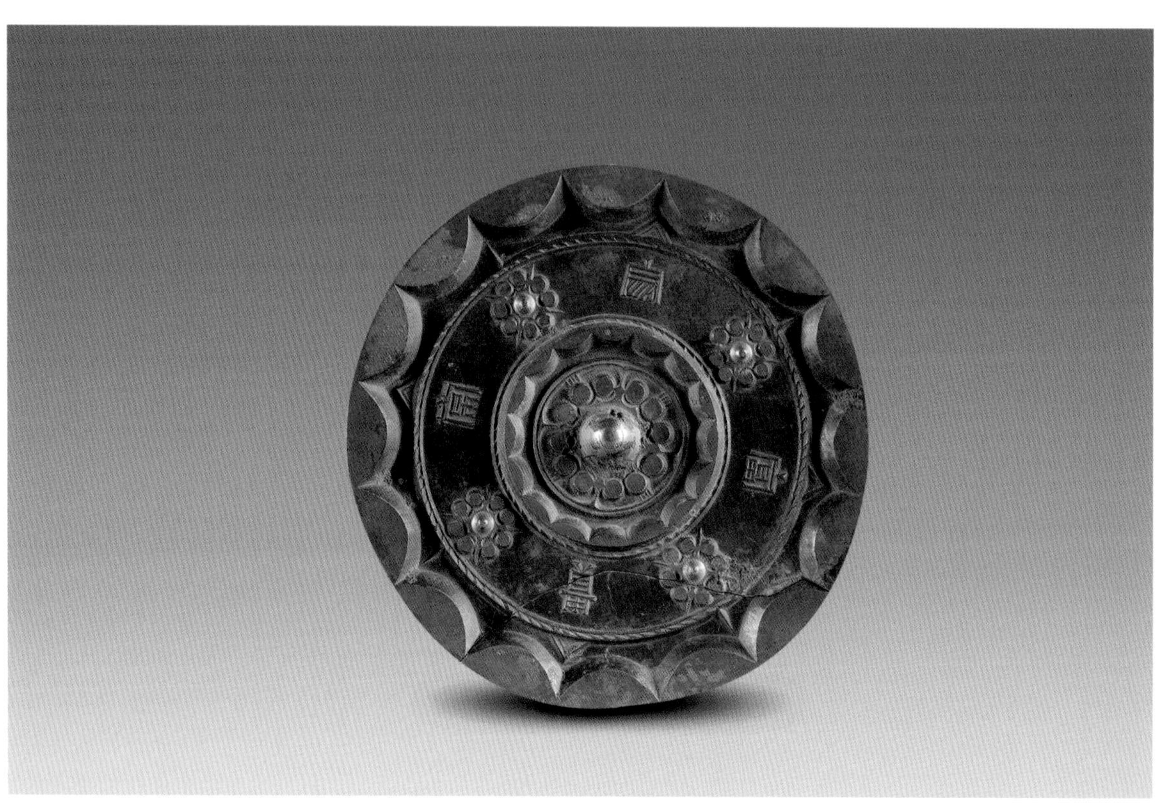

家常贵富镜

西汉

青铜质

直径 18 厘米

"Jia Chang Gui Fu" Mirror

Western Han Dynasty

Bronze

Diameter 18 cm

半圆钮，连珠纹钮座。内区为内向十六连弧纹，外区有铭“家常贵富”四字，每字之间置乳钉并配以连珠纹。外缘为内向十六连弧纹。1962 年山西右玉大川出土。

山西省右玉县博物馆藏

In the middle of the mirror is a semicircular knob with concatenate Buddha pearls pattern on the base of the knob. There are 16-concatenated-arc patterns within the inner zone of the mirror, and four inscriptions “Jia, Chang, Fu, Gui” on the outer zone of the mirror. Between each character is decorated with nipple nail pattern and concatenated-prayer beads pattern. There are also 16-concatenated-arc patterns on the outer edge. This piece was unearthed from Dachuan Town in Youyu County, Shanxi Province in 1962.

Preserved in Youyu Museum of Shanxi Province

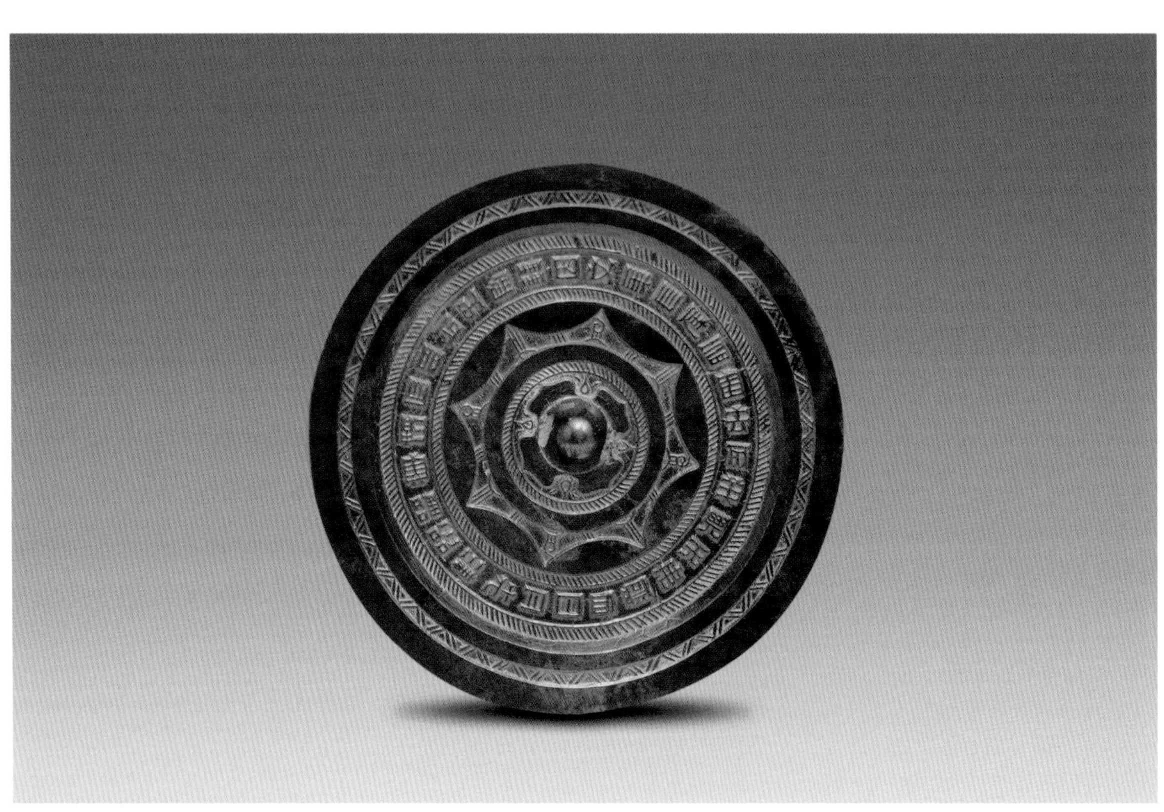

炼冶铜华镜

西汉

青铜质

直径 18.7 厘米

"Ye Lian Tong Hua" Mirror

Western Han Dynasty

Bronze

Diameter 18.7 cm

圆钮，四叶柿蒂纹钮座。内区饰斜线纹一周，其外为八连弧纹。外区二周斜线纹之间饰铭文："炼冶铜华清而明，以之为镜因文章，延年益寿去不祥，与天無丞而日月光"。1973 年江苏扬州东风砖瓦厂出土。

扬州博物馆藏

In the middle of the mirror is a circular knob with a four leaf-calyx kaki pattern beneath the base of the knob. A slash pattern circles the inner zone, while an eight-concatenated-arc pattern circles the outer zone. On the outer zone are two circles of slash patterns with inscriptions between them. The inscriptions mean that the mirror was made of first-class copper and was a mascot for the person to use it daily. This piece was unearthed from Dongfeng brickyard in Yangzhou, Jiangsu Province in 1973.

Preserved in Yangzhou Museum

華

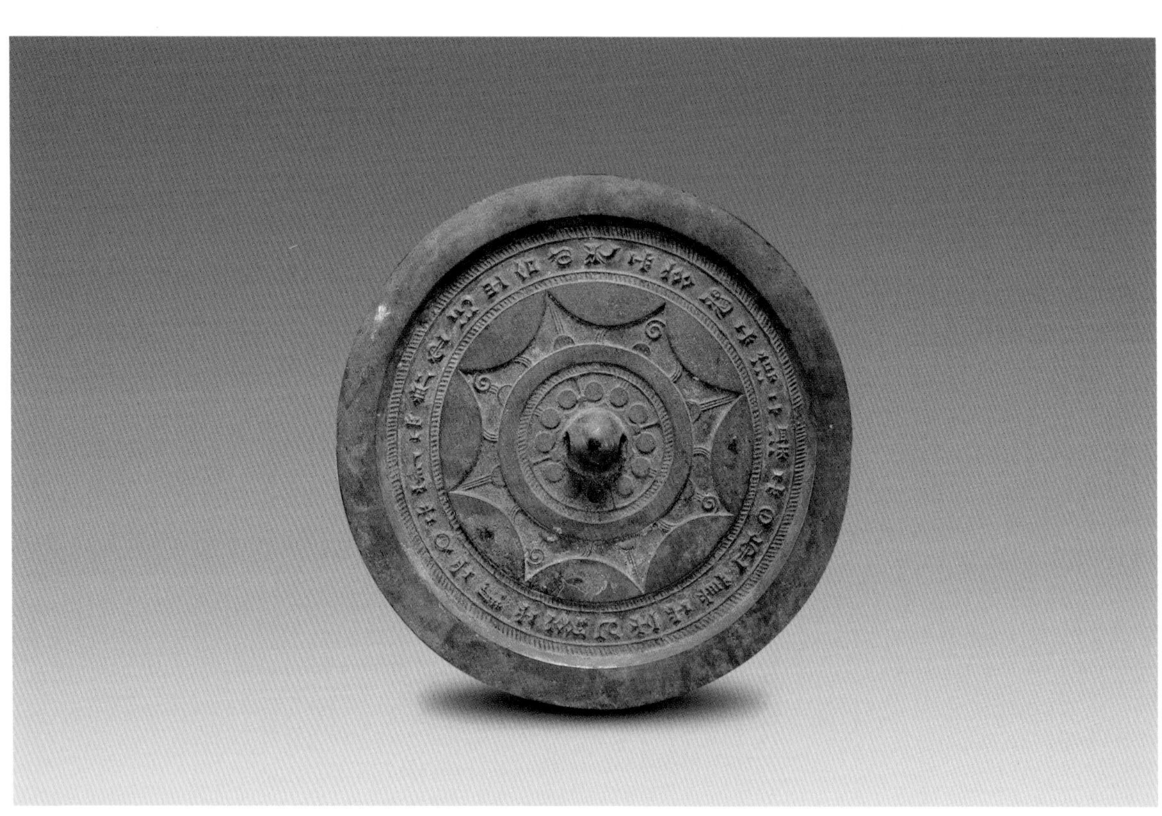

洁清白镜

西汉

铜质

直径 18.5 厘米

“Jie Qing” Mirror

Western Han Dynasty

Copper

Diameter 18.5 cm

圆钮，连珠纹钮座。内区为内向八连弧纹，外区有铭文二十一字："洁清白事君，志污之合明，光玄而流泽，日忘美不已"。每两字之间多有符号，宽缘。江苏扬州出土。

扬州博物馆藏

In the middle of the mirror is a circular knob patterned with concatenate Buddha pearls on the base. An eight-concatenated-arc pattern is decorated on the inner zone and 21 inscriptions are listed on the outer zone. The inscriptions mean that the mirror can help the owner to know right from wrong as well as to help the owner to dress up. There are symbols among the inscriptions. The edge of the mirror is wide. This piece was unearthed from Yangzhou, Jiangsu Province.

Preserved in Yangzhou Museum

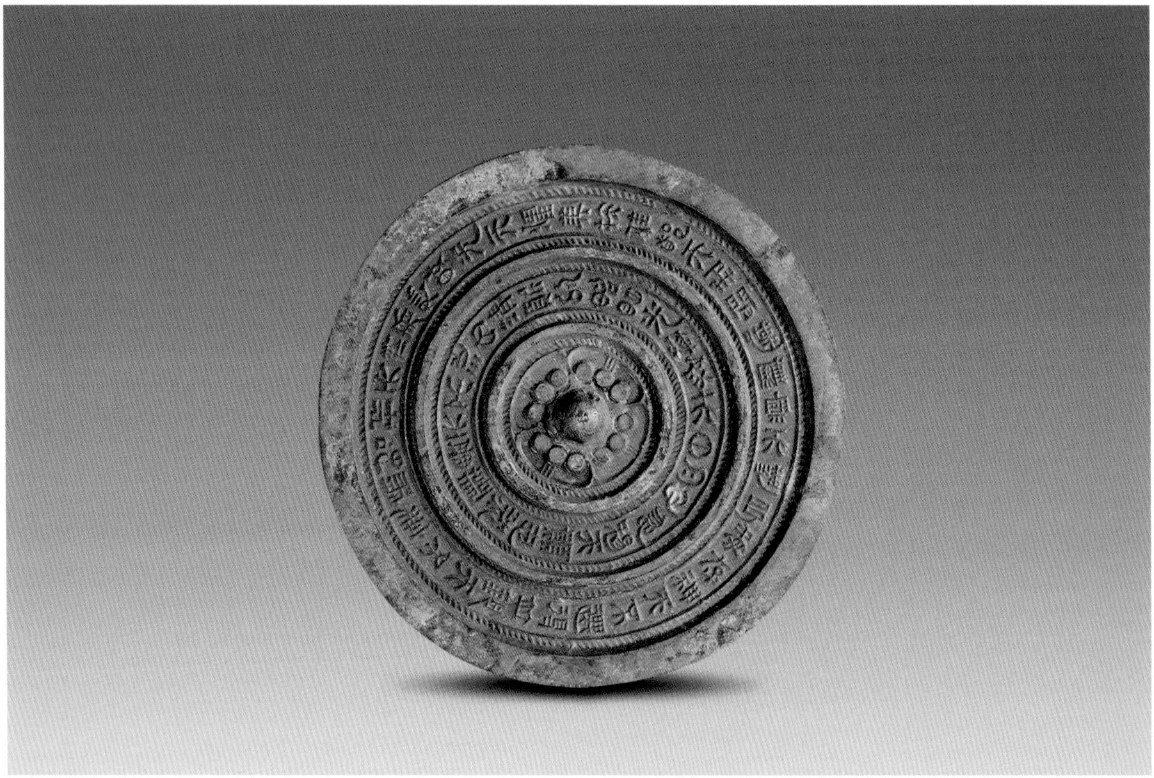

内清镜

西汉

青铜质

直径 19.2 厘米

“Nei Qing” Mirror

Western Han Dynasty

Bronze

Diameter19.2 cm

圆钮，连珠纹钮座。其外围内圈铭文共二十四字:“内清质以昭明，光辉象夫日月，心忽扬而愿忠，然雍塞而不泄”。外圈铭文三十六字：“如皎光而耀美，挟佳都而無间，……”。内外圈由凸起的圆带纹相隔。宽平缘。1982 年山西朔州出土。

山西省平朔考古队藏

In the middle of the mirror is a circular knob patterned with alignment lines on the base. On the inner track are 24 inscriptions and on the outer track 36 inscriptions. There is a circular-belt pattern between the inner and the outer track. The inscriptions mean that the mirror can help the owner to dress up as well as to introspect. The edge of the mirror is wide and flat. This piece was unearthed from Shuozhou, Shanxi Province in 1982.

Preserved in Pingshuo Archaeological Team of Shanxi Province

華

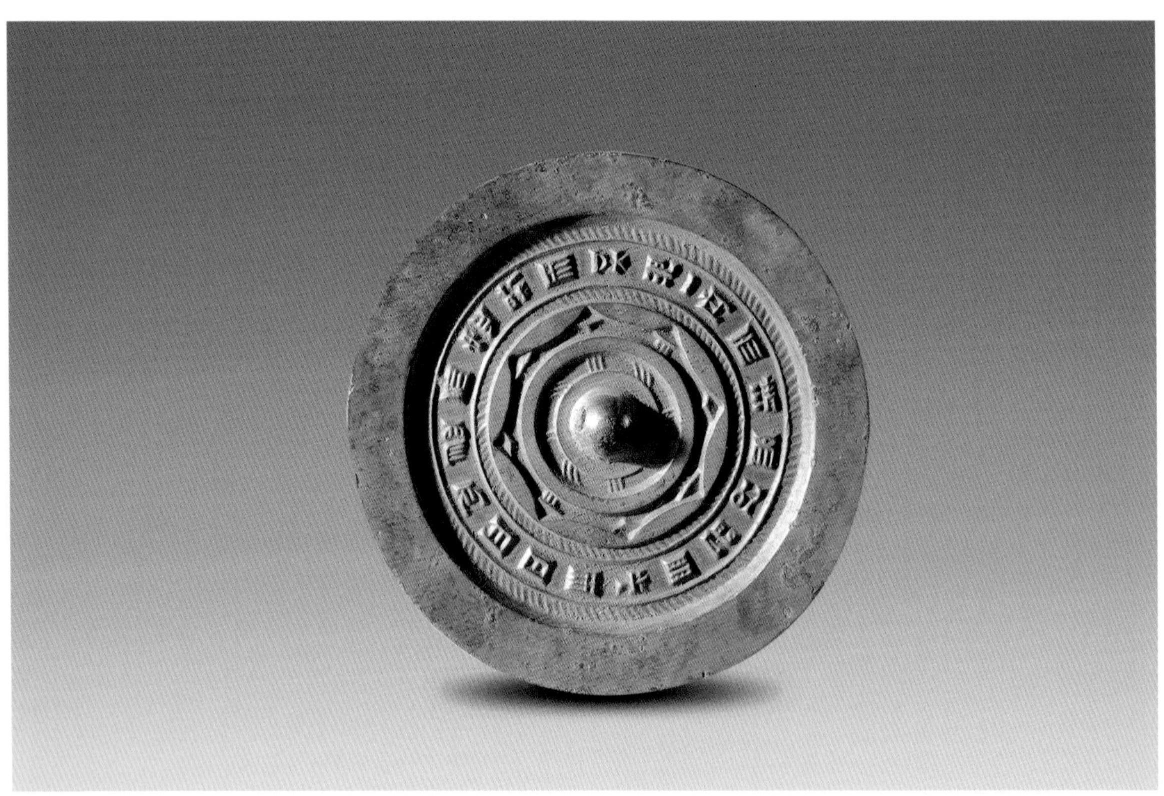

内清镜

西汉

青铜质

直径 7.8cm

"Nei Qing" Mirror

Western Han Dynasty

Bronze

Diameter 7.8 cm

圆钮，圆钮座。内区为一周连弧纹，外区为“内清以昭明，光日月不息……”铭文一周。河南洛阳四〇一工区出土。

洛阳市文物工作队藏

In the middle of the mirror is a circular knob with a base. The inner track is circulated by a concatenated- arc pattern. The outer track is engraved with a circle of inscriptions which mean the mirror can help the owner to introspect. The piece was unearthed in the 401 working area of Luoyang, Henan.

Preserved in Luoyang Municipal Institute of Archaeology and Cultural Relics

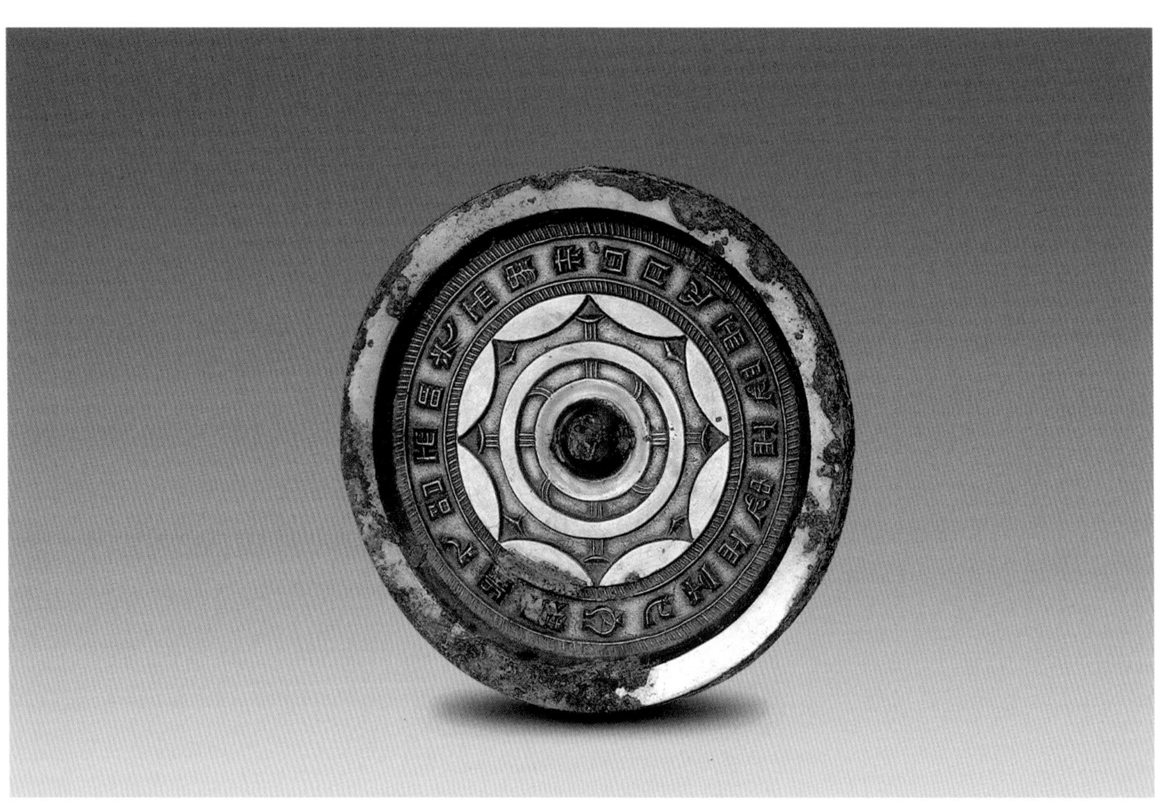

内清连弧纹镜

西汉

青铜质

直径 12.8 厘米

“Nei Qing” Mirror with a Concatenated-Arc Pattern

Western Han Dynasty

Bronze

Diameter 12.8 cm

圆钮。内区饰一周环带纹和八瓣连弧纹。外区为二十一字铭文一周："内清质以昭而明，光而象夫日月，心而厚而患而不泄"。1997 年陕西西安汉陵陪葬墓出土。

陕西省考古研究院藏

There is a circular knob in the middle of the mirror. The inner track is decorated with a circular-belt pattern and eight-concatenated-arc pattern. The outer track is inscribed with 21 Chinese characters which mean that the mirror is like the sun and the moon to help the owner to behave like gentlemen. This piece was unearthed from the subordinate tomb of the Han Mausoleum in Xi'an, Shaanxi in 1997.

Preserved in Shaanxi Provincial Institute of Archaeology

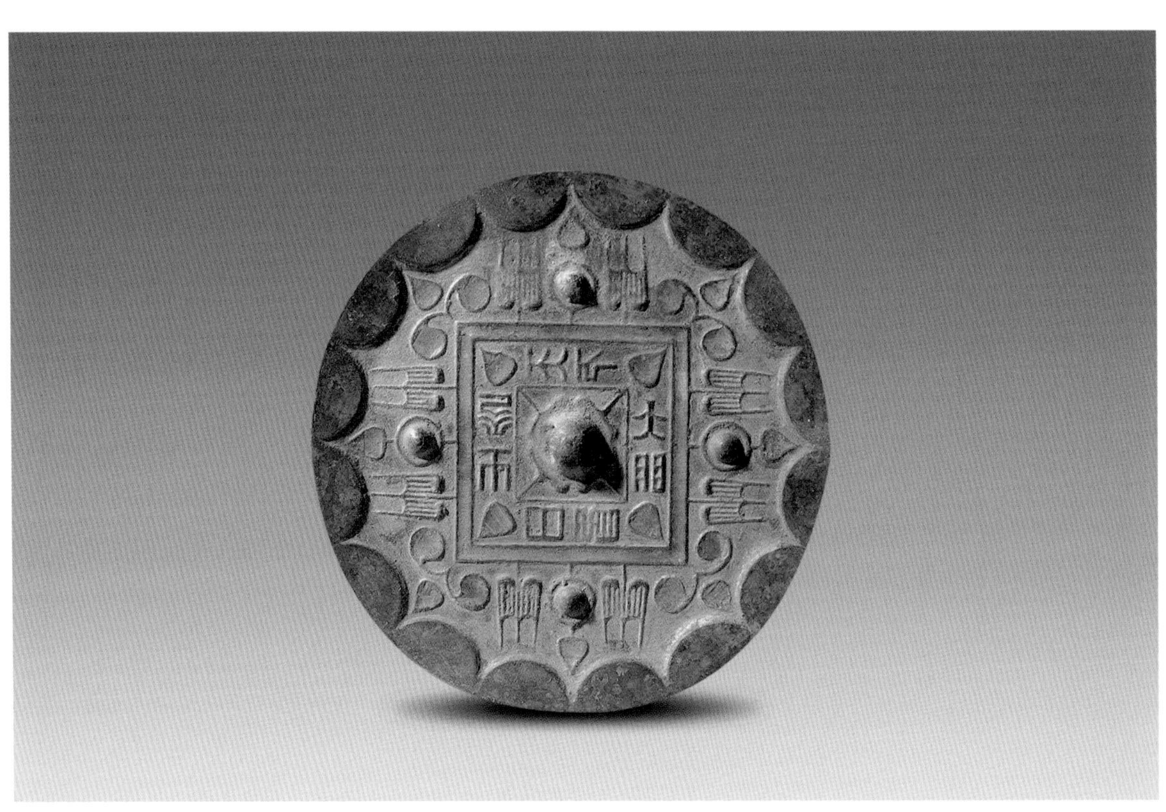

见日之光连弧纹镜

西汉

青铜质

直径 10.5 厘米

“Jian Ri Zhi Guang”Mirror with Concatenated-Arc Patterns and Characters

Western Han Dynasty

Bronze

Diameter 10.5 cm

圆钮，方形钮座。内区为双线方框，框内有八字铭文:“见日之光，天下大明”。外区饰四乳钉及草叶纹。边缘饰十六内向连弧纹。河南洛阳涧西防洪渠出土。

洛阳市文物考古研究院藏

There is a circular knob with a square base in the middle of the mirror. The inner track is ornamented with a double-line square and eight inscriptions which mean that the mirror is like the sun and the moon to shine the earth. There are hour nipple nails and grass-blade patterns on the outer track. The edge of the mirror is patterned with an introvert 16 concatenated-arc. This piece was unearthed from Jianxi flood control channels in Luoyang, Henan province.

Preserved in Luoyang Municipal Institute of Archaeology and Cultural Relics

華

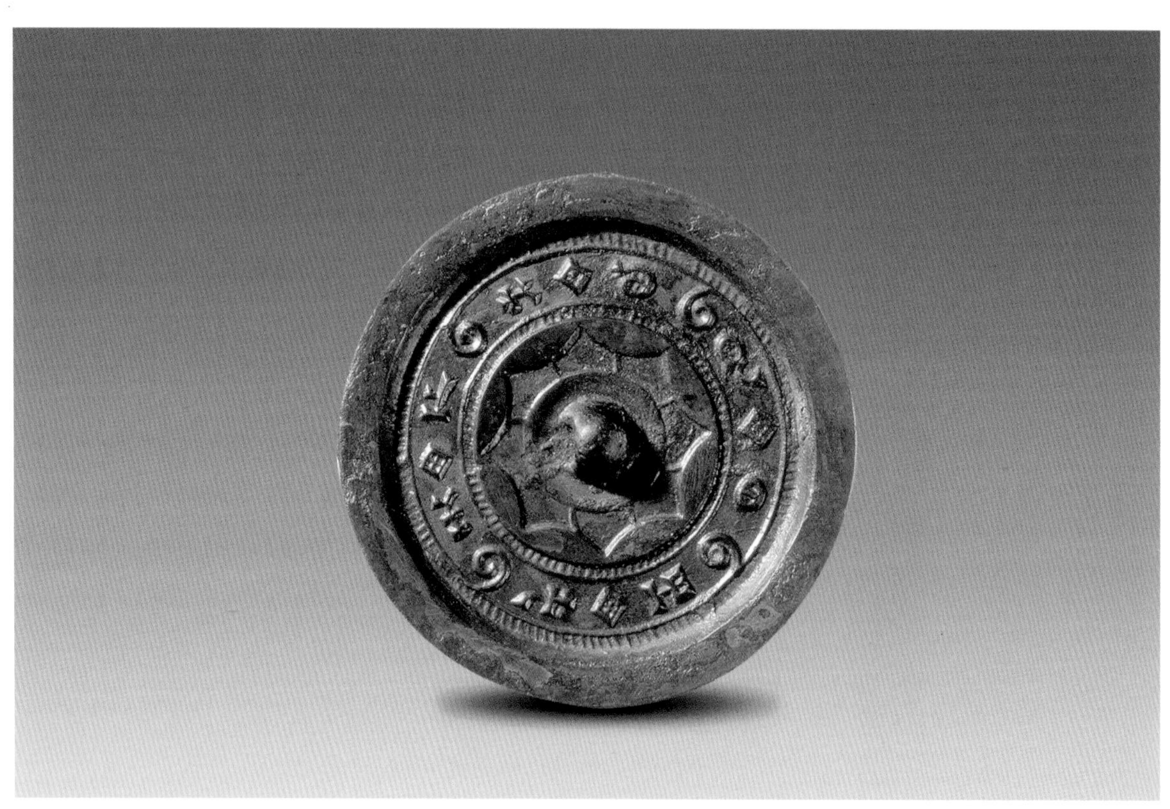

见日之光透光镜

西汉

青铜质

直径 7.4 厘米

"Jian Ri Zhi Guang"Transmitting Mirror

Western Han Dynasty

Bronze

Diameter 7.4 cm

半圆钮，圆形钮座。内区为内向八连弧纹，外围带状八字铭文："见日之光，天下大明"。此镜在阳光或直束光线照射下，能映出与镜背纹饰相对应的纹样，故名。经研究，发生这种现象是由于在铸造冷却过程和加工研磨中产生的应力，使镜面产生了与镜背纹饰相应的微小凹凸变化，从而导致透光效果。

上海博物馆藏

There is a semicircular knob with a circular base in the middle of the mirror. The inner track is patterned with an eight-concatenated-arc and eight inscriptions "Jian Ri Zhi Guang Tian Xia Da Ming" which mean the sun brings light to human. The mirror can reflect a corresponding pattern of the back of the mirror in the sunlight or straight beam. Hence it got the name. Research shows that this phenomenon is caused by the stress during the process of cooling and grinding, which lead to some small changes in the mirror so that it can transmit light.

Preserved in Shanghai Museum

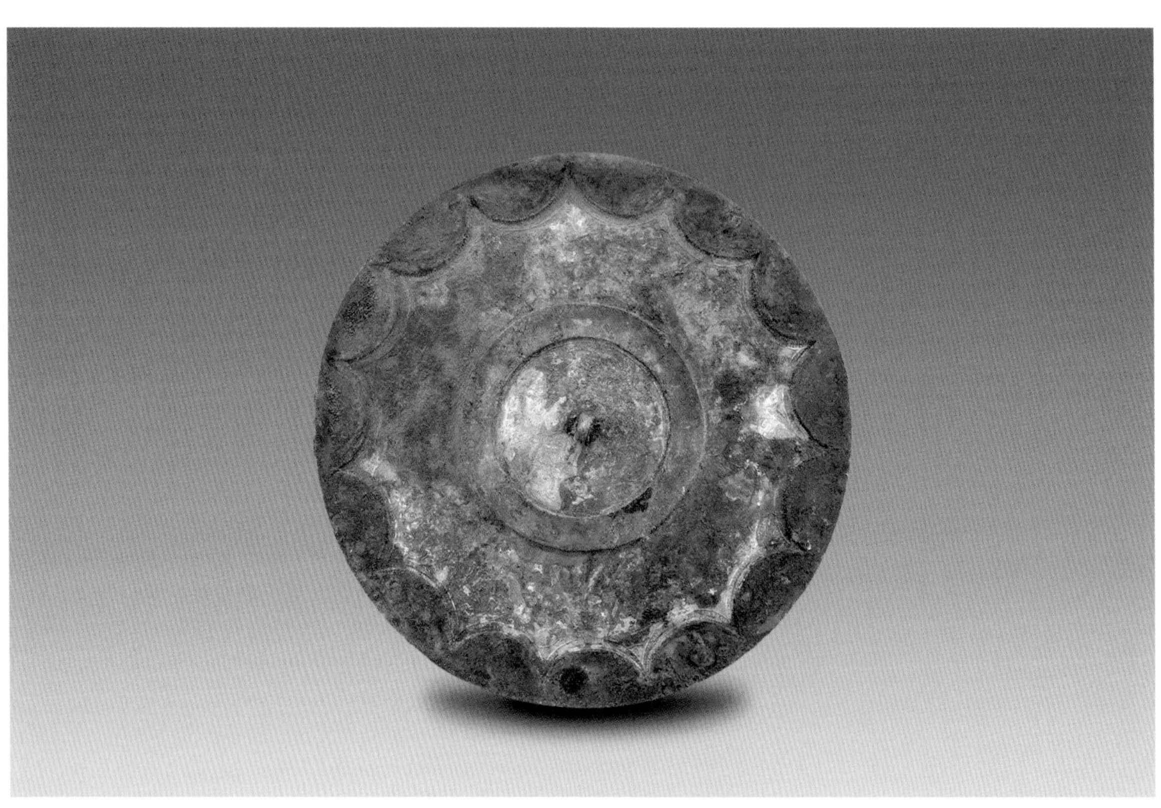

彩绘人物镜

西汉

青铜质

直径 41 厘米

Mirror with Color-Decorated Figures

Western Han Dynasty

Bronze

Diameter 41 cm

桥形钮。浅弧形圆圈带将纹饰分为内外两部分，内区绘卷云纹，外区绘人物，因锈蚀仅一组可辨，中间两人作击剑状，左右两边各有四人，一人在前引导，三人拱手而立。1983 年广东广州象岗山南越王墓出土。

西汉南越王博物馆藏

There is a bridge knob in the middle of the mirror. A shallow arc-shaped circle belt divides the mirror into two parts. The inner part is decorated with a rolling-cloud pattern. There are figures on the outer zone, only one group of which can be identified because of the rustiness. Two fencing men stand in the middle while another four stand on the left and right. One of them is guiding, and the other three men are standing there with one hand in the other submissively. This piece was unearthed from King Nanyue Mausoleum on Xianggang Mountain in Guangzhou, Guangdong Province in 1983.

Preserved in Museum of the Western Han Dynasty Mausoleum of King Nanyue

華

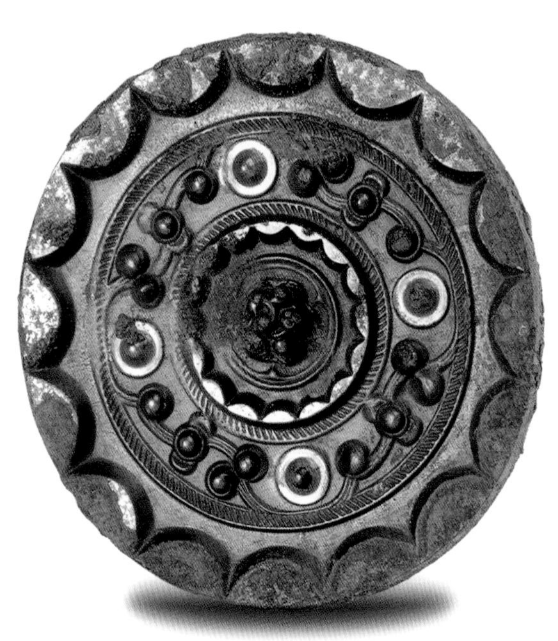

星云纹镜

西汉

青铜质

直径 13.2 厘米

Mirror with Nebula Patterns

Western Han Dynasty

Bronze

Diameter 13.2 cm

连峰钮，圆钮座。内区饰弦纹和连弧纹。外区四方饰四枚大乳钉，其间饰用弧线相连的小乳钉。边缘饰连弧纹一周。1997年陕西西安汉陵陪葬墓出土。

陕西省考古研究院藏

There is a knob made of a series of peaks with a circular base in the middle of the mirror. The inner track is patterned with string and concatenated-arc patterns. Four big nipple nails are decorated on the four sides of the outer track with small nipple nails connected with arc. The edge is a circle of concatenated-arc pattern. This piece was unearthed from the subordinate tomb of the Han Mausoleum in Xi'an, Shaanxi Province in 1997.

Preserved in Shaanxi Provincial Institute of Archaeology

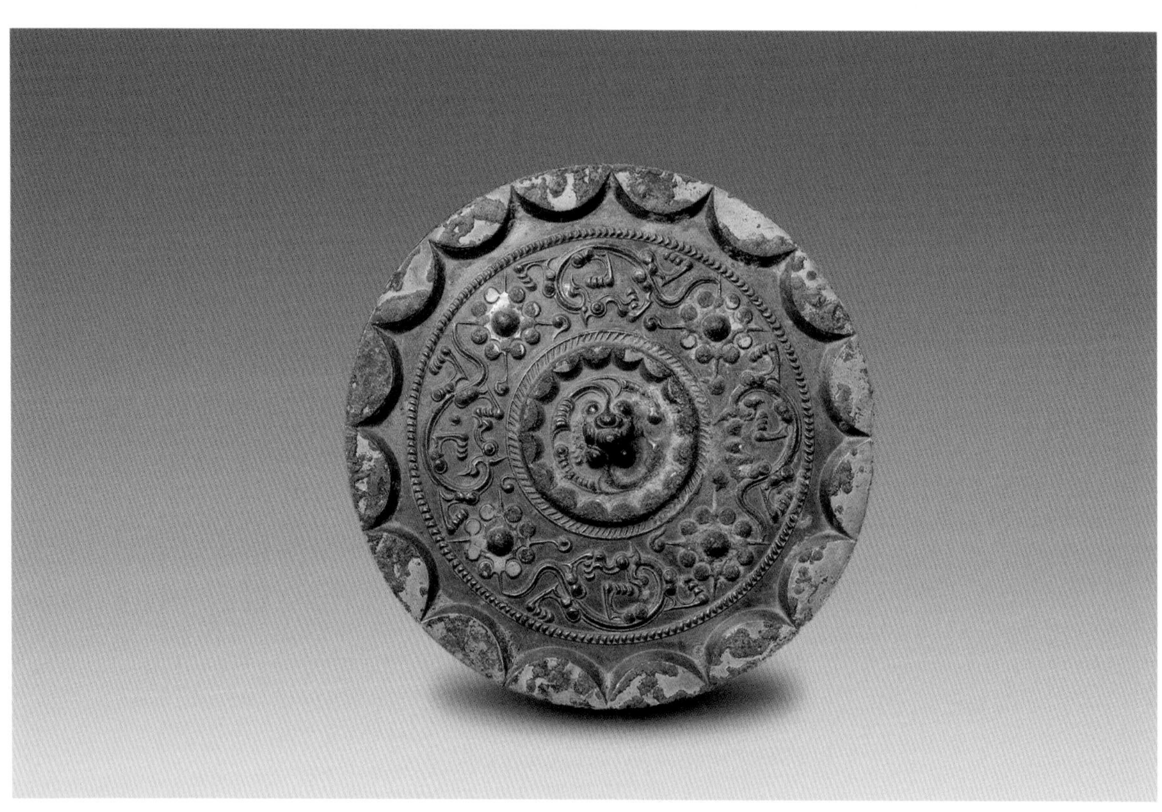

四龙连弧纹镜

西汉

青铜质

直径 17 厘米

Mirror with Four-Dragon and Concatenated-Arc Patterns

Western Han Dynasty

Bronze

Diameter 17 cm

连峰钮，圆钮座。钮座外饰乳钉纹一周。内区饰四组乳钉纹，每组中间一枚大乳钉，周围饰八枚小乳钉。四组龙纹饰于乳钉纹之间，边缘饰连弧纹一周。1952 年陕西西安出土。

陕西历史博物馆藏

There is a knob made of a series of peaks with a circular base in the middle of the mirror. A circular of nipple nails patterns is decorated round the base. The inner track is ornamented with four groups of nipple nail patterns. In each group eight small nails surrounds a big one in the center. Meanwhile, four groups of dragon patterns intertwine with the nipple nails patterns. The rim of the mirror is a circle of concatenated-arc pattern. This mirror was unearthed from Xi'an, Shaanxi Province in 1952.

Preserved in Shaanxi History Museum

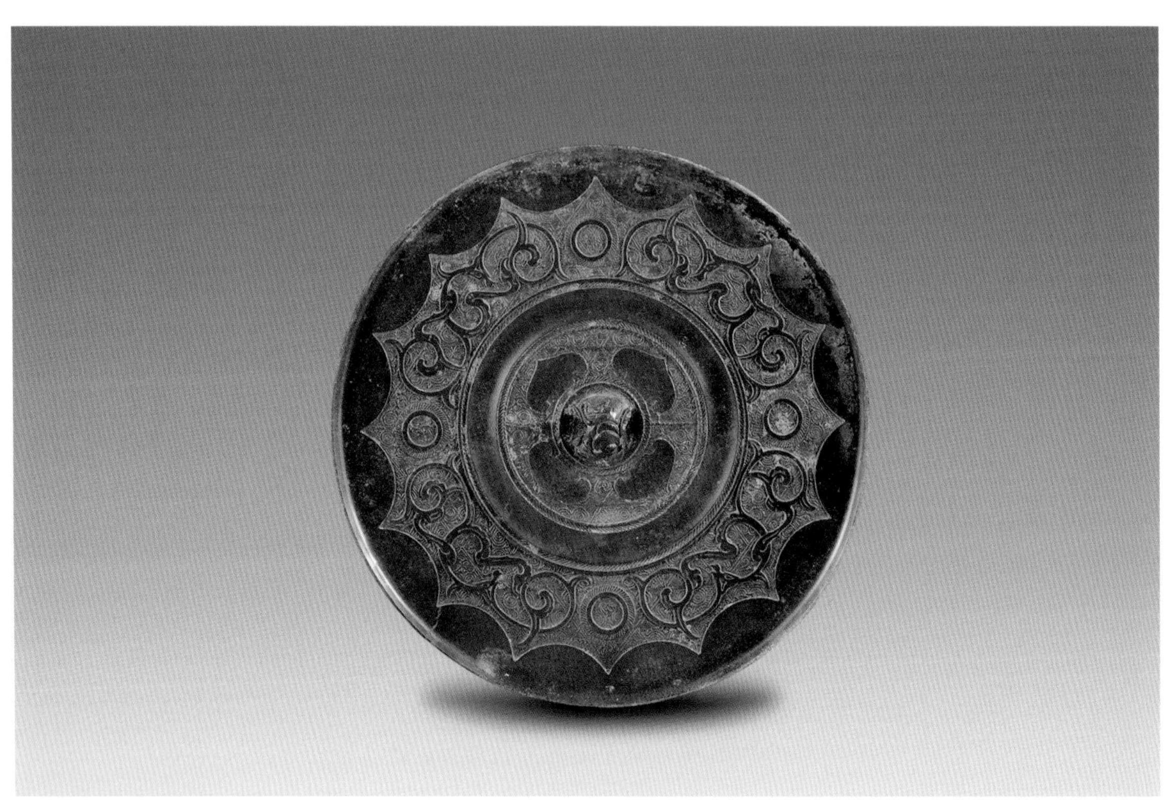

四龙连弧纹镜

西汉

青铜质

直径 17.1 厘米

Mirror with Four-Dragon and Concatenated-Arc Patterns

Western Han Dynasty

Bronze

Diameter 17.1 cm

兽钮，圆钮座。钮座外为四柿蒂形叶，圆框外饰四组蟠龙纹，间饰以圆圈，整个纹饰均以云雷纹为地。镜缘饰十六内向连弧纹。

上海博物馆藏

There is an animal knob and a circular knob base in the middle of the mirror. The knob base is circled by four kaki calyx leaf patterns. Outside the shallow round frame are four groups of dragon patterns that interphase with circle patterns, all of which are shaded with cloud-thunder patterns. The rim is ornamented with a 16 concatenated-arc pattern directed inward.

Preserved in Shanghai Museum

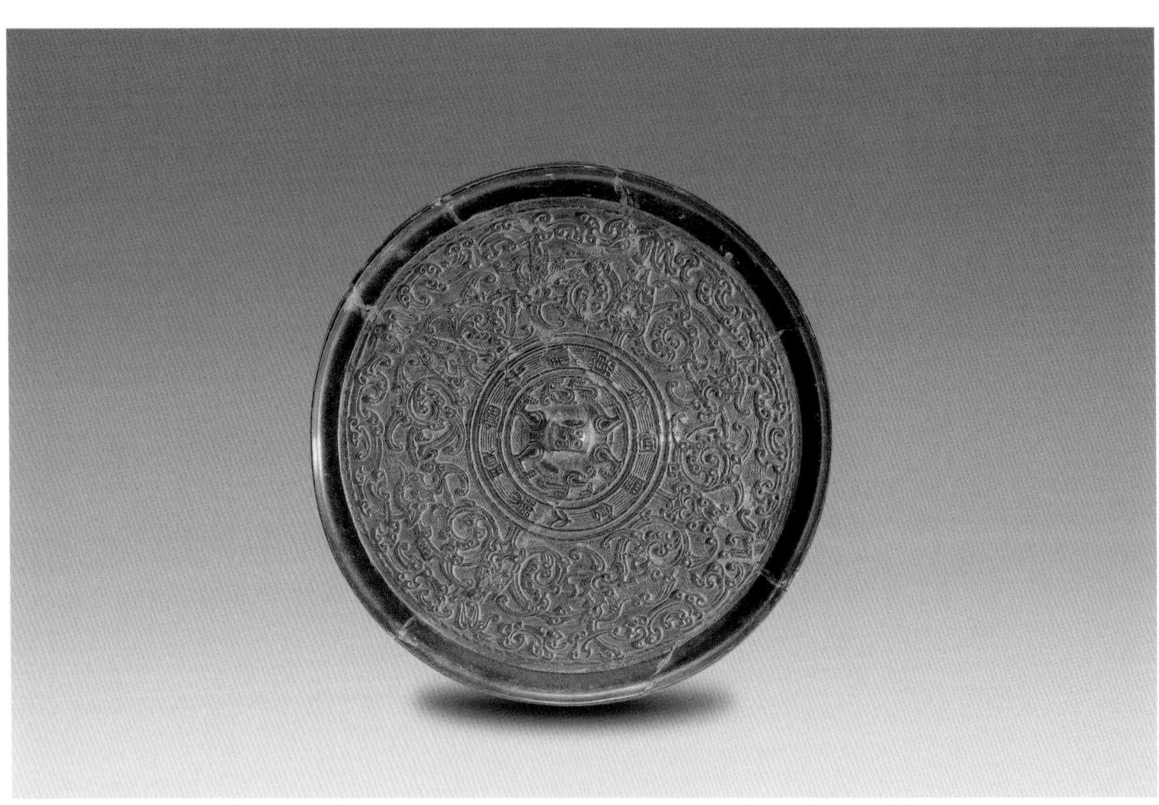

大乐贵富蟠龙纹镜

西汉

青铜质

直径 14.3 厘米

"Da Le Gui Fu" Mirror with Dragon Patterns

Western Han Dynasty

Bronze

Diameter 14.3 cm

兽钮，圆钮座。钮座之外有一周铭文："大乐贵富，千秋万岁，宜酒食"。主题纹饰为繁缛的蟠龙纹，龙身由三线或四线组成。1955 年湖南长沙燕子嘴 17 号墓出土。

湖南省博物馆藏

There is an animal knob with a circular base in the middle of the mirror. Around the base is a group of inscriptions which mean forever happy, noble, and wealthy. The topical pattern is one of overelaborated curled-up dragon whose body consists of three or four lines. This piece was unearthed from Changsha Yanzizui No.17 tomb in Hunan Province in 1955.

Preserved in Hunan Provincial Museum

華

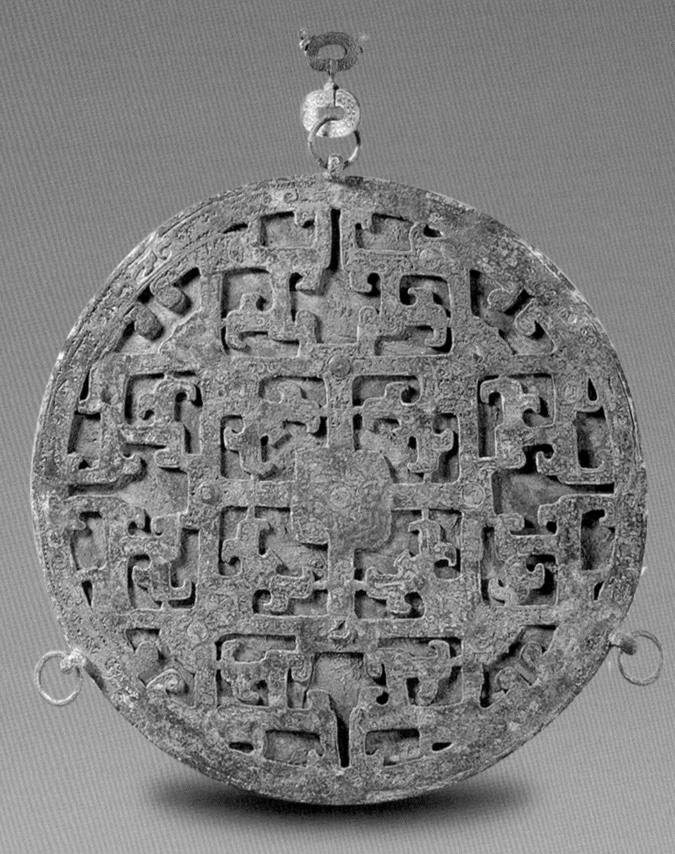

透雕龙纹三钮镜

西汉

青铜质

直径 29 厘米

Mirror with Three Button and Openwork Carving Dragon Patterns

Western Han Dynasty

Bronze

Diameter 29 cm

圆钮，椭方形钮座。由一方框划分内外两区，内区饰四龙纹，外区饰一周变形龙纹，间填鎏银小泡。整个纹饰均镂空。镜缘有小环三个，其中一个缀连两个椭圆形小玉璧。此镜面、背分铸再合二为一，形制别致。1965 年江苏涟水三里墩出土。

南京博物院藏

There is a circular knob with an oval square base in the middle of the mirror. The mirror is divided into two parts by a block. The inner zone is ornamented with four-dragon patterns, and the outer zone a circle of transformative dragon pattern. The dragon patterns are filled with silver gilding bubbles. All the patterns are hollow. On the rim are three small annulet with each linked to two oval jade discs. The surface and the back of the mirror were casted individually and then were combined into one. The shape and structure are very unconventional. This piece was unearthed from Sanlidun in Lianshui County, Jiangsu Province in 1965.

Preserved in Nanjing Museum

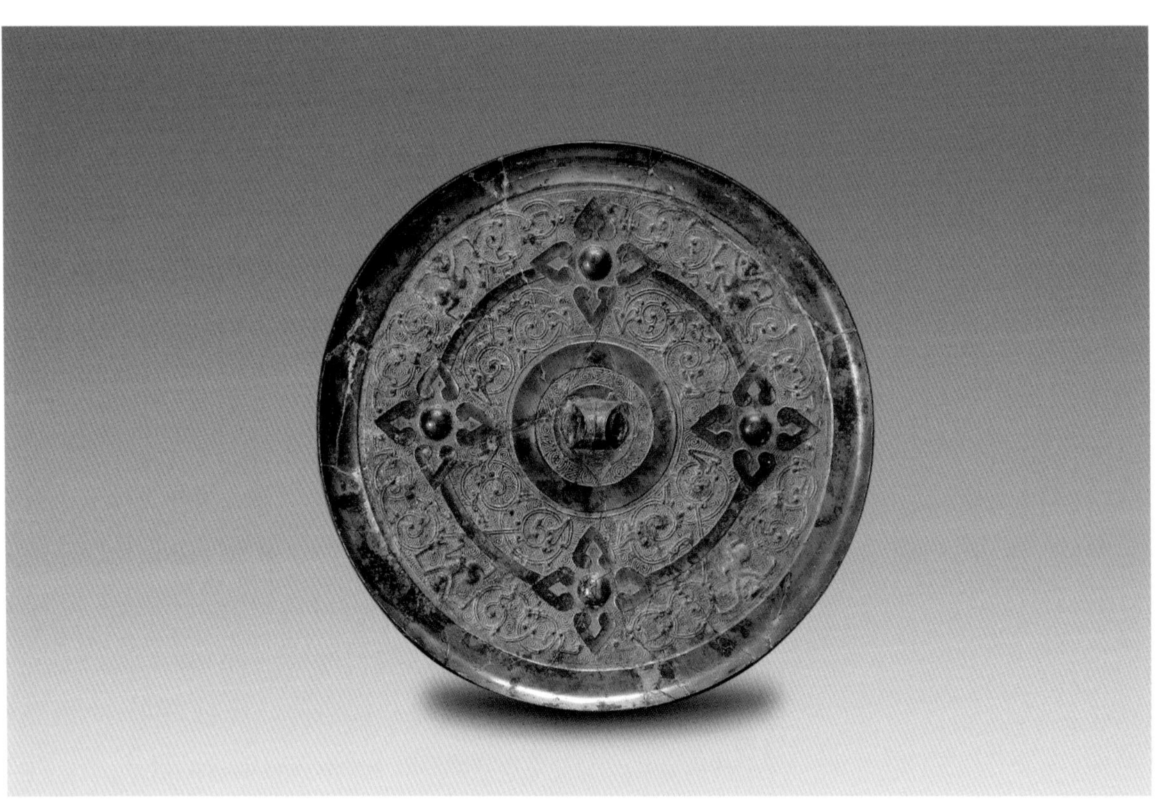

四猴蟠龙纹镜

西汉

青铜质

直径 25.4 厘米

Mirror with Patterns of Four Monkeys and Curled-up Dragons

Western Han Dynasty

Bronze

Diameter 25.4 cm

三弦钮，圆钮座。其外是二周浅凹弧形圆圈带将镜背分为内外二区，外圈带饰四乳钉将其四等分，乳钉外有四花瓣。内外区均配置四组蟠龙纹，外区每组蟠龙纹中间饰一正面形的猴子，宽额，长臂舒展而下垂，曲足作腾跃状，形象生动。1968 年河北满城汉墓出土。

河北博物院藏

There is a three-string knob with a circular base in the middle of the mirror. The mirror is divided into the inner zone and the outer zone by two scrobicula circular arcs. The outer zone is decorated with four nipple nails which divide the belt into four parts. There are also four petals around each nail. There are four curled-up dragon patterns on both inner and outer zones. On the outer zone a positive vivid monkey centers on each dragon pattern. The monkey has a wide forehead, long arms which stretch down, and the feet are wrapped like it would curvet. This piece was unearthed from Han tomb in Man City, Hebei Province in 1968.

Preserved in Hebei Museum

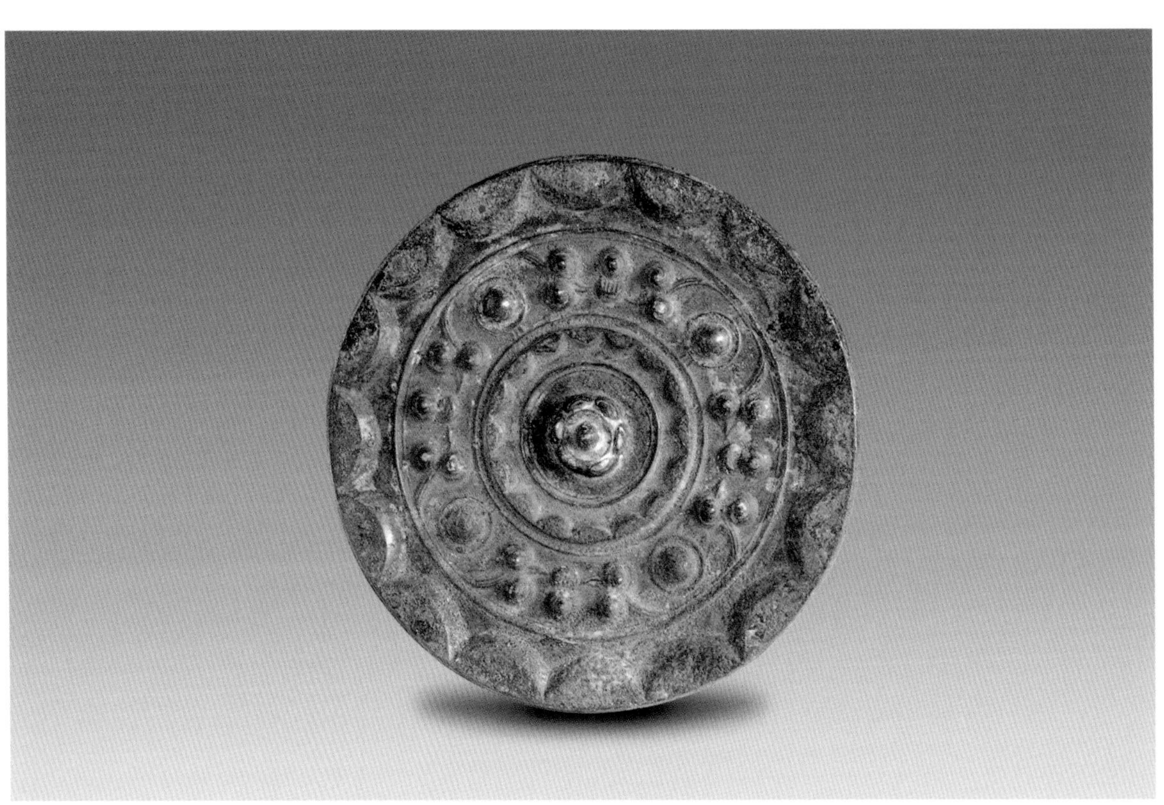

四乳四曜镜

西汉

青铜质

直径 13.5 厘米

Mirror with Four Yao and Four Nipple Nail pattern

Western Han Dynasty

Bronze

Diameter 13.5 cm

百乳状为钮，圆形座，座外为连弧纹，中间纹饰为四乳纹，间以相连的小乳纹，镜外缘为连弧纹。

刘板泮藏

There is a nipple knob with a circular base in the middle of the mirror. The base is circled by a concatenated-arc pattern. There are four nipple-like patterns in the middle of the mirror with small nipple patterns among them. The rim is also circled by a concatenated-arc pattern.

Collected by Liu Banpan

華

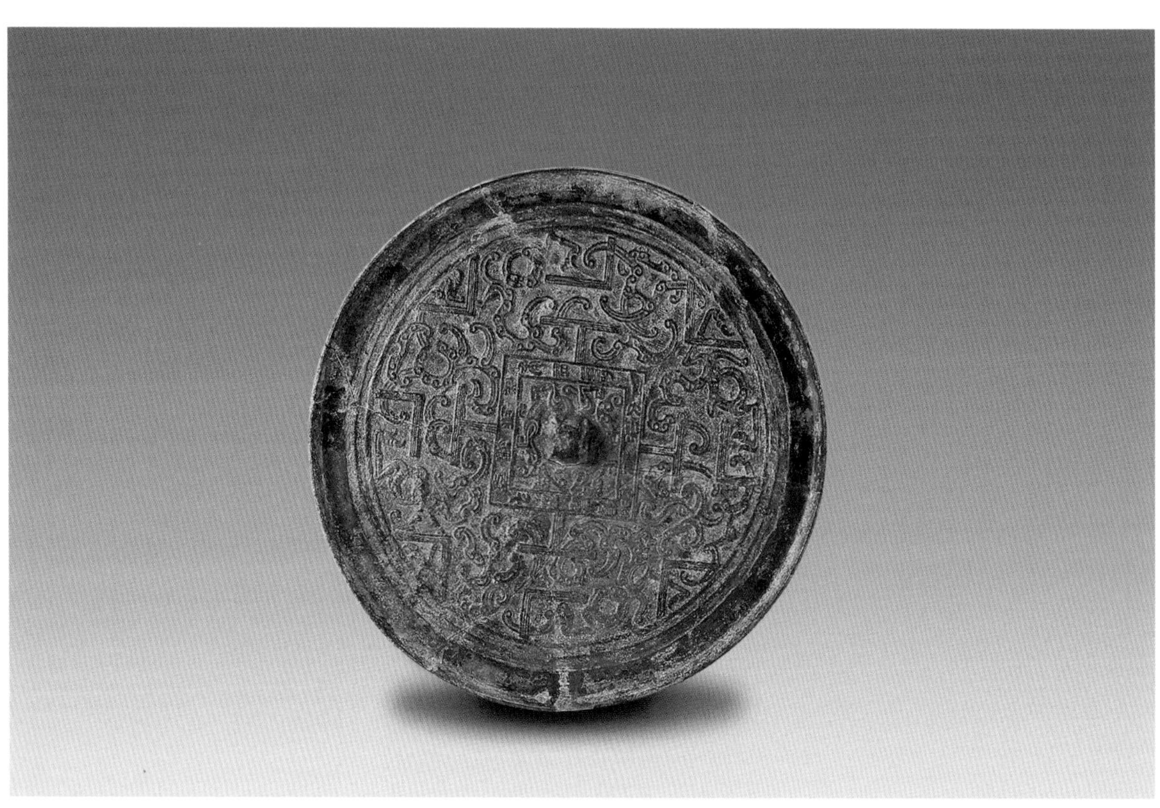

蟠螭纹规矩镜

西汉

青铜质

直径 18.4 厘米

TLV Mirror with Panchi Pattern

Western Han Dynasty

Bronze

Diameter 18.4 cm

桥形钮，方形钮座，座内二龙环绕，雷纹地，地上浮雕繁缛的蟠螭纹，间以规矩纹。纽座外两凸弦纹之间有铭文“大乐贵富，得所好，千秋万岁，延年益寿”十五字。这是目前所知年代最早的规矩镜。

河北博物院藏

There is a bridge knob with a square base in the middle of the mirror. Two dragons intertwine within the base shaded by thunder patterns interphase with TLV. Overelaborated Panchi (a mythical dragon in ancient China) patterns are also embossed on the base. On the two convex string patterns, there are 15 inscriptions which mean forever wealthy and noble. The piece is the oldest TLV mirror we have known for now.

Preserved in Hebei Museum

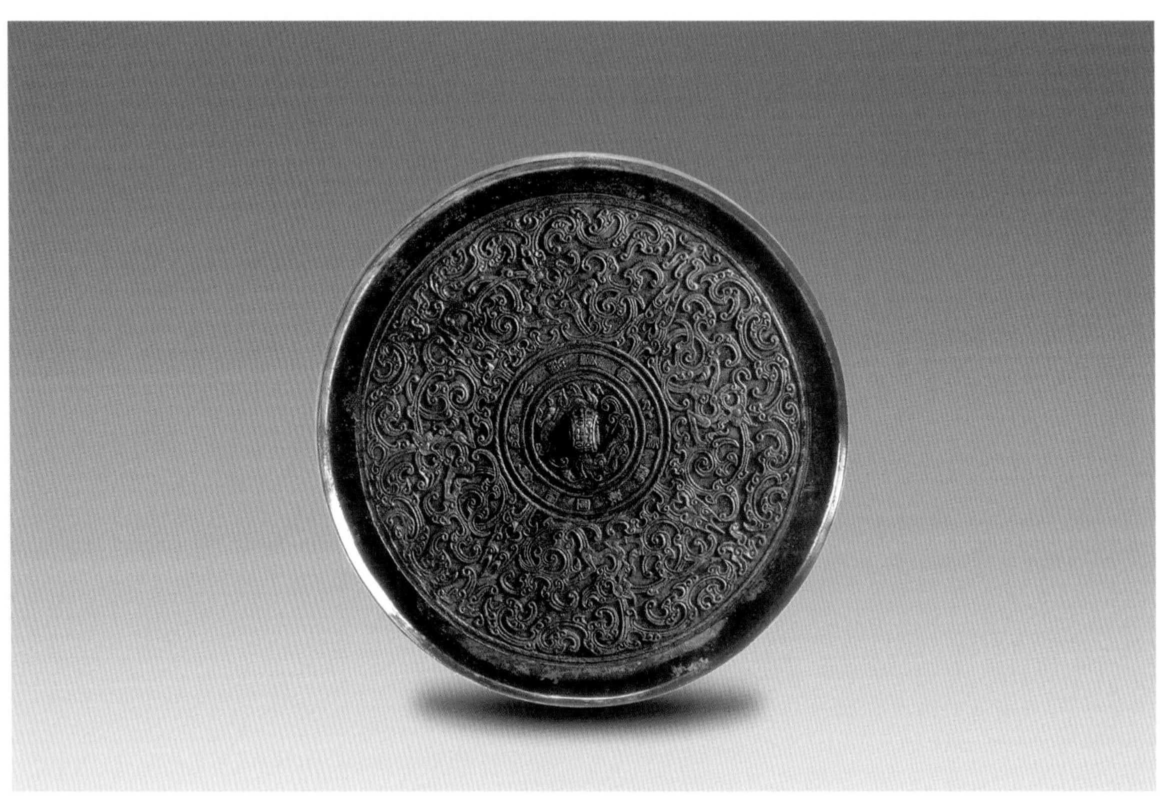

蟠螭纹铜镜

西汉

青铜质

直径 23.2 厘米

Copper Mirror with Panchi Patterns

Western Han Dynasty

Bronze

Diameter 23.2 cm

圆形。半环形兽面纹钮，双龙纹钮座。座外有二道弦纹。弦纹外有一圈铭文，铭文："大乐贵富千秋万岁宜酒食"。铭文外又有二道弦纹，外弦为绳纹。镜面云雷纹地，主题纹饰为变形蟠螭纹缠绕环转。主纹分四组，每组以火焰纹间隔。该铜镜具有战国晚期西汉早期风格，为扬州馆藏铜镜中所罕见。2001 年扬州市郊西湖镇蚕桑砖瓦厂西汉墓出土。

扬州考古队藏

The mirror is circular. There is a semicircular animal face knob with a double-dragon pattern base in the middle of the mirror. There are double-string pattern outside the knob, and a circular of inscriptions outside the patterns which are "Da Le Gui Fu, Qian Qiu Wan Sui, Yi Jiu Shi" which mean good wishes. Outside the inscriptions is another double-string pattern and the second string is in rope shape. The shading pattern of the mirror surface is cloud-thunder patterns. The topical pattern is transformative Panchi pattern (a mythical creatures in ancient China) which circles around. The main pattern is divided into four groups which interphase with flame patterns. This mirror has the style between the late Warring States Period and early Western Han Dynasty. It is really rare in Yangzhou Museum. This piece was unearthed from a Western Han tomb in silkworm bricks and tiles plant in West Lake Town, Yangzhou City.

Preserved in Yangzhou Archaeological Team

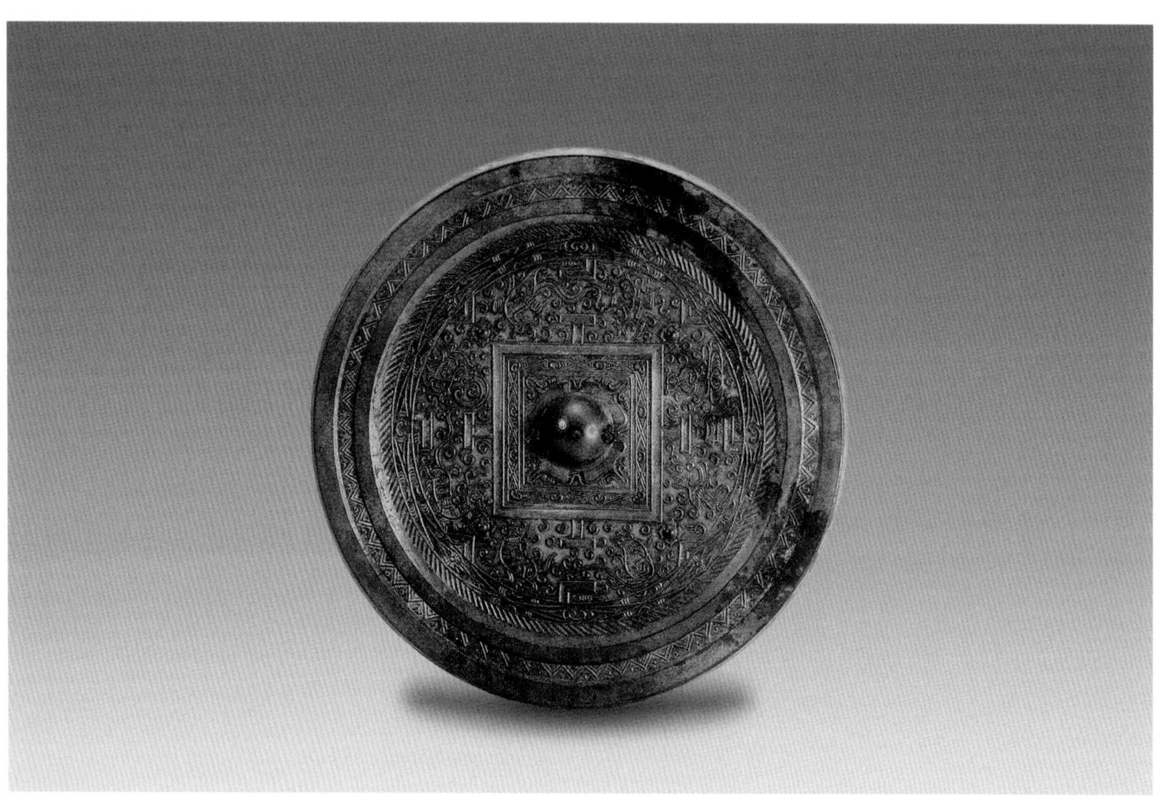

神人瑞兽铜镜

西汉

青铜质

直径 18 厘米

Copper Mirror with Immortal and Auspicious Beast

Western Han Dynasty

Bronze

Diameter 18 cm

镜作圆形，圆钮，柿蒂纹钮座，周围饰草叶。其外饰三层：在双线方栏与单线方栏间饰菱形几何纹；外为双线方栏；方栏外饰柿蒂、四乳与规矩纹，其间饰以狮子、羽人、道人、鸨羊、雏凤等人物禽兽纹和菱形几何纹。其外饰以射线和两周宽平素纹相间的双线波折纹。1986 年扬州市西郊蜀岗大队五号墓出土。

扬州博物馆藏

In the middle of the circular mirror is a circular knob with a calyx kaki base circled with grass-blade pattern. There are three zones around the base: rhombus patterns are between the double-line square and the single-line square; a double-line square is outside the rhombus patterns; outside the double-line square are kaki-calyx patterns, four nipple patterns, and Guiju patterns. There are also lions, feather men, Taoist priest, bustard sheep, immature phoenix, and some human-beast patterns as well as rhombus patterns. The rim is ornamented with double-line twists and turns patterns which include ray patterns and two circles of arcs. This piece was unearthed from Shugang Team No.5 Tomb in western Yangzhou in 1986.

Preserved in Yangzhou Museum

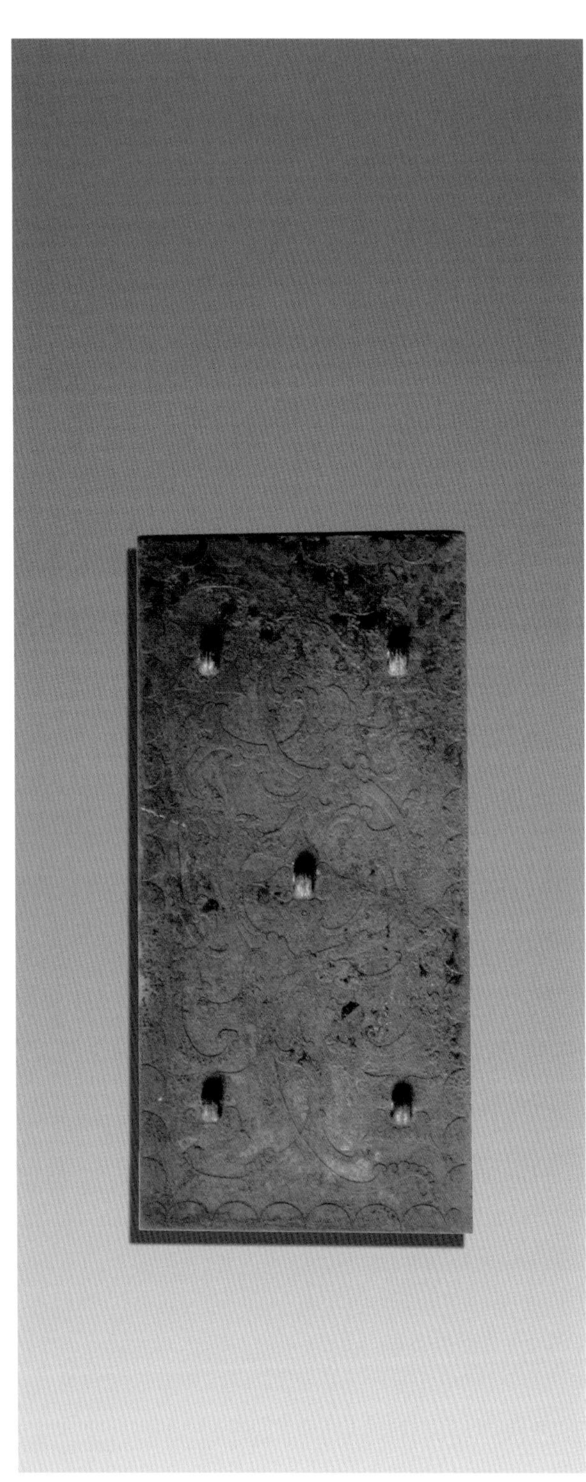

龙凤纹矩形铜镜

西汉

青铜质

长 115.1 厘米，宽 57.7 厘米，重 56500 克

钮长 5 厘米，宽 3.5 厘米，高 3.2 厘米

Rectangular Copper Mirror with Dragon-Phoenix Patterns

Western Han Dynasty

Bronze

Length 115.1 cm/ Width 57.7 cm/ Weight 56,500g

The knob: Length 5 cm/ Width 3.5 cm/ Height 3.2 cm

长方形，正面平整，背面四角及中间有 5 个拱形三弦钮。其间饰龙纹，四边饰垂帐纹。龙首较长，长角，张口吐舌，身细长而卷曲，四足有力，尾分双叉，栩栩如生。

山东省淄博市博物馆藏

The mirror is rectangular. Its surface is smooth. There are five arc three-string knobs on the four corners and in the middle of the back. There is a knob base with calyx kaki patterns interphase with a dragon pattern. The four sides are decorated with drooping curtain patterns. The dragon has a long head, long corners, and a big open mouth with its tongue stretching out. The dragon's body is slender and wrapped. It has four strong feet and its tail branches off in the end. The dragon is as natural as it is alive.

Preserved in Zibo Museum of Shandong Province

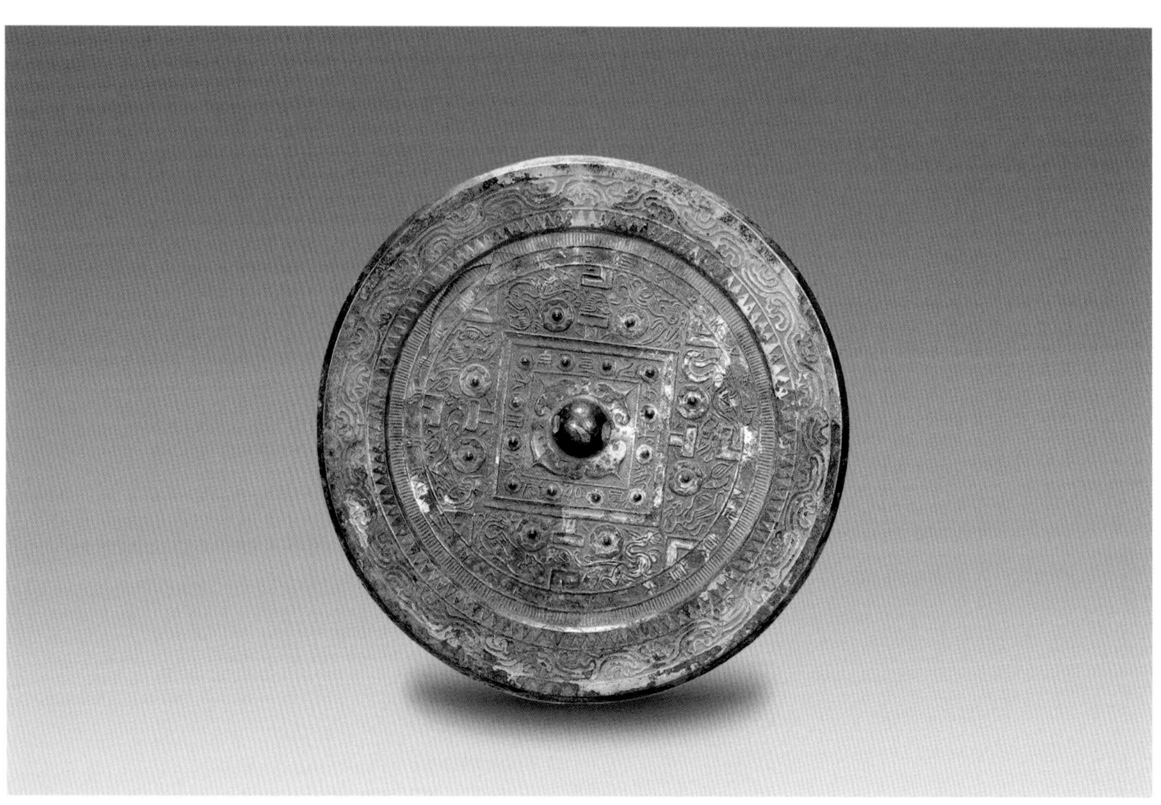

尚方鸟兽纹镜

新莽

青铜质

直径 18.5 厘米

Shangfang Mirror with Bird-Animal Patterns

Xinmang Dynasty

Bronze

Diameter 18.5 cm

圆钮，柿蒂纹钮座。座外方框内饰乳钉，乳钉间有十二地支铭文。方框外饰乳钉及规矩纹，其间饰鸟兽纹，外镌铭文一周。边缘饰锯齿纹、云气纹各一周。河南洛阳同乐寨 15 号墓出土。

洛阳博物馆藏

There is a circular knob with calyx kaki base in the middle of the mirror. Nipple nails and inscriptions of Chinese era among the nails are ornamented in the square outside the base. Outside the square are nipple nails and Guiju patterns interphase with bird-animal patterns Outside the patterns are a circle of inscriptions. The rim is circled by sawtooth patterns and cloud-air patterns. This piece was unearthed from Tonglezhai No.15 Tomb in Luoyang, Henan Province.

Preserved in Luoyang Museum

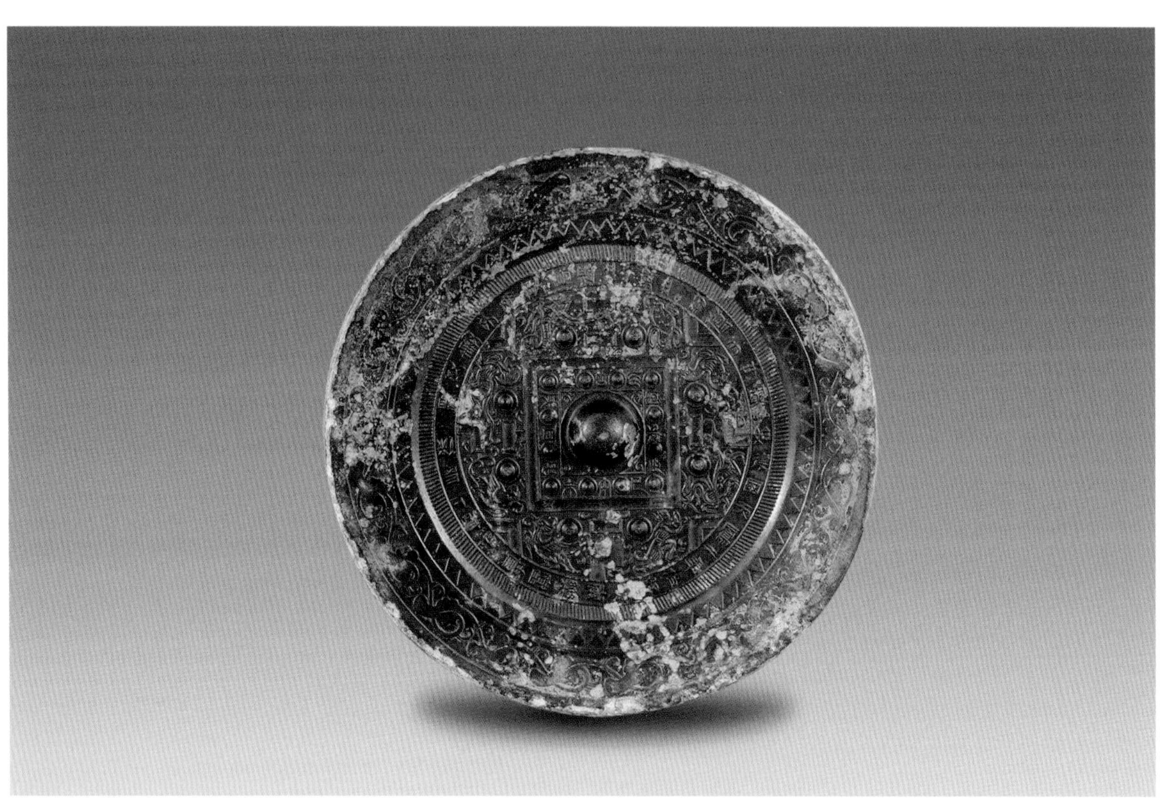

天凤二年常乐富贵镜

新莽

青铜质

直径 16.6 厘米

Chang Le Fugui Mirror in the 2nd Year of Tianfeng

Xinmang Dynasty

Bronze

Diameter 16.6 cm

圆钮，方钮座区域内有十二字铭，间以十二个乳钉纹。内区有博局、四灵及羽人、蟾蜍、羊等纹样。外区有铭文三十八字。镜缘内侧饰一周锯齿纹，外侧饰缠枝叶纹。天凤二年，为公元 15 年。

上海博物馆藏

There is a circular knob with a square base in the middle of the mirror. Twelve inscriptions interphase with 12 nipple nails patterns within the knob base. On the inner zone are patterns like Boju, Siling, feather man, bufonid, and sheep (all of them were mythical creatures in ancient China). There are 38 inscriptions on the outer zone. Inside the rim are a circle of sawtooth patterns and entangled-foliage patterns outside. The 2nd year of Tianfeng stands for the year of 15 A.D.

Preserved in Shanghai Museum

華

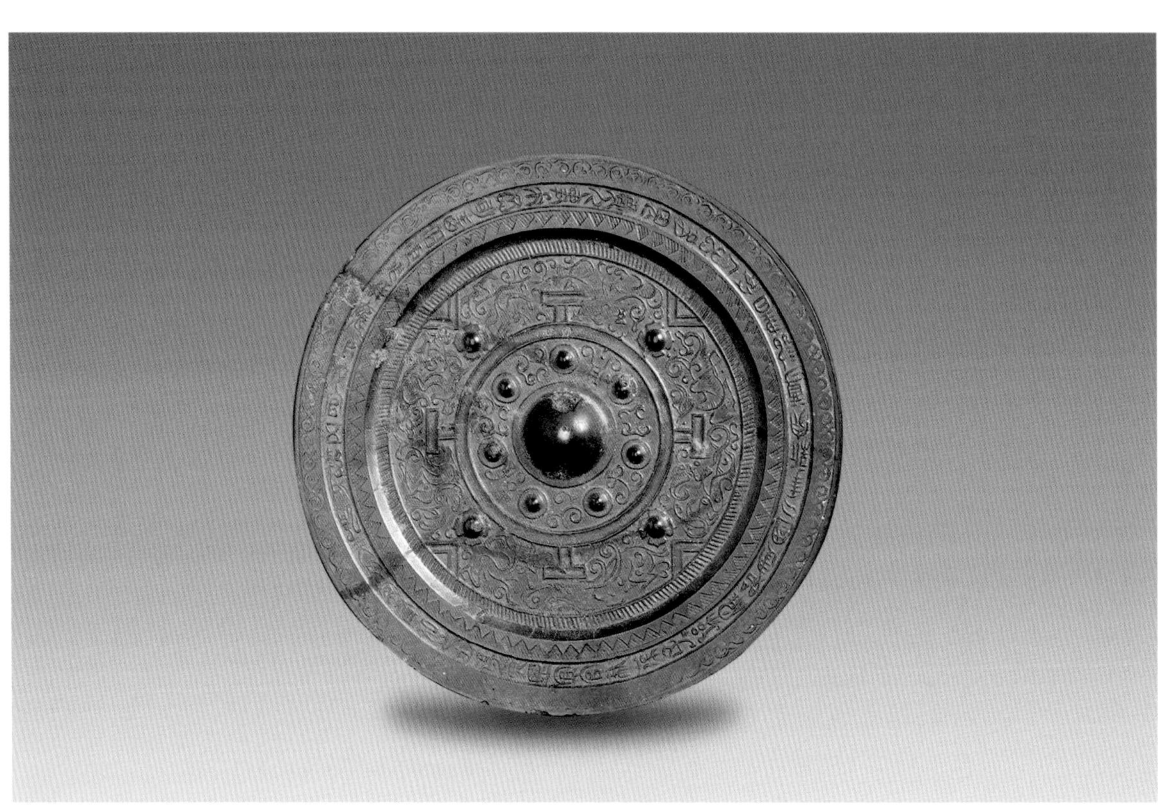

始建国二年新家镜

新莽

青铜质

直径 16.1 厘米

New House Mirror in the 2nd Year of the Shijianguo

Xinmang Dynasty

Bronze

Diameter 16.1 cm

圆钮，圆钮座。钮座外七乳钉环绕，乳钉间有“宜子孙”三字，另饰四组卷草纹。外围双线轮带，轮带外为简化博局，另缀四乳，把纹饰分成八区，分别饰以鸟、兽、羽人、仙人等图案，外有栉纹、锯齿纹各一周。锯齿纹带外有铭文一周五十二字。始建国二年，为公元 10 年。

中国国家博物馆藏

There is a circular knob with a circular base in the middle of the mirror. The base is circled by seven nipple nail patterns with three characters “Yi, Zi, Sun” among the nails. which mean good wishes. It is decorated with four groups of wrapped-grass patterns. On the outer zone are double-line arc with simplified chess games. Four nails divide the pattern zone into eight parts which are decorated with bird, beast, feather man, and immortal. Outside the patterns is a circle of comb and sawtooth patterns. Outside the sawtooth pattern belt is a circle of 52 inscriptions. The 2nd Year of the Shijianguo stands for the year of 10 A.D.

Preserved in National Museum of China

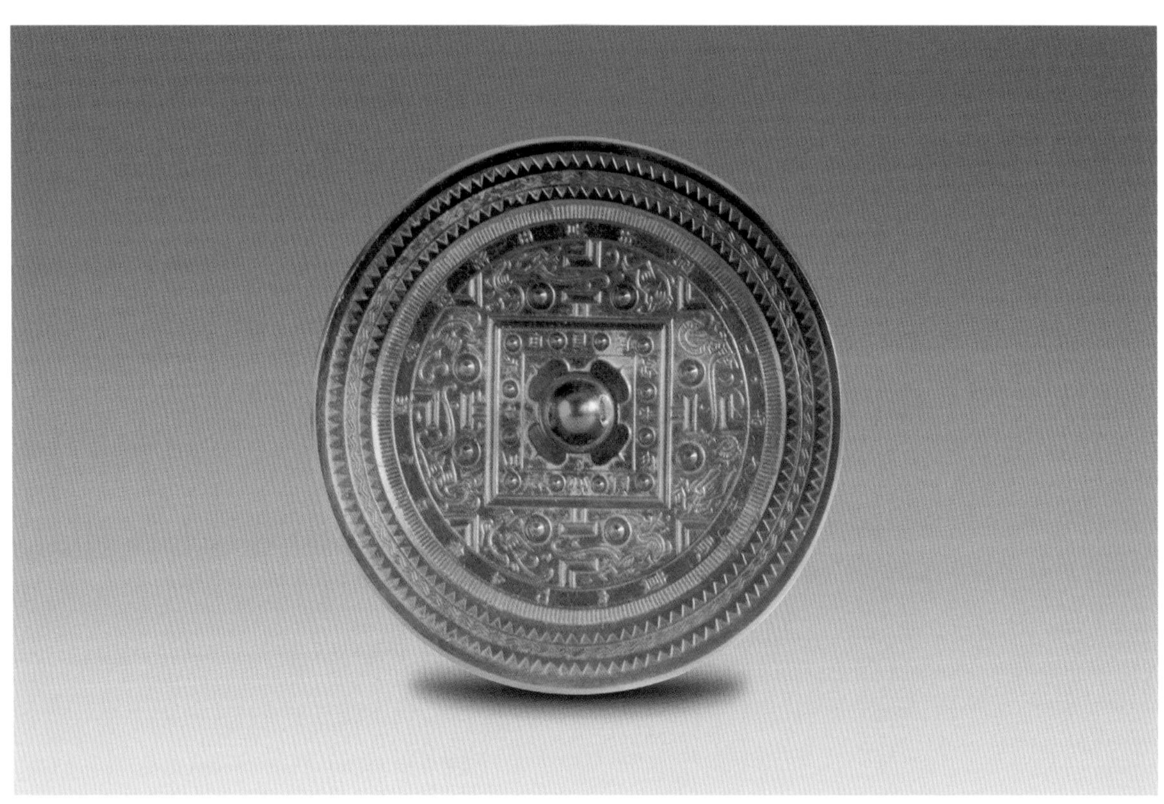

乳纹规矩四神镜

东汉

青铜质

直径 17.2 厘米

TLV Mirror with Pattern of Nipple and Four Mythical Creatures

East Han Dynasty

Copper

Diameter 17.2 cm

西汉末至东汉中期流行的规矩镜。纹饰精细，镜内有铭文：“尚方作镜真大巧……”。“尚方”是当时制造皇室器物的机构，秦始置，汉沿袭继承制镜因此而得名。

梁戊年藏

The piece is a TLV mirror which gets popular from The late Western Han Dynasty to the middle of the East Han Dynasty. It has elaborate patterns with inscriptions “Shang Fang Zuo Jing Zhen Da Qiao” inside the mirror, which praise the mirror-making skills of Shang Fang Shang Fang is the institution which made the royal artifacts. It was established by Qin Dynasty, and inherited by the Han Dynasty the to produce mirrors, Hence the mirror got its name.

Collected in Liang Wunian

華

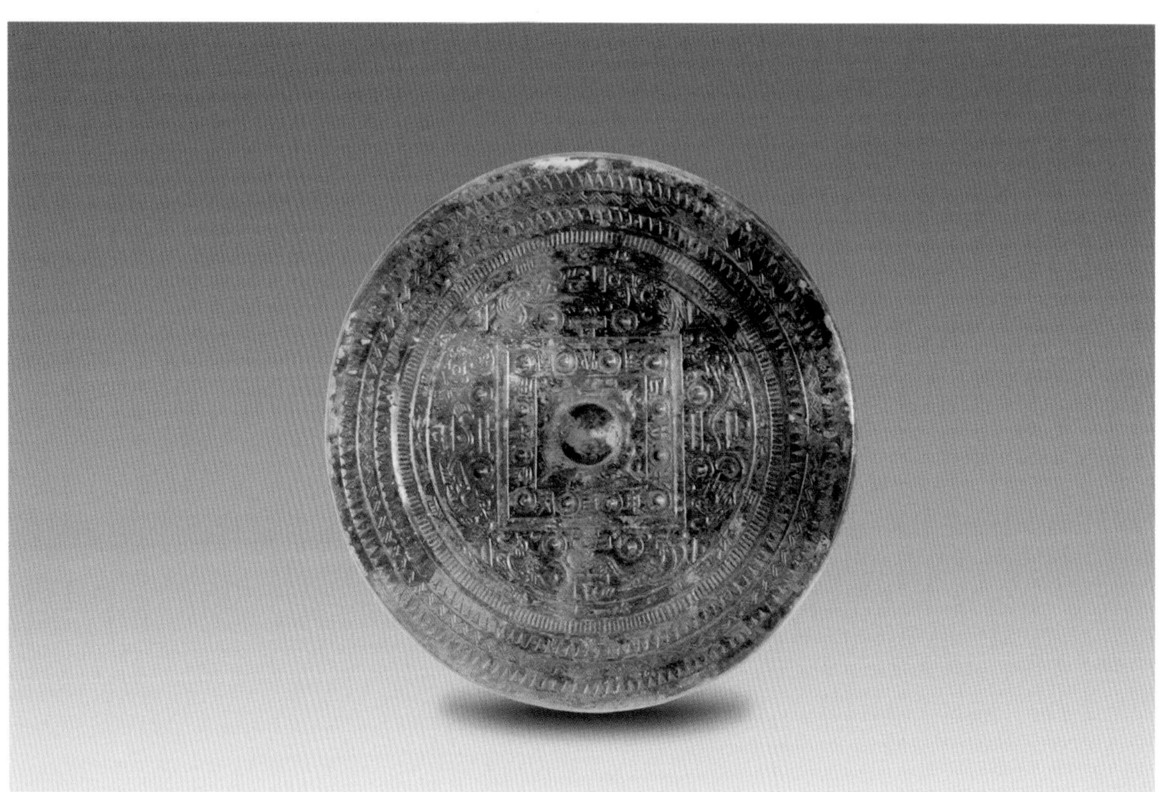

乳纹规矩四神镜

东汉

青铜质

直径 18.3 厘米

TLV Mirror with Pattern of Nipple and Four Mythical Creatures

East Han Dynasty

Bronze

Diameter 18.3 cm

东汉中期，尚方出产规矩镜，图纹精美。镜沿边有铭文曰“尚方作镜真大巧……”。从该镜的质量可见当地所产铜镜是上乘之作。

李庆全藏

Shangfang produced TLV mirrors with exquisite patterns in the Mid Han Dynasty. The inscriptions on the rim are “Shang Fang Zuo Jing Zhen Da Qiao…” The quality of this mirror proves that Shang Fang was a place to produce mirrors with superior quality.

Collected by Li Qingquan

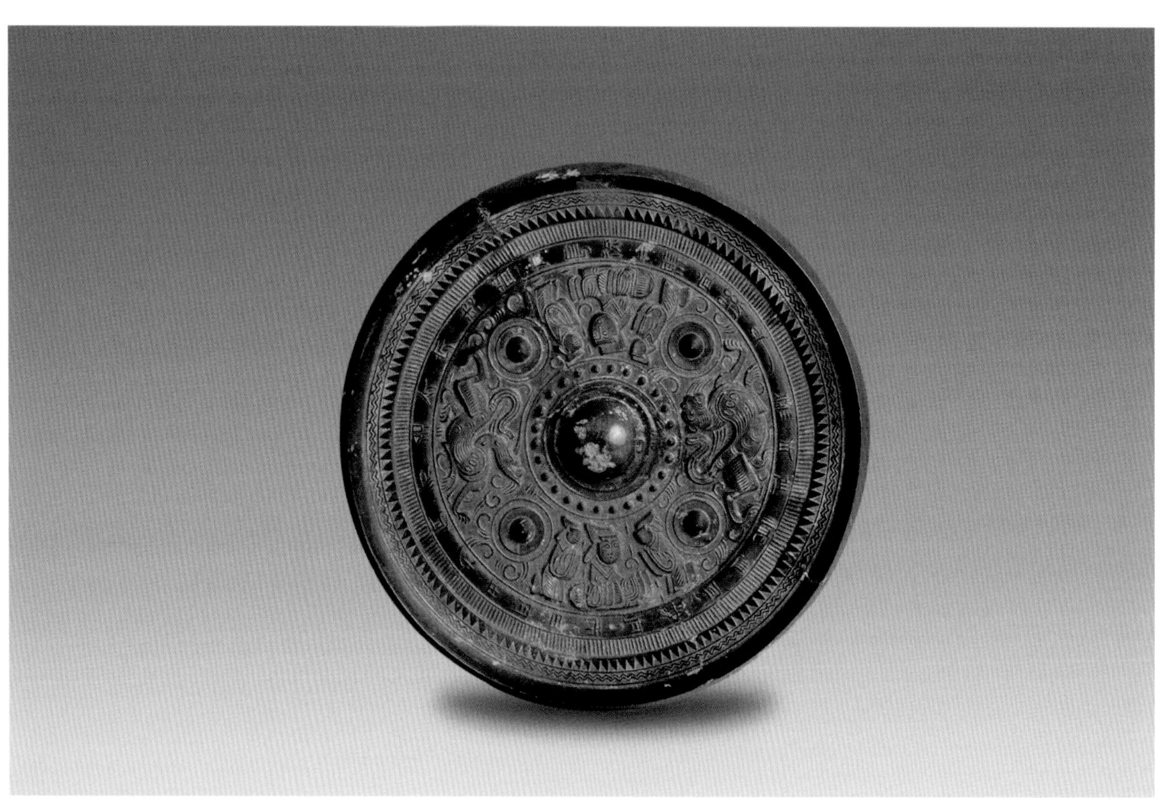

神人龙虎画像镜

东汉

青铜质

直径 18 厘米

TLV Mirror with Image of God-Man, Dragon and Tiger

East Han Dynasty

Bronze

Diameter 18 cm

圆形，扁圆钮。钮座外有四枚乳钉将镜背纹饰分为四区。其中两区为神人形象，另两区分别为一龙一虎。外围饰一周铭文带。镜缘饰三角锯齿纹和波状纹。南京南郊出土。

南京博物院藏

The mirror is circular with a flat circular button. Four nipple nails divide the mirror into four quarters. Two quarters are decorated with God-Man images and the other two are in the design of a dragon and a tiger respectively. Circling the four quarters is a decorative inscription. The rim is in the design of triangle sawtooth and wave patterns. This piece was unearthed in the southern suburbs of Nanjing.

Preserved in Nanjing Museum

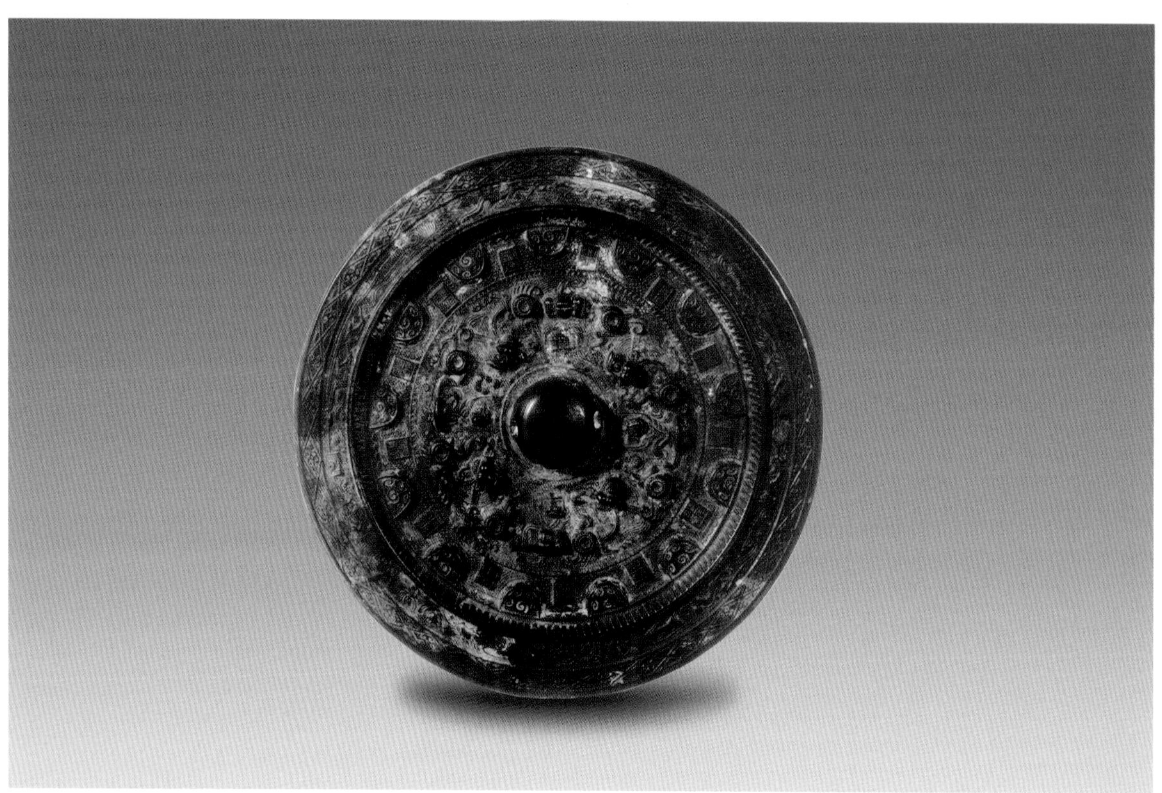

神兽纹铜镜

东汉

青铜质

直径 19.2 厘米

Copper Mirror with Immortal and Animal Pattern

East Han Dynasty

Bronze

Diameter 19.2 cm

该镜为传世品。扁圆钮，圆钮座。背面纹饰分为内区和外区两部分。内区以高浮雕相间配置四神四兽，四神似为东王公、西王母等。神兽外有半圆形和方枚一周，每一方枚内有“天王日月”四字铭文。内外区以锯齿纹一周分开。外区为画文带、神兽等形象，斜平缘，缘部饰菱形连珠纹。

高邮市博物馆藏

As a historical legacy, the mirror has a flat circular button with a circular button base. The decorative patterns divide the rear of the mirror into two parts: the inner part and the outer part. They are separated by a circle of sawtooth pattern. The inner part is decorated with four gods and four beasts in high relief. The four gods resemble Tung Wang Kung (God of the Immortals), Xi Wang Mu (Queen Mother of the West), etc. The pattern is circled by semicircular and square points and four Chinese character inscription "Tian Wang Ri Yue" are engraved on each square points. The outer part is decorated with the image of text drawing and sacred animals. The rim is slanting flat and decorated with a string of beads in diamond pattern.

Preserved in Gaoyou Museum

華

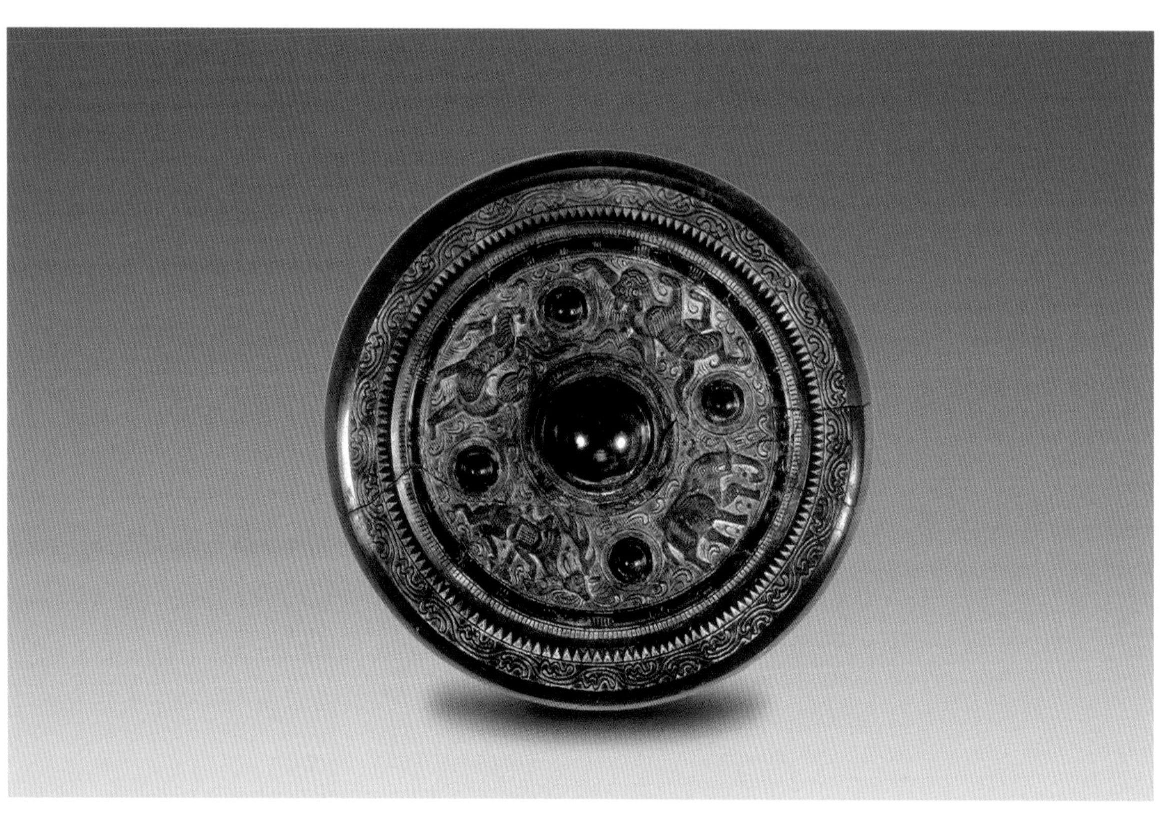

瑞兽纹铜镜

东汉

青铜质

直径 18.4 厘米，厚 0.7 厘米

Copper Mirror with Auspicious Animal Pattern

East Han Dynasty

Bronze

Diameter 18.4 cm/ Thickness 0.7 cm

此镜圆钮，钮座圆形。四乳钉之间饰浮雕，象、豺、虎、鹿等动物作为主纹，其间辅饰花草纹。外区铭文带为："王氏作竟真大工，上有仙人不知老，食饮玉泉饥食枣兮。"镜缘饰锯齿和云气纹带，之间以弦纹一道分隔，此镜纹饰饱满，工艺考究，铸造精良，是画像镜中之精品。1978 年邗江区西湖槐柳出土。

扬州博物馆藏

The mirror has a circular button with a circular base. Among the four nipple nails is the main pattern in relief such as elephant, jackal, tiger, and deer complemented by flower and grass pattern. The inscription on the outer part aims to praise the mirror maker. The rim is decorated with sawtooth and cloud-qi patterns. They are separated by a circle of string pattern. The mirror is fully patterned with exquisite craftsmanship and fine casting. Hence it belongs to a boutique of portrayal mirror. It was unearthed in Xihu Huailiu, Hanjiang District in 1978.

Preserved in Yangzhou Museum

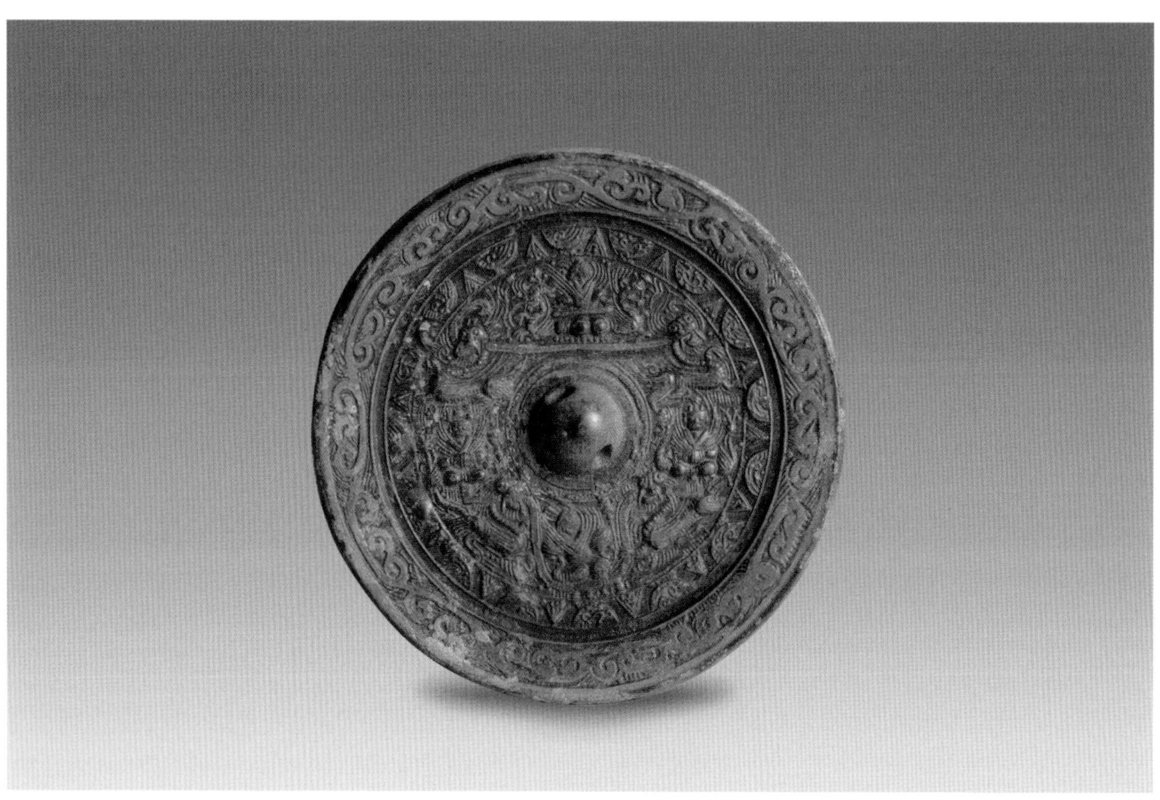

重列式神兽镜

东汉

青铜质

Mirror with Arrayed Immortal and Animal Patterns

East Han Dynasty

Bronze

圆钮，圆钮座。主要纹饰自上而下分为三段。最上段正中为神人，两侧各为一兽；第二段在镜钮左右分饰神人；下段中为神人，左右各配一兽，纹饰采用高浮雕方式；排列有序。外区作半圆形弧纹和三角形几何纹，缘部饰连续的云气纹。

南京博物院藏

The mirror has a circular knob with a circular base. The topical patterns divide the mirror into three parts from top to base. The upper part is centered by an immortal with two animals on each side. In the middle part, two immortals are respectively engraved on the left and right side of the knob. The lower part is centered by an immortal with two animals on each side. The decorative patterns are in high relief and orderly arrayed. The outer zone is decorated with semicircular string patterns and triangle geometric pattern. The rim design consists of consecutive cloud-qi patterns.

Preserved in Nanjing Museum

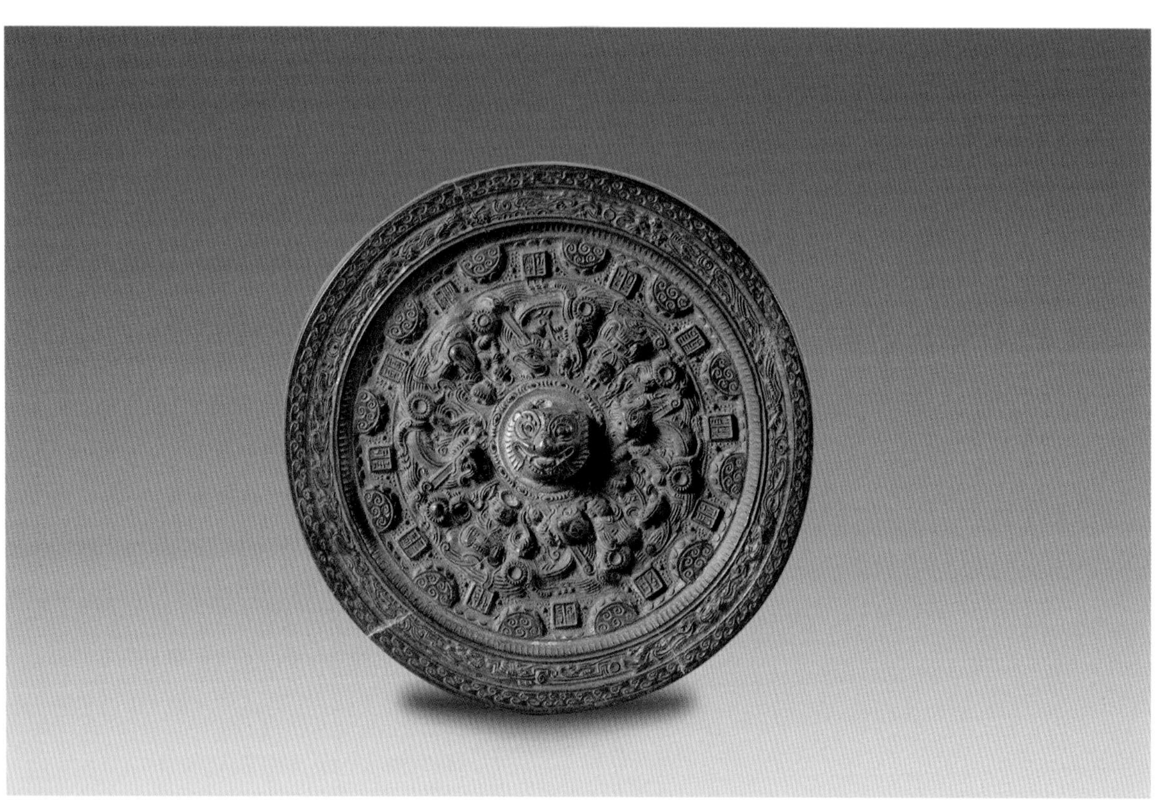

神兽镜

东汉

青铜质

直径 14 厘米

Mirror with Immortal and Animal Patterns

East Han Dynasty

Bronze

Diameter 14 cm

兽首钮，连珠纹钮座。内区有八枚，每枚上有神人，左右有神兽，皆作环状排列。外圈各有十二方枚与半圆块，方枚每块二字，半圆块饰卷云纹。镜缘内圈饰神人车马，外缘为卷云纹。浙江绍兴漓渚出土。

浙江省博物馆藏

The mirror has an animal head knob with a base ornamented with the pattern of a string of beads. There are a circle of eight leads beads with an immortal on each. The immortal is decorated with two sacred animals engraved on each side. In the outer arc twelve squares with each engraved with two characters and twelve semicircles decorated with rolling-cloud pattern. There are carriages, horses, and immortals inside the rim. The outer rim is in the design of rolling-cloud patterns. This piece was unearthed in Lizhu District located in Shaoxing, Zhejiang.

Preserved in Zhejiang Provincial Museum

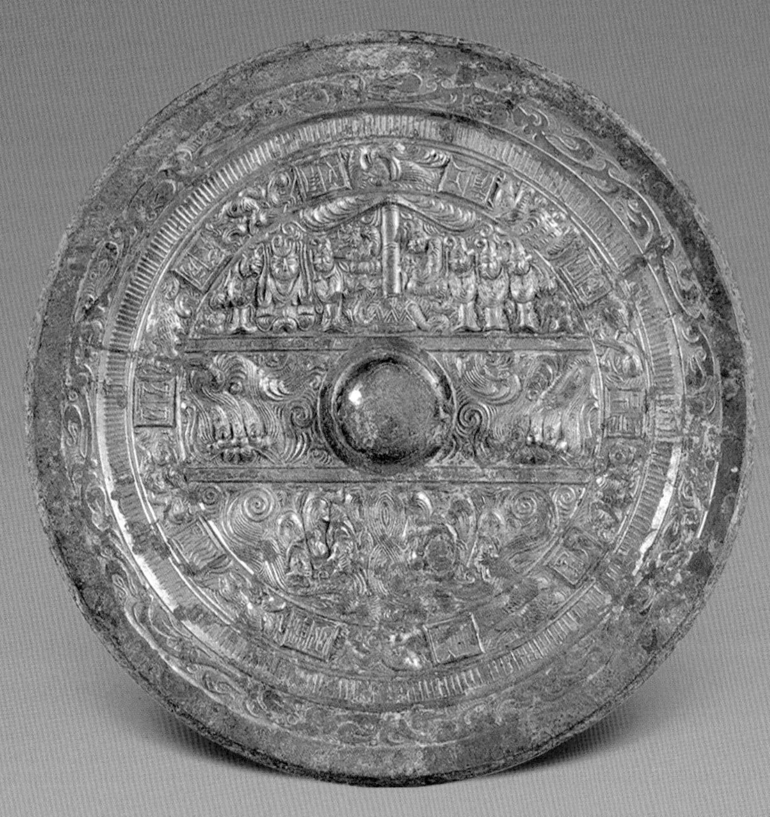

八子神兽镜

东汉

青铜质

直径 16.7 厘米

Mirror with Sacred Animal and Eight-Immortal Patterns

East Han Dynasty

Bronze

Diameter 16.7 cm

半圆钮，圆钮座。内区纹饰由两条平行线分为上中下三组。上组中为鼍礎华盖，两旁各一神人，一舞蹈，一端坐。左侧为一神人三侍从，右侧为四神人侧立。中组为天禄、辟邪。下组纹饰倒置，两神相对侧坐。外圈置十块方枚与动物纹相间。镜缘作缠枝纹。

上海博物馆藏

The mirror has a semicircular knob with a circular base. The inner part is divided by two parallel lines into three subdivisions. The upper is decorated with an alligator sinensis canopy with an immortal standing on each side. One is dancing and the other is sitting straightly. There are one immortals and three servants on the left part of the upper subdivision. There are four immortals standing laterally on the right side. The middle subdivision is decorated with Tianlu and Bixie (two sacred animals in ancient legend). The lower subdivision is decorated with reversing patterns and two laterally sitting immortals facing each other. Ten squares interphase with animal patterns in the outer part. The rim is patterned with flowers twining around branches.

Preserved in Shanghai Museum

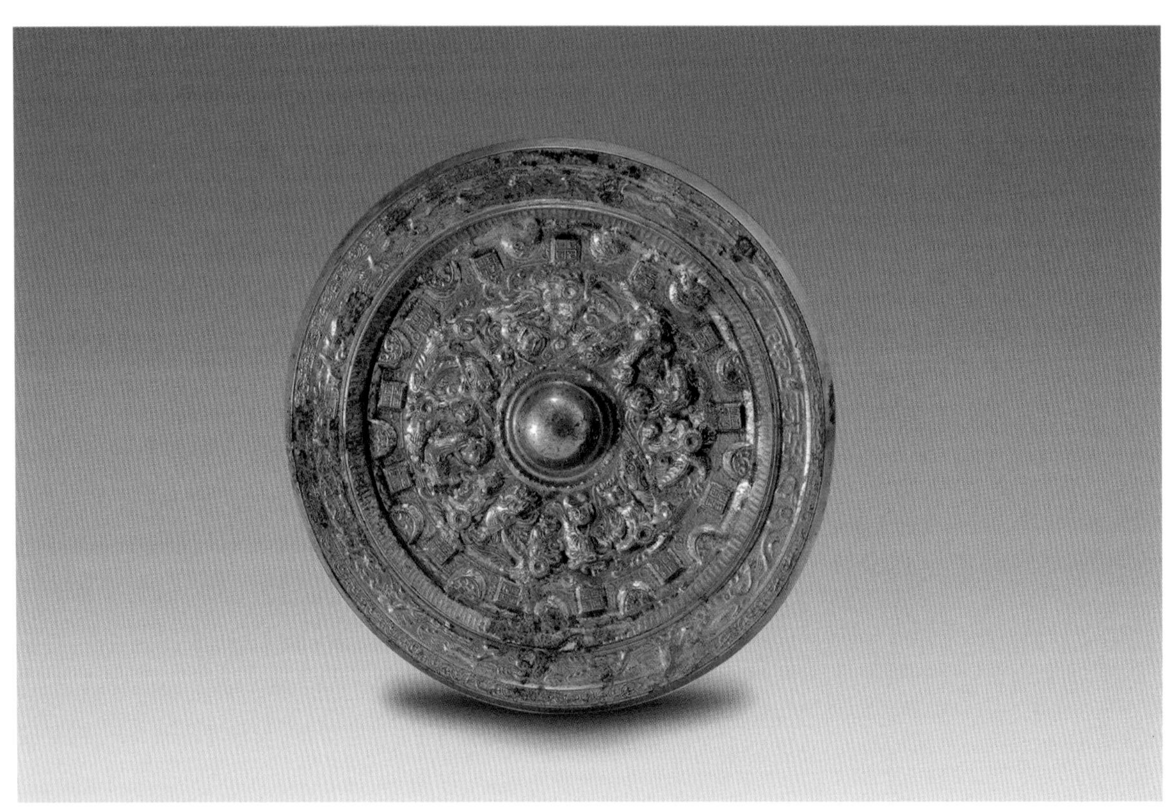

天王日月神兽镜

东汉

青铜质

直径 14.3 厘米

Mirror with Pattern of Immortal, Animal, Heaven King, Sun and Moon

East Han Dynasty

Bronze

Diameter 14.3 cm

半圆钮，连珠纹钮座。内区饰神人四组，下方为东王公，上方为西王母，两神人左右各有天禄和辟邪，还有两个神人、神兽。外区有相间的方枚与半圆块，各十二块。边缘纹饰分两圈，内圈为六龙驾云车，车上有神人、羽人，后面有三羽人各跨一青鸟，外圈饰菱形云纹。1982 年河南洛阳金谷园出土。

洛阳市文物考古研究院藏

The mirror has a semicircular knob with a base decorated with the pattern of a string of beads. The inner part is decorated with four groups of immortals, with Tung Wang Kung (God of the Immortals) on the top and Xi Wang Mu (Queen Mother of the West) on the base. On each side of them, there are Tianlu, Bixie (two sacred animals in ancient legend), two immortals, and sacred animals. The outer part is decorated with twelve interphase squares and semicircles. The decorative patterns on the rim consist of two tracks. The inner track is decorated with six dragons riding the cloud-like carriage along with immortals and feather men. Behind them are three feather men and each rides a bird messenger of Fairy God-Mother. The outer track is decorated with diamond-like cloud patterns. This piece was unearthed in Jingu Garden in Luoyang, Henan.

Preserved in Luoyang Municipal Institute of Archaeology and Cultural Relics

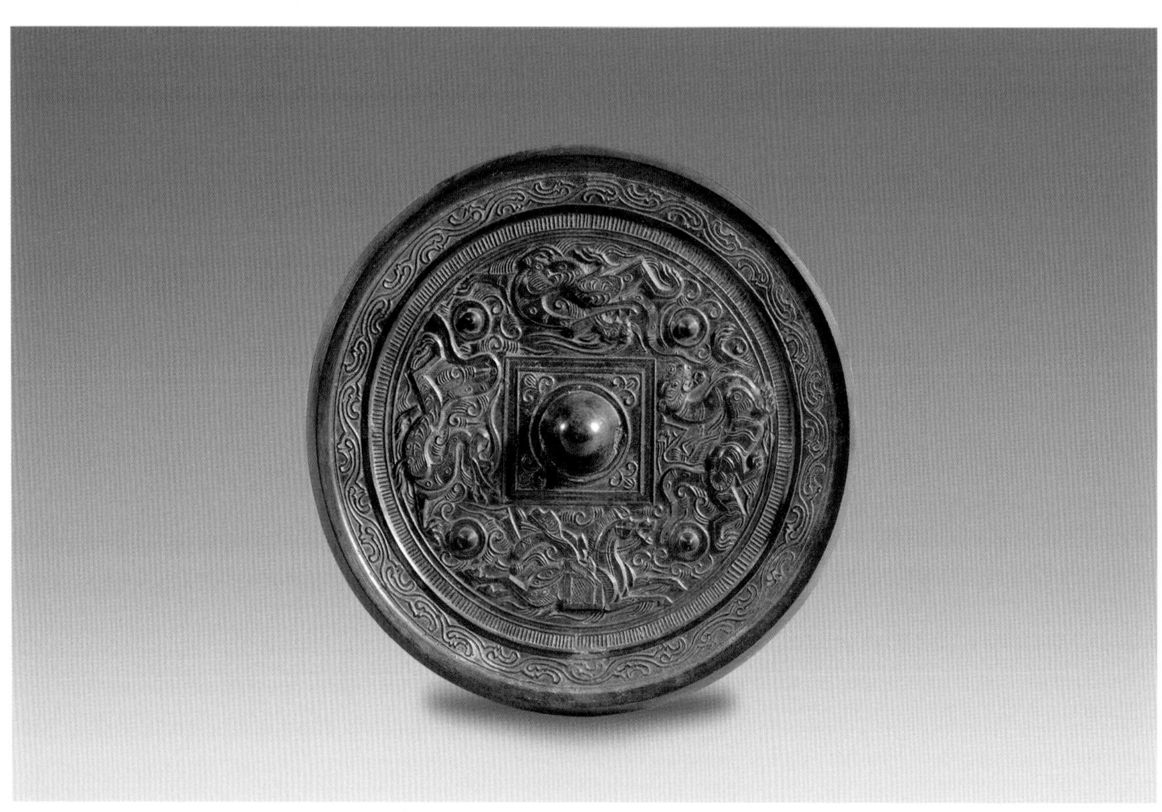

仙人骑马神兽镜

东汉

青铜质

直径 18.5 厘米

Mirror with Pattern of Sacred Animal and Immortals Riding Horses

East Han Dynasty

Bronze

Diameter 18.5 cm

圆钮，双线方框钮座。主题纹饰为仙人骑马及龙、虎、神兽，间饰四乳钉，边缘饰云纹。浙江绍兴赵建村出土。

绍兴博物馆藏

The mirror has a circular knob with a double-line square base. The topical pattern is immortals riding horses, dragons, tigers, and sacred animals. Among these patterns, four nipple nails are decorated. The rim is decorated with cloud-like patterns. This piece was unearthed in Zhaojian District in Shaoxing, Zhejiang.

Preserved in Shaoxing Museum

華

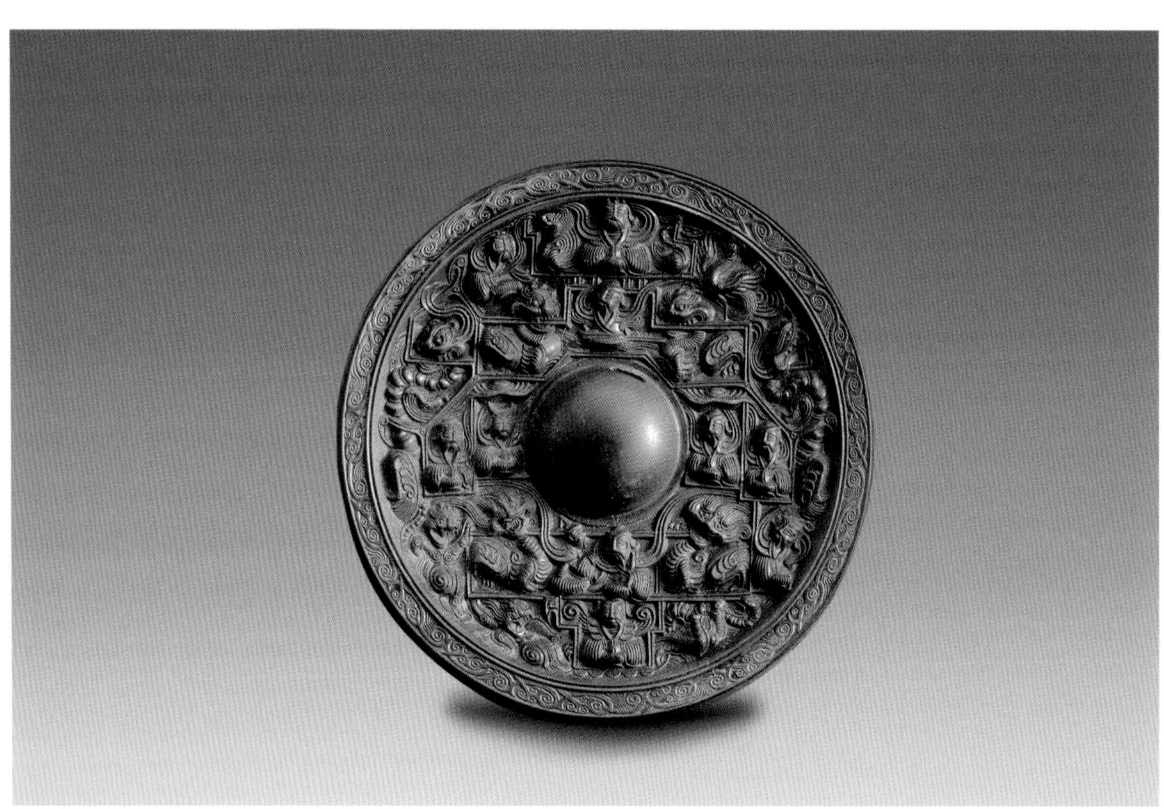

神兽镜

东汉

青铜质

直径 16.6 厘米

Mirror with Immortal and Sacred Animal Patterns

East Han Dynasty

Bronze

Diameter 16.6 cm

圆钮，圆钮座。纹饰横列成五排。第一排神人正面坐，左青龙右白虎，第二排神人面略向左侧，双手置于案上，两侧有神兽、神鸟、小神人，第三排在钮的两侧端坐四个神人，第四排两神人相对而坐，两侧共有一神人三神兽，第五排中间神人正面坐，左侧为玄武右侧为白虎。镜缘饰云纹图案。此镜纹饰极为精细。

日本千石唯司藏

The mirror has a circular knob with a circular base. The decorative patterns are arranged in five horizontal rows. The first row of immortal are in the sitting position with the azure dragon on the left and the white tiger on the right. The second row is decorated with immortals with their heads facing slightly toward left and two hands putting on the board. On both sides of this row, there are sacred animals, supernatural birds, and little immortals. On both sides of the knob in the third row, four immortals are sitting decorously. The fourth row is decorated with two immortals sitting face to face with one immortal and three sacred animals on both sides. An immortal is sitting in a positive position in the middle of the fifth row with a tortoise on the left and a white tiger on the right. The rim is decorated with cloud-like patterns. The decorative patterns of this mirror is extremely fine and exquisite

Preserved by Sengoku Tadashi Museum Japan

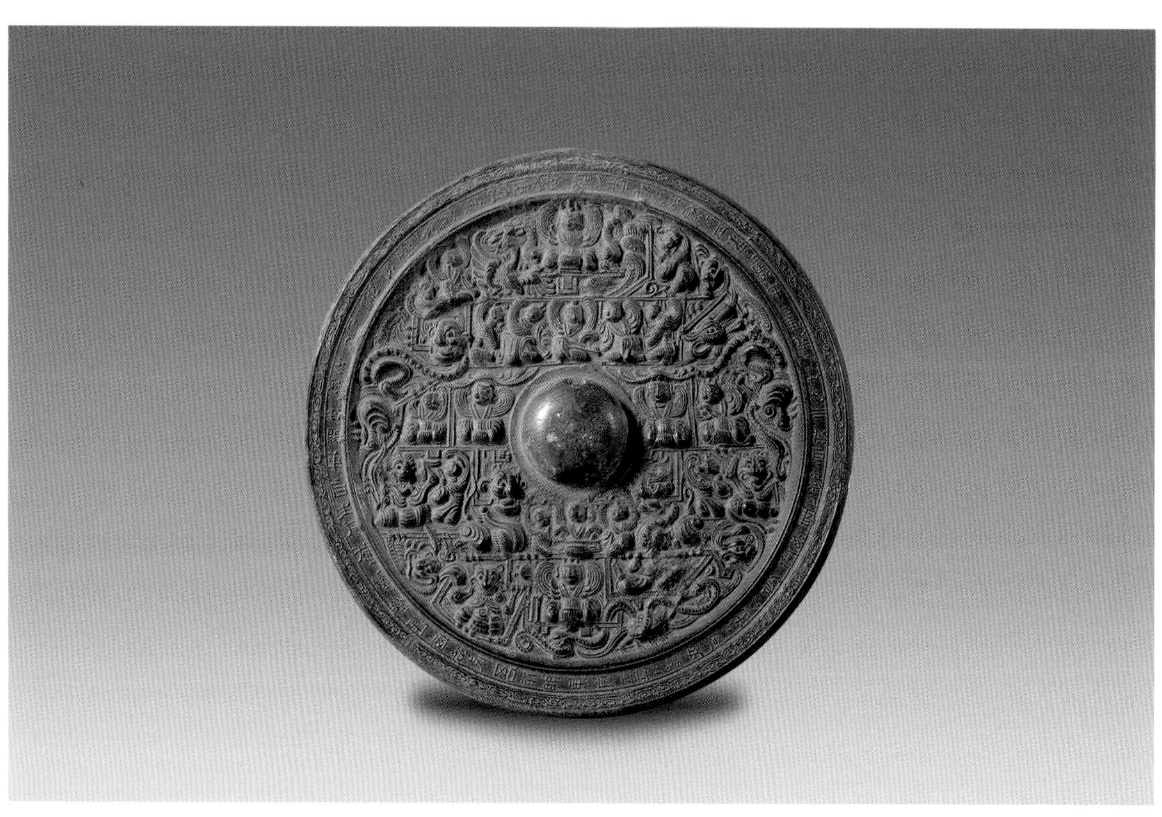

吾作神兽镜

东汉

青铜质

直径 13 厘米

Self-made Mirror with Immortal and Animal Patterns

East Han Dynasty

Bronze

Diameter 13 cm

扁圆钮，圆钮座。纹饰横列成五排。有神人、神兽、羽人等。外圈有铭文一周六十四字。镜缘饰云纹。

浙江省博物馆藏

The mirror has a flat circular knob with a circular base. The decorative patterns, such as the immortals, the acred animals, and the feather men, are arranged in five horizontal rows. Sixty four Chinese characters are inscribed on the outer track. The rim is decorated with cloud-like patterns.

Preserved in Zhejiang Provincial Museum

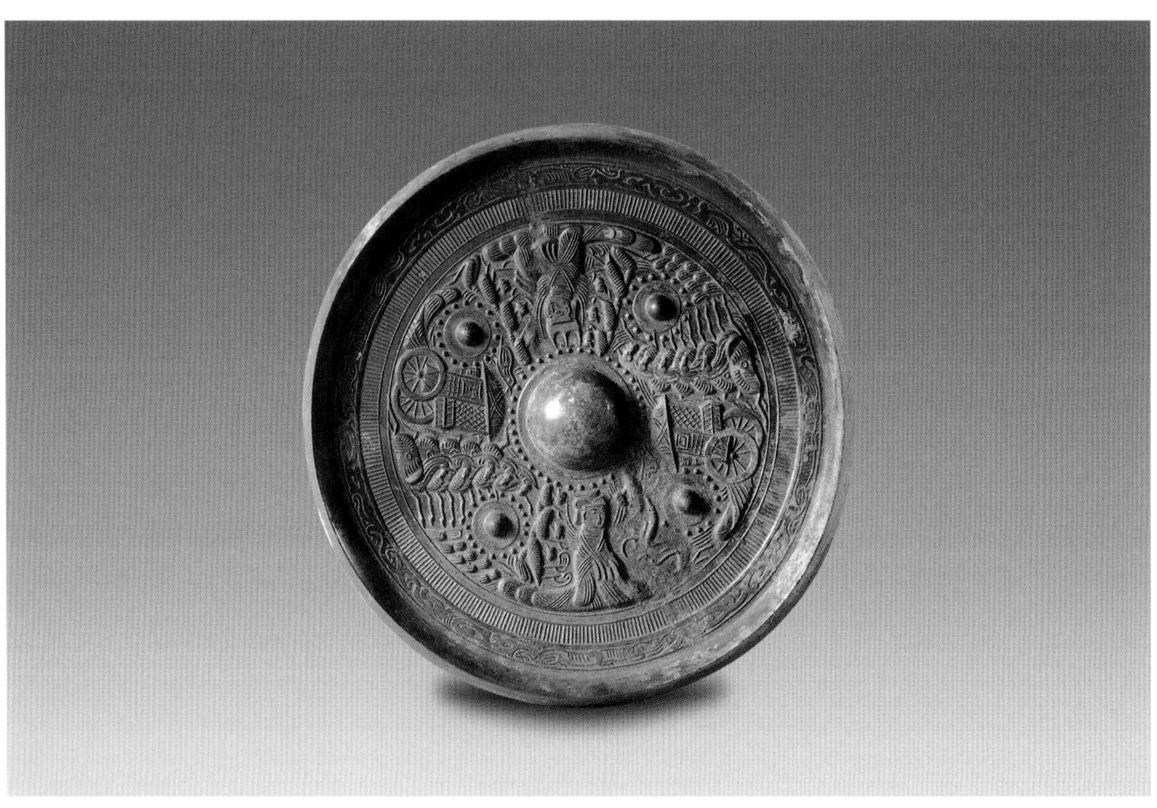

神人车马镜

东汉

青铜质

直径 23 厘米

Mirror with Pattern of Immortals and Carriages and Horses

East Han Dynasty

Bronze

Diameter 23 cm

圆钮，圆钮座。四乳钉将纹饰分为四组，两组为六马驾车，两组为一神人端坐。镜缘饰一周云纹。1976 年浙江绍兴出土。

浙江省博物馆藏

The mirror has a flat circular knob with a circular base. Four nipple nails divide the decorative patterns into four groups. Two groups are in the decoration of six horses pulling a carriage. The other two groups are decorated with an immortal sitting decorously respectively. The rim is decorated with cloud-like patterns. This piece was unearthed in Shaoxing, Zhejiang in 1976.

Preserved in Zhejiang Provincial Museum

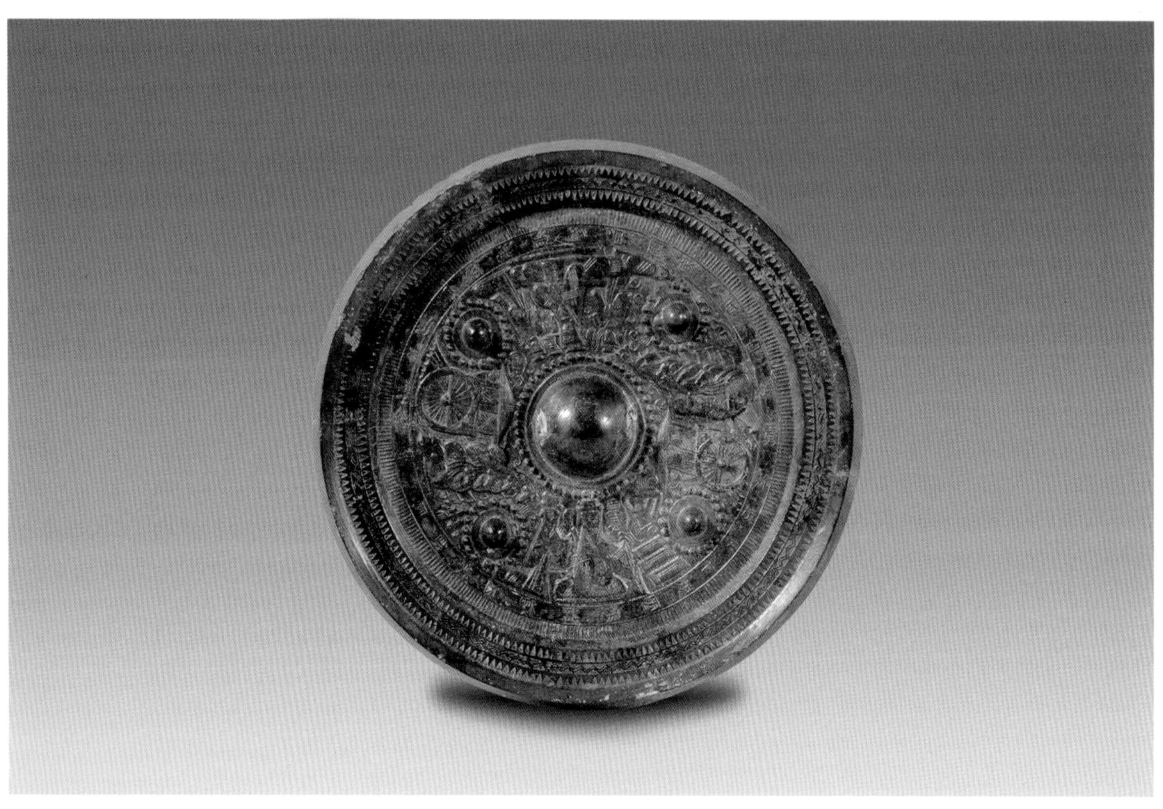

周氏神人车马镜

东汉

青铜质

直径 22.1 厘米

Zhou Family Mirror with Pattern of Immortals and Carriages and Horses

East Han Dynasty

Bronze

Diameter 22.1 cm

圆钮，圆钮座。四乳钉纹将纹饰分为四组。一组六马驾车。一组五马驾车，车中站一人。一组端坐一神，有两侍女，另有二羽人舞剑，一羽人戏丸。一组端坐一神，有三侍从，另有羽人。外圈有铭文一周四十五字。镜缘饰锯齿纹和波纹。浙江绍兴出土。

绍兴博物馆藏

The mirror has a circular button and a circular button base. Four nipple nails divide the decorative patterns into four groups. The first group is in the decoration of six horses pulling a carriage. The second group is decorated with five horses pulling a carriage with a person standing inside. The third group is decorated with an immortal sitting decorously with two maidservants, two feather men doing sword dance and one feather man playing with a ball. The fourth group is decorated with an immortal sitting decorously with three maidservants and feather men. Forty five Chinese characters are inscribed on the outer track. The rim is decorated with sawtooth and wave patterns. This piece was unearthed in Shaoxing, Zhejiang.

Preserved in Shaoxing Museum

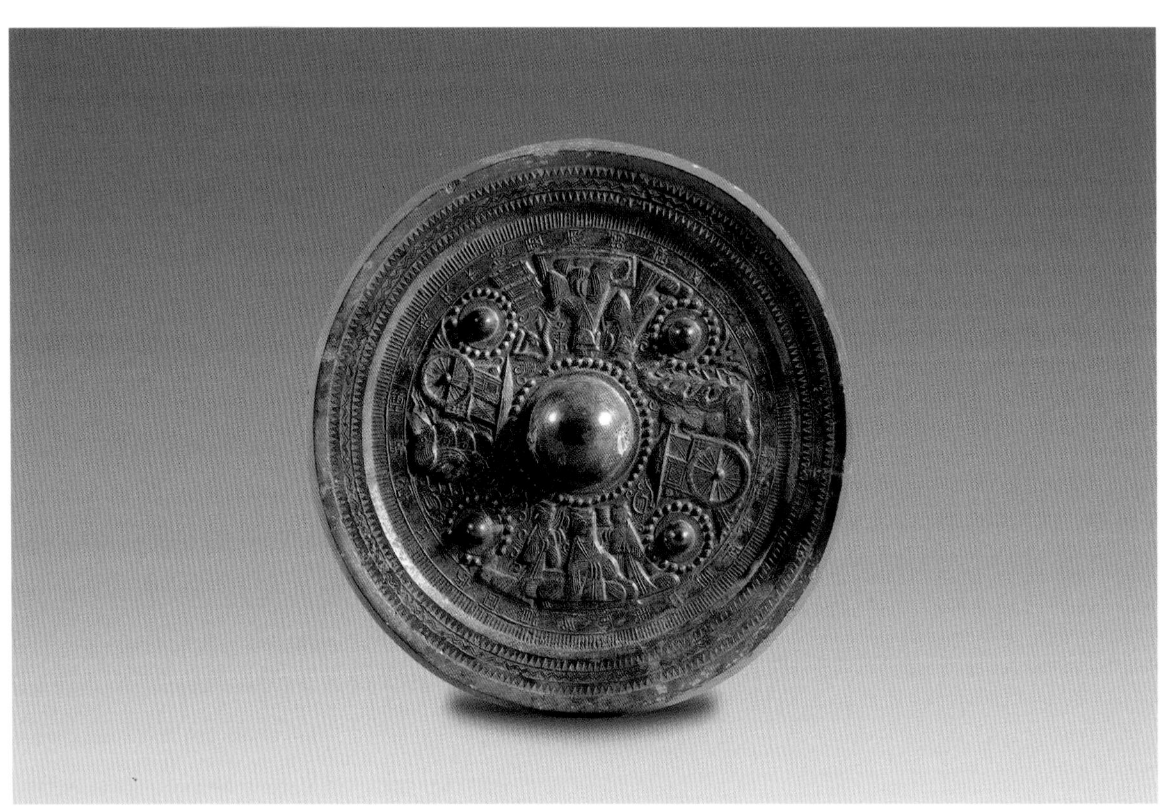

騶氏神人车马镜

东汉

青铜质

直径 22.5 厘米

Zou Family Mirror with Pattern of Immortals and Carriages and Horses

East Han Dynasty

Bronze

Diameter 22.5 cm

圆钮，连珠钮座。内区饰驷车与神人，间饰带座四乳及雀鸟，边饰铭文一周。边缘饰锯齿纹带及水波纹带。浙江绍兴娄宫出土。

绍兴博物馆藏

The mirror has a circular knob with a circular base decorated with a string of beards. Circled by inscription, the inner area is patterned with four-horse-driving carriages and immortals interphase with birds. The rim is decorated with sawtooth and wave patterns. This piece was unearthed in Lougong District located in Shaoxing, Zhejiang.

Preserved in Shaoxing Museum

華

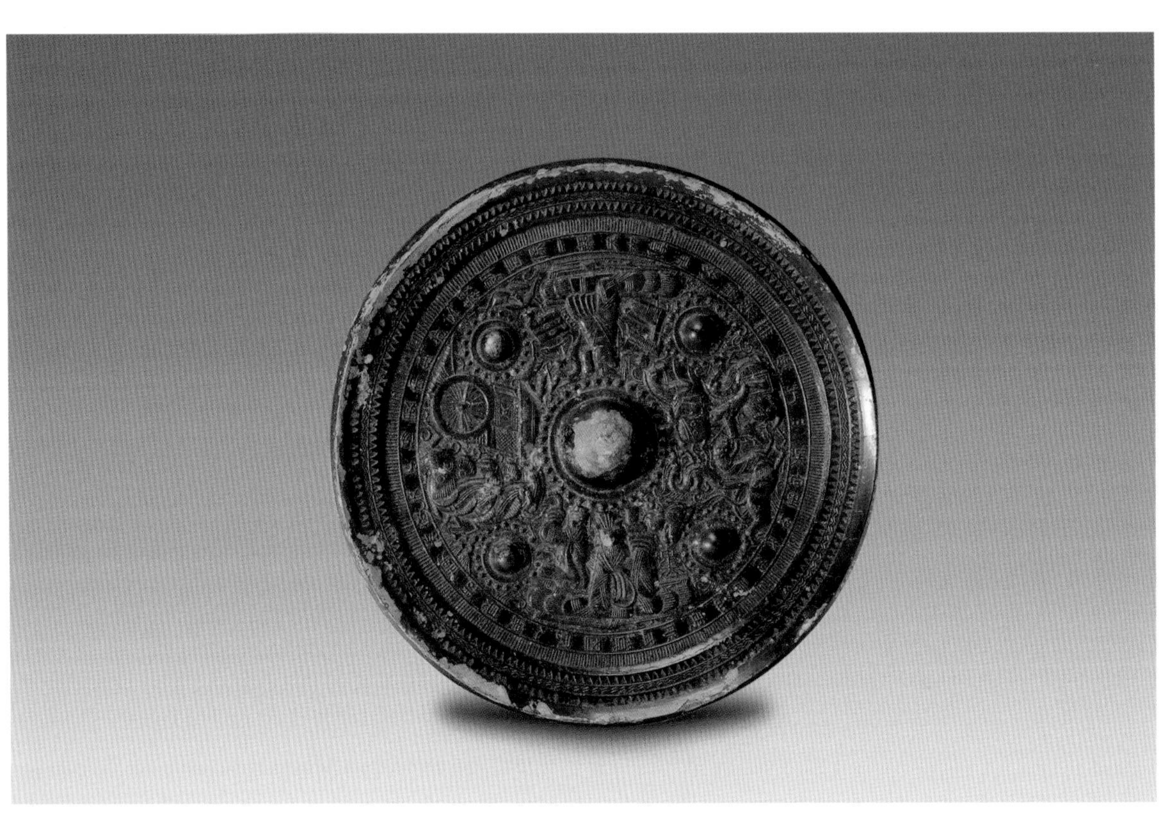

柏氏神人车马镜

东汉

青铜质

直径 20.1 厘米

Bo Family Mirror with Pattern of Immortals and Carriages and Horses

East Han Dynasty

Bronze

Diameter 20.1 cm

圆钮，连珠纹钮座。四枚乳钉把纹饰分成四区，一区为四马驾车，车后拽有长帛，两马昂首，两马回头。一区为狩猎纹，两人跃马并列飞驰，一人回首手持长矛刺一翔龙，另一人回首手持弓箭射一奔跑猛虎。一区为东王公趺坐，左右各一侍者。一区为西王母趺坐，左侧一羽人跪地吹笙奏乐，右有一羽人倒立起舞。外有四十五字铭文一周，铭文带外饰栉纹和锯齿纹。传浙江绍兴出土。

中国国家博物馆藏

The mirror has a circular knob with a base decorated with a string of beads. Four nipple nails divides the decorative patterns into four subdivisions. In the first subdivision, four horses, two of which are raising their heads and the other two are looking back, are pulling a carriage with a long silk cloth attached to it. The second subdivision is decorated with hunting patterns. Two men are riding horses side by side, one of which is looking back with his hands holding a spear to stab a dragon and the other one is also looking back with his hands holding a bow and arrow to shoot a running fierce tiger. In the third subdivision, Tung Wang Kung (God of the Immortals) is sitting crosslegged with two servants on both sides. In the third subdivision, Xi Wang Mu (Queen Mother of the West) is sitting cross-legged. On her left side, one feather man is playing music while kneeling down; on her right side, a feather man is dancing in the position standing upside down. Forty five Chinese characters are inscribed on the outer track. The rim is decorated with comb and sawtooth patterns. This piece was unearthed in Shaoxing, Zhejiang.

Preserved in National Museum of China

華

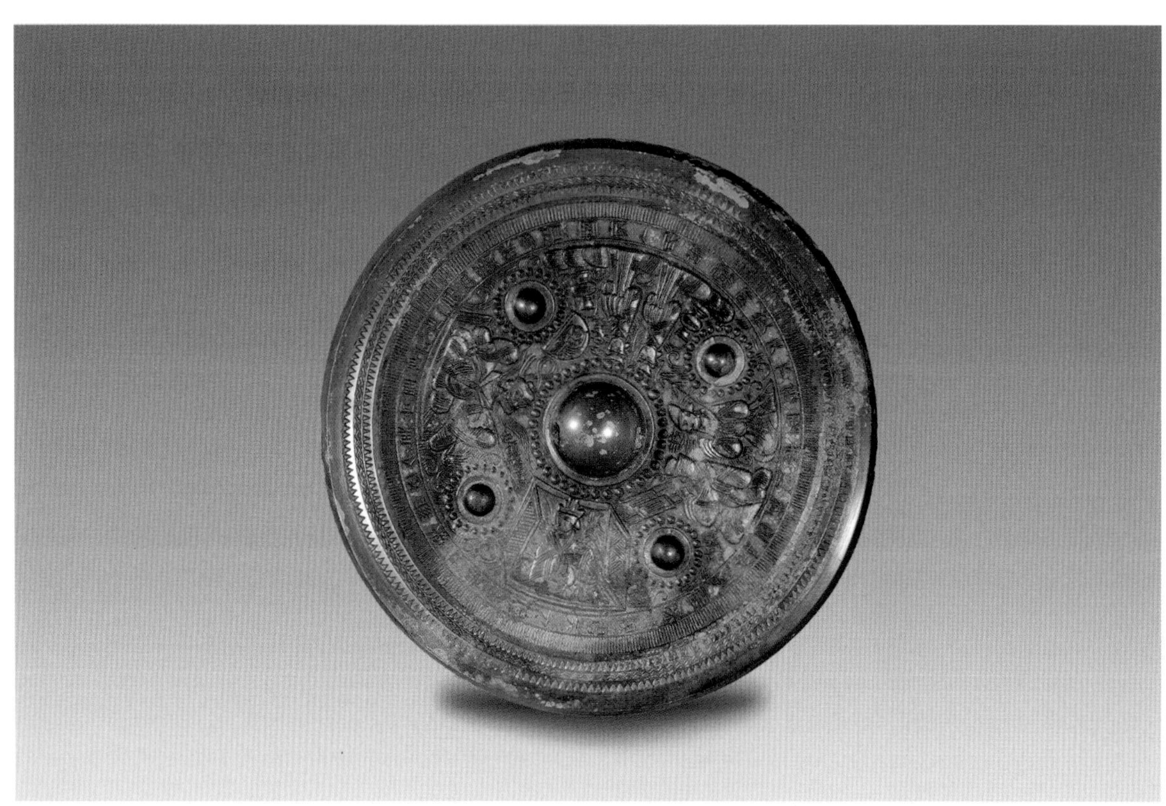

柏氏伍子胥镜

东汉

青铜质

直径 20.7 厘米

"Wu Zixu" Mirror from Bo Family

East Han Dynasty

Bronze

Diameter 20.7 cm

圆钮，圆钮座。四乳钉纹将纹饰分四组，吴王夫差端坐在帷幕中，右旁有“吴王”两字。左面是伍子胥仗剑作自刭状，左上角有“忠臣伍子胥”五字。右面越王执节而立，范蠡席地而坐，并有“越王”及“范蠡”字样。吴王对面两女并列，有“玉女两人”字样。外圈铭文一周四十五字。

上海博物馆藏

The mirror has a circular knob with a circular base. Four nipple nails divides the decorative patterns into four sections. In one section, Fuchai, the empire of Wu State, is sitting behind a curtain decorously with two characters “Wu Wang” engraved on his right. On the left, Wu Zixu is cutting his own throat with a sword and five characters “ Zhong Chen Wu Zixu” (means the loyalty Wu Zixu) engraved on the left right corner. On the third section, the empire of Yue State is standing still with a tally in his hands and Fanli is sitting on the ground accompanied with inscription “Yue Wang” and “Fanli”. Two paralleling maid servants are facing the empire of Wu State with inscriptions “Yu Nv Liang Ren”. Forty-five characters are inscribed along the outer circle.

Preserved in Shanhai Museum

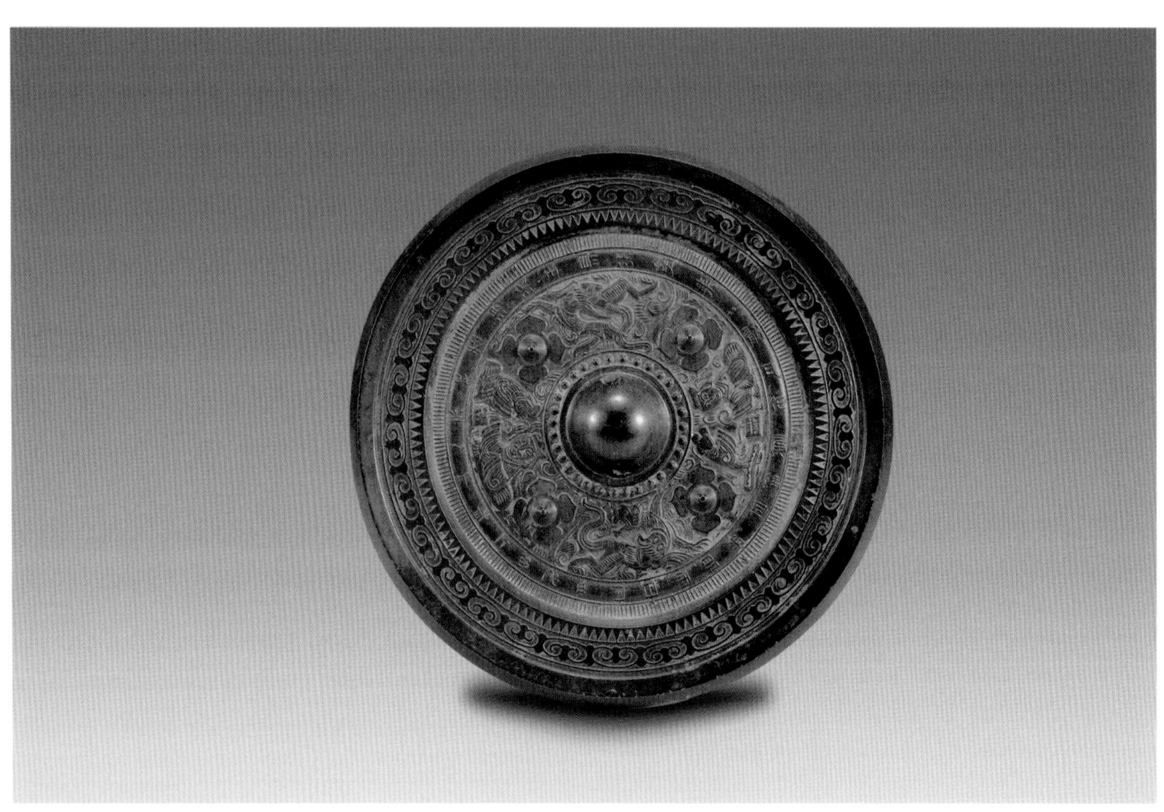

龙氏神兽镜

东汉

青铜质

直径 18 厘米

Long Family Mirror with Pattern of Immortal and Sacred Animals

East Han Dynasty

Bronze

Diameter 18 cm

圆钮，圆钮座。座外一周弦纹，内填一圈小乳钉。四枚柿蒂座大乳钉将主纹等分成四组神人神兽纹，神人相对，内容相同，性别相异；神兽为龙虎相对。铭文二十八字，其外一周直线纹。镜边饰锯齿纹、流云纹各一周。1972 年安徽寿县仇集出土。

安徽博物院藏

The mirror has a circular knob with a circular base. The base is patterned by a circle of string embedded with a circle of little nipple nail pattern. Four big nipple nails with persimmon calyx base equidistantly divides the topical patterns into four groups of immortals and sacred animals. The immortals with opposite genders are facing each other; the sacred animals are dragons facing tigers. Twenty-eight characters are inscribed on the outer track which is circled by straight line patterns. The rim is decorated with sawtooth flowing cloud patterns in two circles respectively. This piece was unearthed in Chouji District located in Shou County, Anhui.

Preserved in Anhui Museum

華

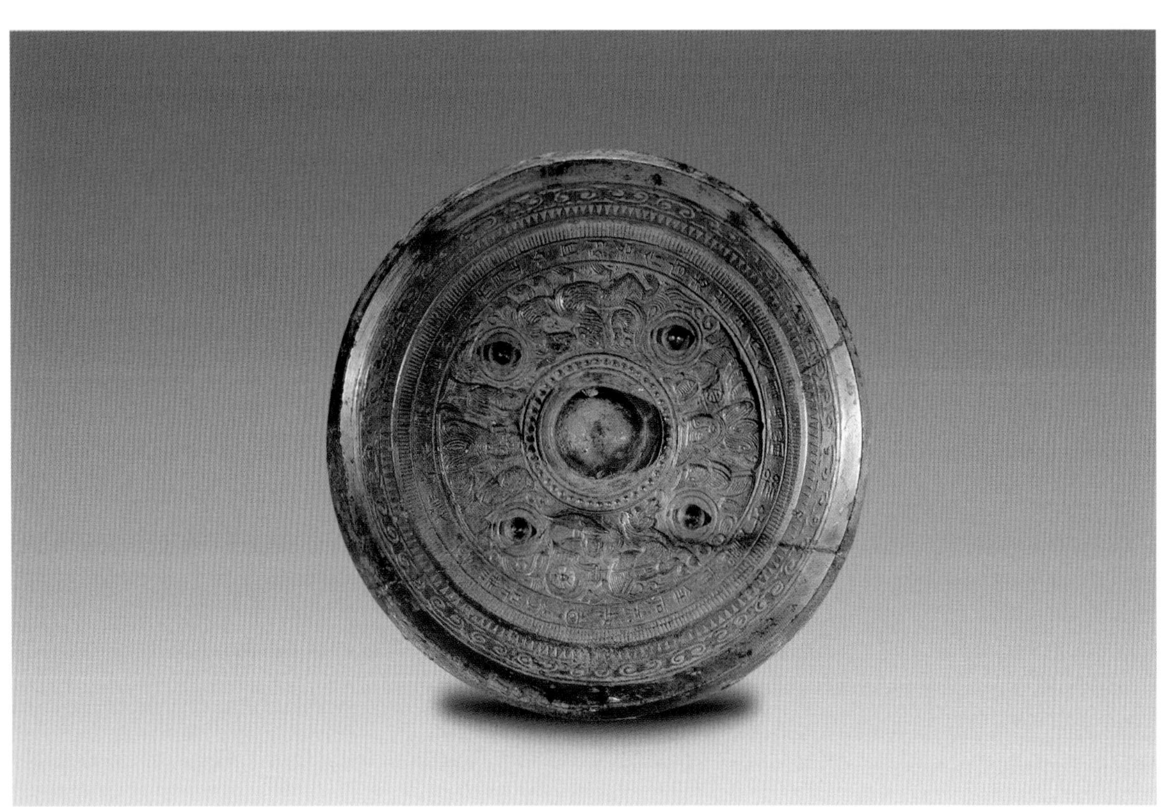

蔡氏神人车马镜

东汉

青铜质

直径 19.2 厘米

Chai Family Mirror with Pattern of Sacred Animals, Carriages and Horses

East Han Dynasty

Bronze

Diameter 19.2 cm

圆钮，连珠纹钮座。内区四乳钉之间饰东王公、西王母及车马、神兽纹。东王公、西王母均戴冠端坐，一旁分别刻“王公”、“王母”，左右两侧均有跪坐侍从。车为双轮，上乘一人，车前一马拉车飞奔。神兽双翼，雄健若狮。外区有“蔡氏作镜佳且好，明而月世少有……”铭文一周，边缘饰云纹和锯齿纹各一周。1955 年河南洛阳邙山出土。

洛阳市文物考古研究院藏

The mirror has a semicircular knob with a base decorated with the pattern of a string of beads. There are four nipple nails in the inner part. Among them, Tung Wang Kung (God of the Immortals), Xi Wang Mu (Queen Mother of the West), carriages and horses as well as sacred animals are decorated. Tung Wang Kung and Xi Wang Mu are sitting decorously with characters "Wang Gong" and 'Wang Mu" engraved besides them. On both sides of each immortal are kneel sitting servants. One person is riding a double wheel carriage being pulled by a dashing horse. The sacred animals, which have double wings, are as strong as the lions. The inscriptions on the outer track highly comment the workmanship of the mirror maker. The rim is decorated with sawtooth cloud patterns in two circles respectively. This piece was unearthed in Mangshan District located in Luoyang, Henan in 1955.

Preserved in Luoyang Municipal Institute of Archaeology and Cultural Relics

華

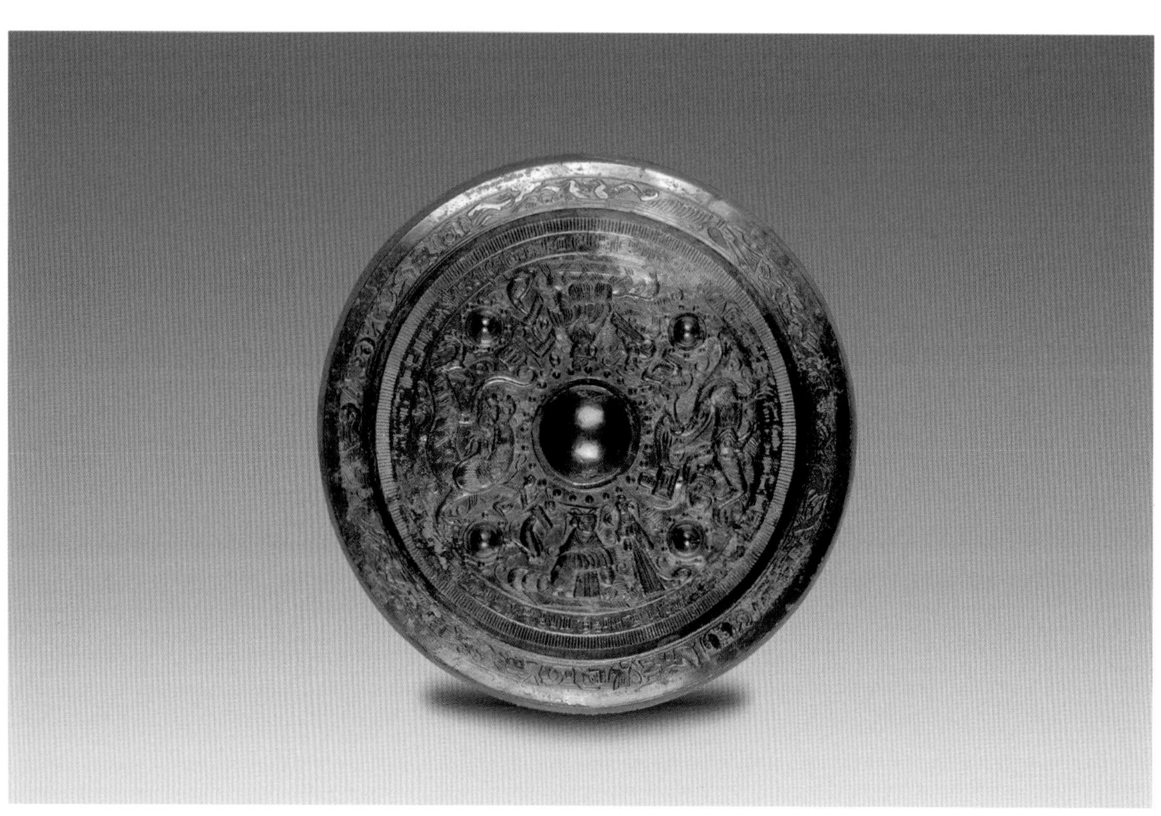

吕氏神兽镜

东汉

青铜质

直径 22.05 厘米

Lv Family Mirror with Pattern of Sacred Animals

East Han Dynasty

Bronze

Diameter 22.05 cm

圆钮，圆形钮座。四乳钉将纹饰分为四组，一组为一人端坐，一人抚琴，二人侍立。一组为一人端坐，二人舞蹈，一人侍立。另外两组为龙、虎各一。外圈铸“吕氏作镜流信德……”铭文一周七十字。镜缘饰以神人鸟兽纹。

故宫博物院藏

The mirror has a circular knob with a circular base. Four nipple nails divides the decorative patterns into four sections. In the first section, one person is sitting decorously and another person is playing zither with two servants beside them. In the second section, one person is sitting decorously and the other two are dancing with one servant beside them. The last two sections are decorated with a dragon and a tiger respectively. Seventy inscriptions on the outer track mean the family is good at making mirror. The rim is decorated with immortals, birds and sacred animal patterns.

Preserved in the Palace Museum

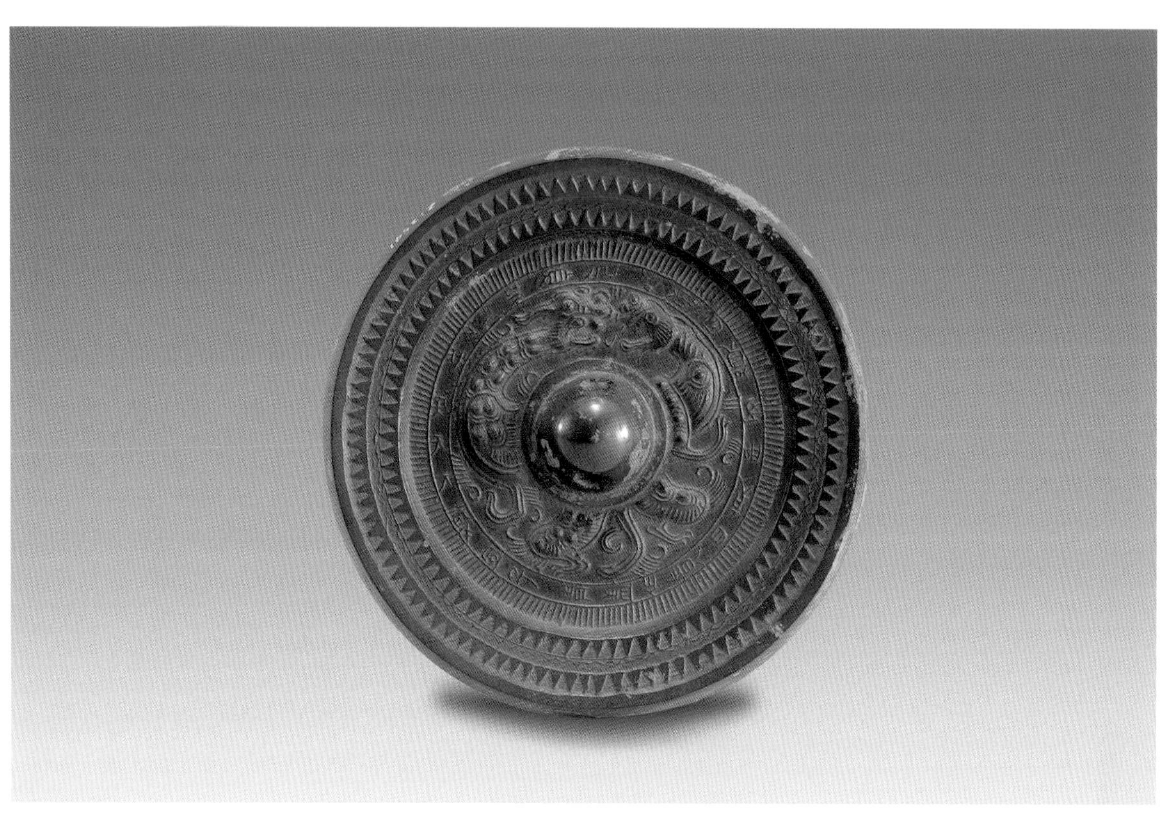

青盖龙虎纹镜

东汉

青铜质

直径 13.5 厘米

Mirror with Dragon-Tiger Pattern and Green Canopy

East Han Dynasty

Bronze

Diameter 13.5 cm

圆钮，圆钮座。钮座外有“青盖作镜四夷服，多贺国家人民息……”铭文一周。内区饰浅浮雕龙虎纹。外区分别为短线、锯齿、水波和弦纹组成的纹带。1955 年湖南长沙丝茅冲 49 号墓出土。

湖南省博物馆藏

The mirror has a circular knob with a circular button base. Around the button base is a circle of inscription which means that this green canopy mirror will bring peace to the country and the people. The inner area is decorated with dragon-tiger patterns in bas-relief. The outer area is decorated with patterns consisting of short line, sawtooth, wave, and string. This piece was unearthed in No. 49 Tomb in Maochong District located in Changsha, Hunan in 1955.

Preserved in Hunan Provincial Museum

華

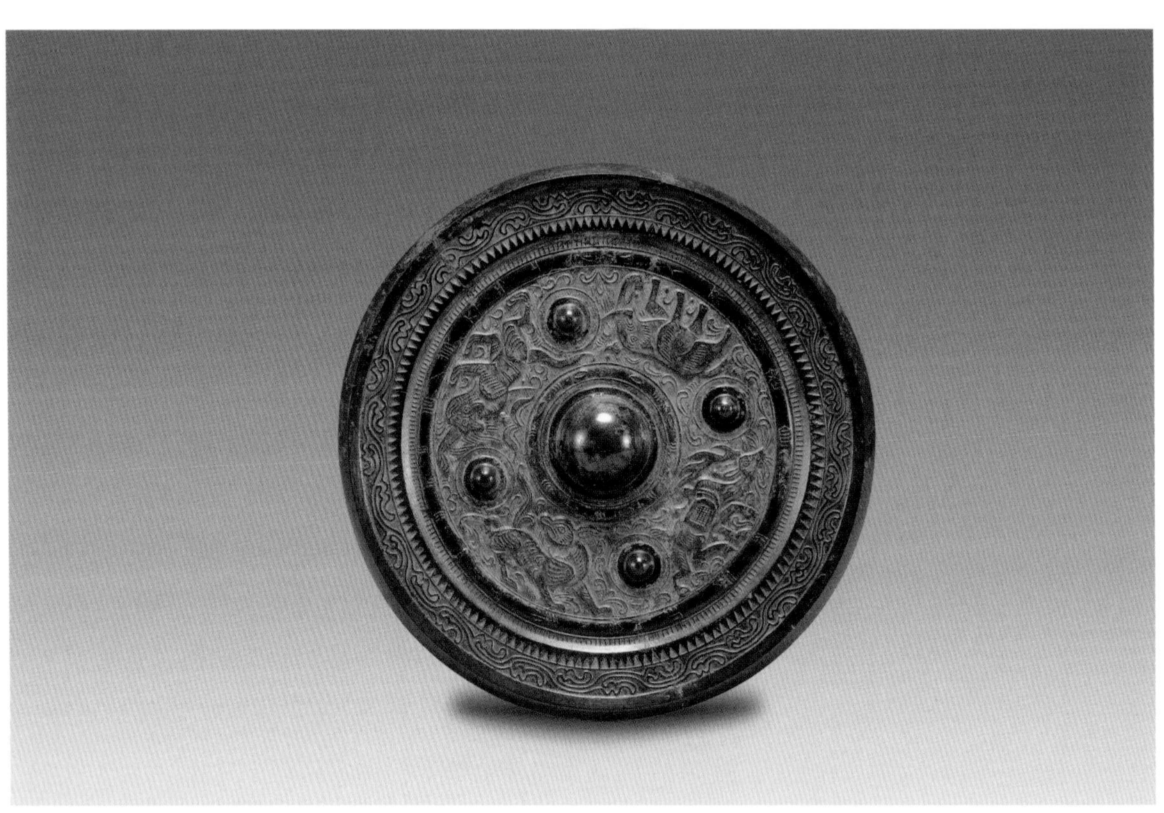

王氏四兽纹镜

东汉

青铜质

直径 18.3 厘米

Wang Family Mirror with Pattern of Four Sacred Animals

East Han Dynasty

Bronze

Diameter 18.3 cm

圆钮，连珠纹钮座。主题纹饰为象、虎、独角兽及鹿纹，间以四乳钉纹。外圈有铭文二十二字："王氏作镜其大巧，上有仙人不知老，渴饮玉泉饥食枣兮"。镜缘饰锯齿纹和云纹。江苏扬州出土。

扬州博物馆藏

The mirror has a circular knob with a button base decorated with the pattern of a string of beads. The topical pattern includes elephants, tigers, unicorns, and deer, which are interphase with four nipple nail patterns. Twenty two inscriptions decorate the outer track which means: Wang family make really nice mirror; and there are immortals living in the Heaven; they drink the jade spring when they are thirsty and eat dates when they are hungry. The rim is decorated with sawtooth and cloud patterns in two circles respectively. This piece was unearthed in Yangzhou, Jiangsu.

Preserved in Yangzhou Museum

華

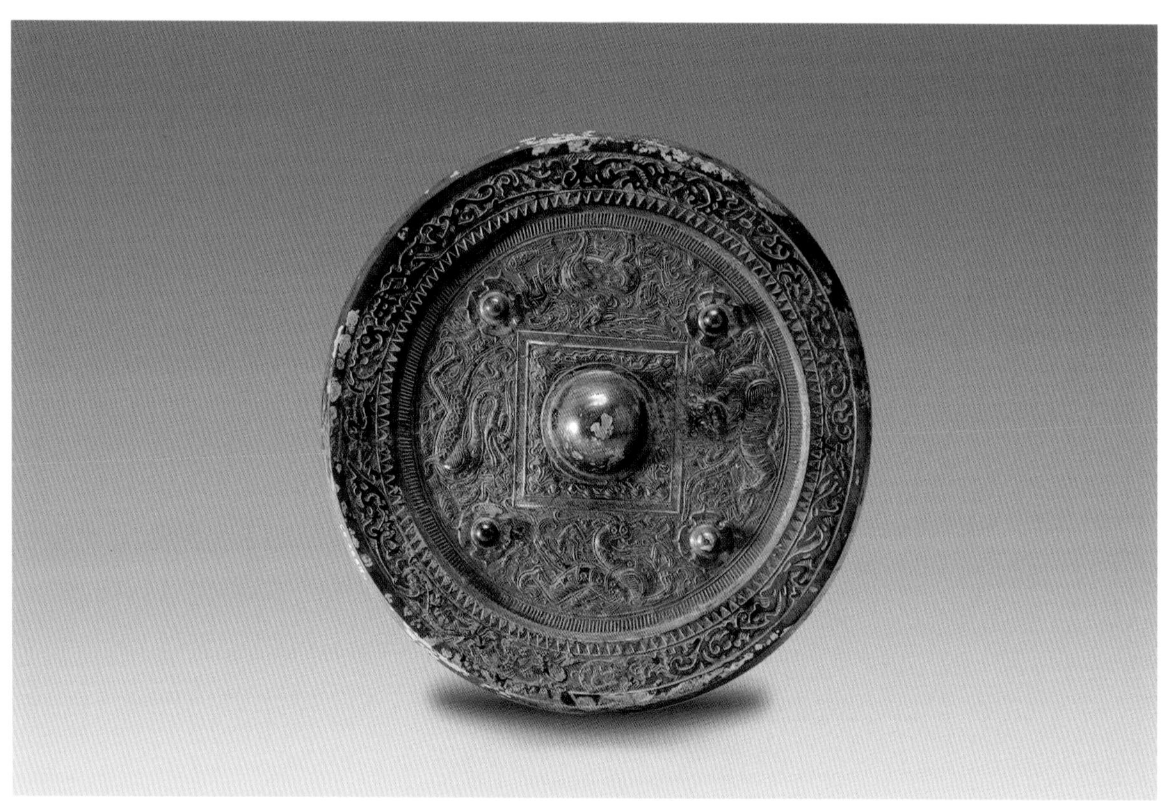

龙虎纹镜

东汉

青铜质

直径 23.8 厘米

Mirror with Dragon-Tiger Pattern

East Han Dynasty

Bronze

Diameter 23.8 cm

圆钮，方形钮座。钮座四角对应四乳钉，将饰纹分为四区，相对两区为羽人骑龙、羽人骑虎，另两区为羽人骑貔、羽人骑梅花鹿，外有羽人钓鱼纹，二羽人手持鱼竿，旁放鱼篓等物，二鱼头露水面已上钩，隙间饰羽人和鱼纹。外饰栉纹、齿纹各一周，外圈为卷草、飞鸟、奔兽组成的纹带。镜形体厚重，纹饰精致。

中国国家博物馆藏

The mirror has a circular knob with a square button base. Four nipple nails lie at the four corners of the square button base. They divide the decoration into four sections. The opposite two sections are decorated with the image of a feather man riding a dragon and a feather man riding a tiger respectively. The other two sections are decorated with a feather man riding a Pi (a mythical bearlike wild animal) and a feather man riding a sika deer. There are also images of fishing feather men: two feather men are holding the fishing rods with creels beside them; two fishes had been caught with their heads on the surface of the water. Among them, the patterns of feather men and fishes are decorated. The outer two tracks are decorated with comb and tooth patterns respectively. The rim is decorated with patterns of scrolled grass, flying birds, and rushing animals. The mirror is massively shaped and exquisitely decorated.

Preserved in National Museum of China

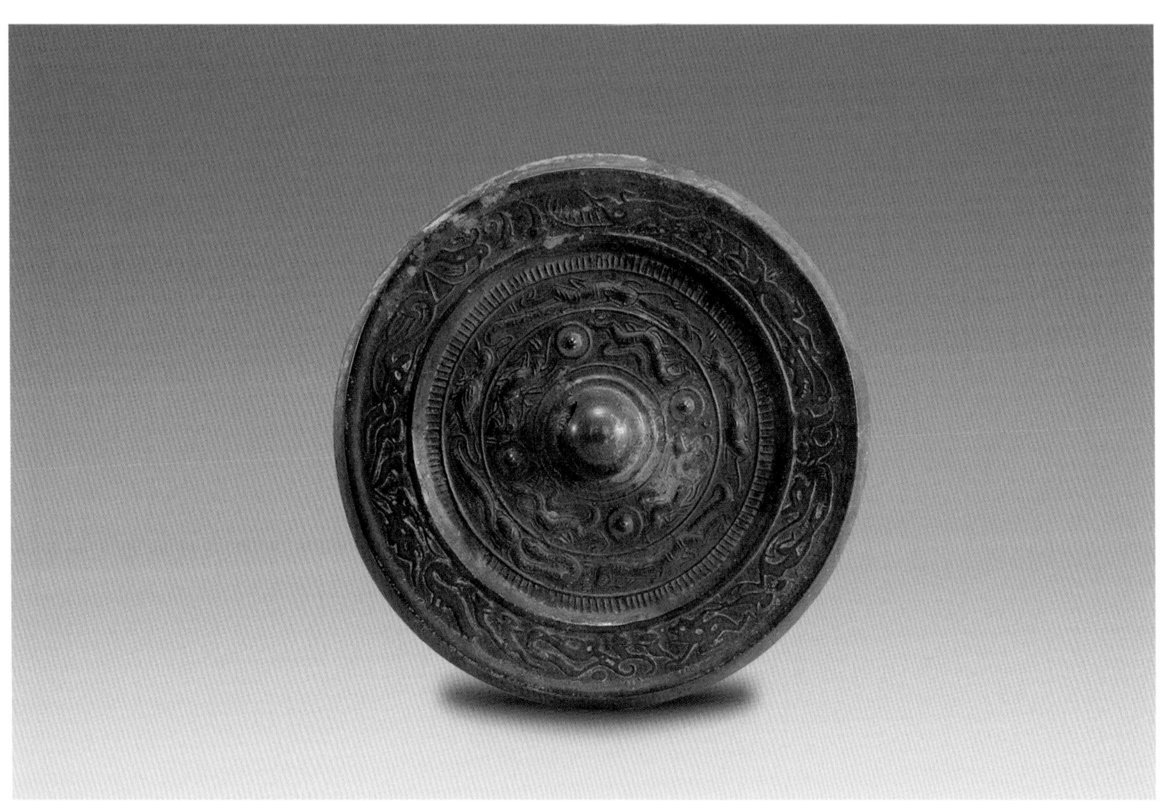

神兽纹镜

东汉

青铜质

直径 13.2 厘米

Mirror with Pattern of Sacred Animals

East Han Dynasty

Bronze

Diameter 13.2 cm

圆钮，圆钮座。主题纹饰为四乳钉纹及神兽纹。边缘饰狐、鹿、兽及鸟纹。1953年湖南长沙南门外月亮山 28 号墓出土。

湖南省博物馆藏

The mirror has a circular knob with a circular button base. The topical patterns include four-nipple-nail and sacred-animal patterns. The rim is patterned with fox, deer, and bird. This piece was unearthed in the 28th tomb in Yueliang Mountain located in the outside of south gate in Changsha, Hunan.

Preserved in Hunan Provincial Museum

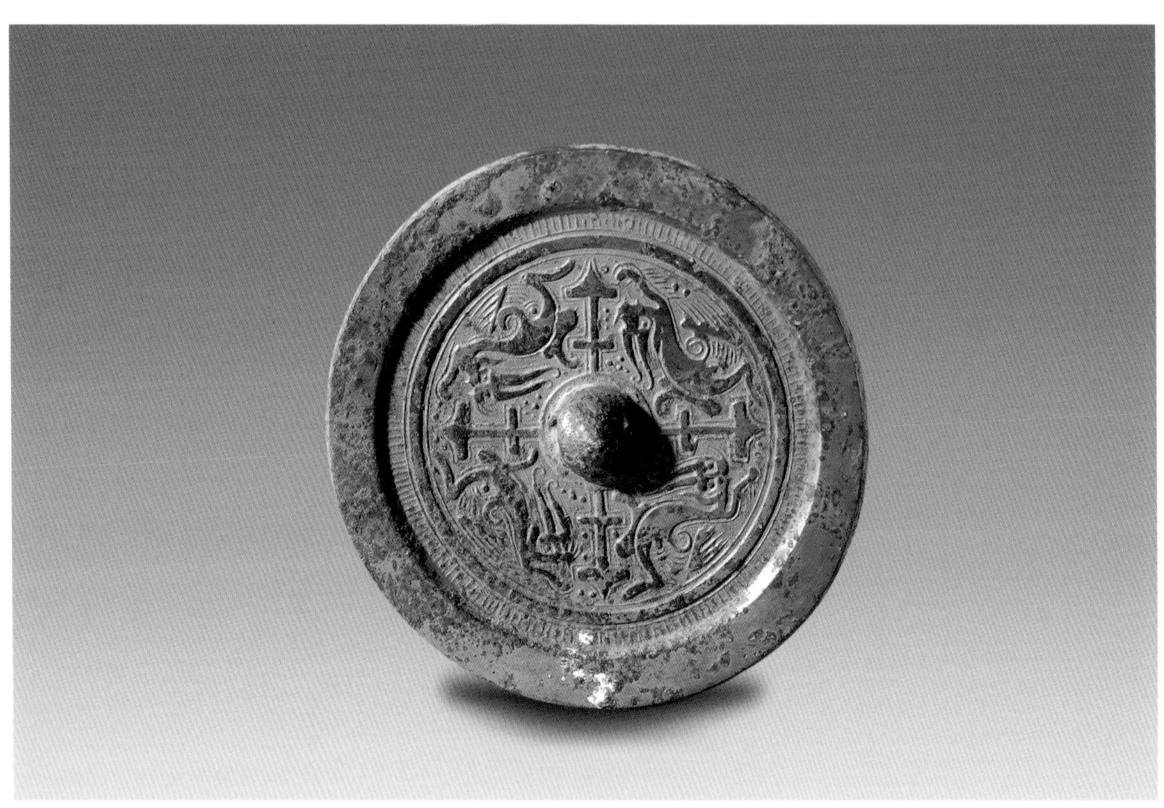

四兽纹镜

东汉

青铜质

直径 12.1 厘米

Mirror with Pattern of Four Sacred Animals

East Han Dynasty

Bronze

Diameter 12.1 cm

圆钮，圆钮座。主题纹饰为四个变形兽纹，两两相对，置于四个小区内，神态各异。河南洛阳岳家村出土。

洛阳市文物考古研究院藏

The mirror has a circular knob with a circular button base. The topical pattern includes four transformed sacred animals with different gestures and expressions. Every two of them are facing each other and all are positioned within the four quarters. This piece was unearthed in Yuejia District located in Luoyang.

Preserved in Luoyang Municipal Institute of Archaeology and Cultural Relics

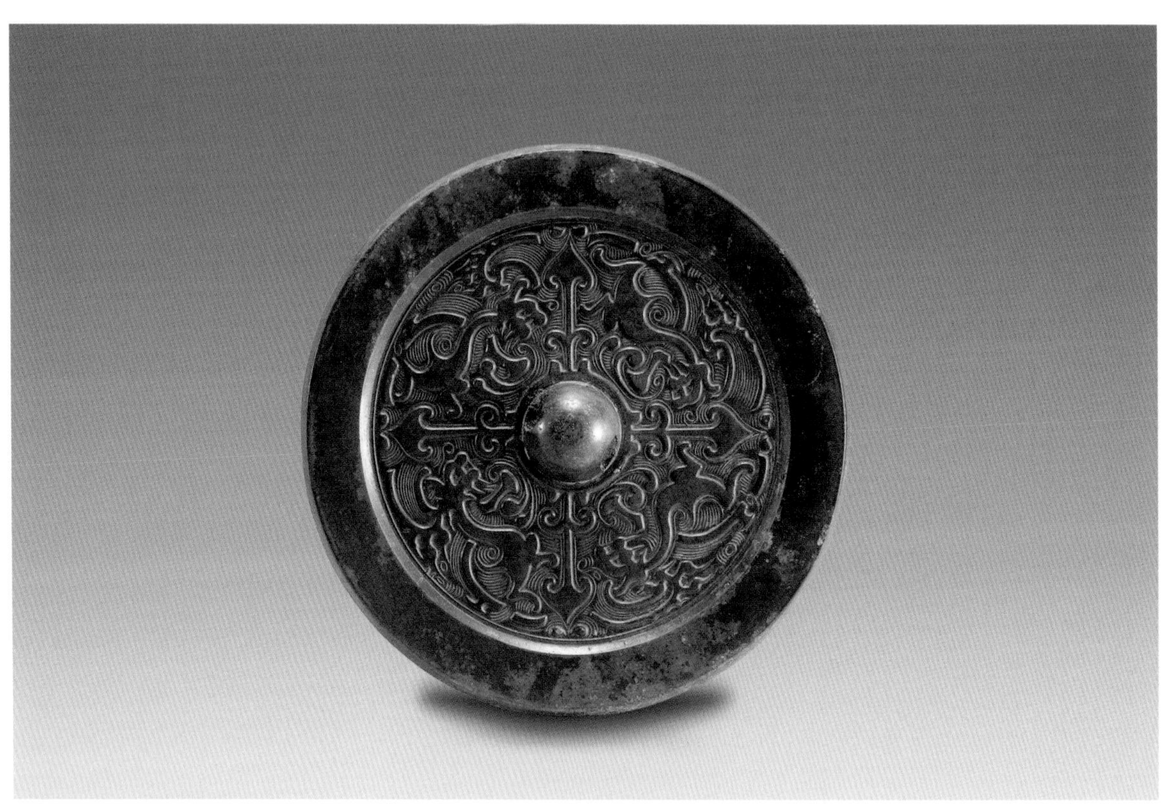

四龙纹镜

东汉

青铜质

直径 15.2 厘米

Mirror with Pattern of Four Dragons

East Han Dynasty

Bronze

Diameter 15.2 cm

圆钮。主纹由放射状四叶分成四区，每区内饰龙纹，以弧线纹为地。宽平缘。1952年长沙蓉园出土。

湖南省博物馆藏

The mirror has a circular knob and a broad rim. The topical patterns are divided by four radiating leaves into four quarters. Each is decorated with dragon patterns shaded by arc patterns. This piece was unearthed from Rong Garden, Changsha.

Preserved in Hunan Museum

華

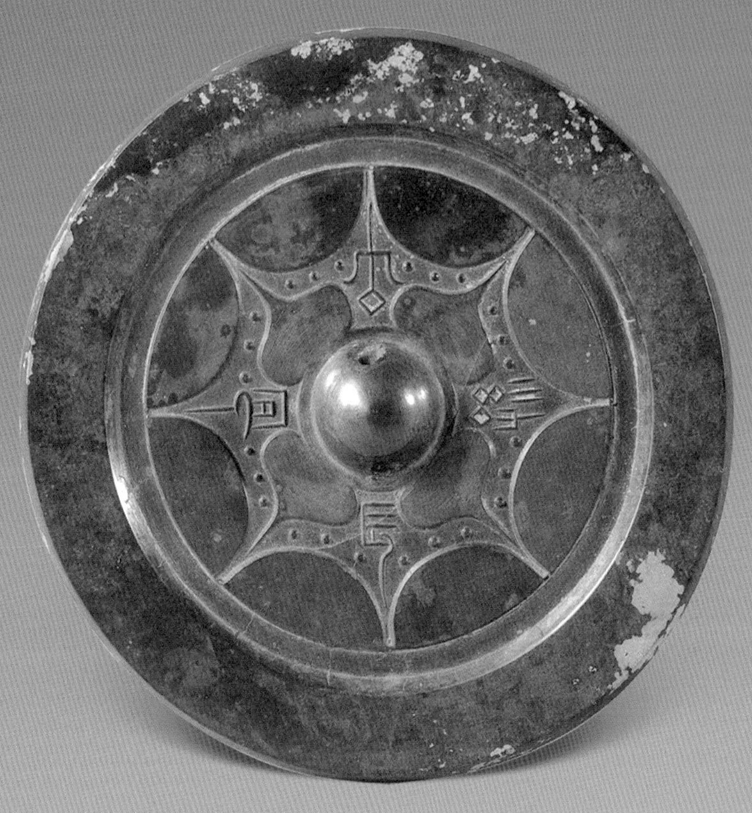

长宜子孙连弧纹镜

东汉

青铜质

直径 13.75 厘米

"Zhang Yi Zi Sun" Mirror with Arc Pattern

East Han Dynasty

Bronze

Diameter 13.75 cm

圆钮，柿蒂形钮座。钮座间有铭文“长宜子孙”四字。其外为内向八连弧纹。外缘平宽。

浙江省博物馆藏

The mirror has a circular button and a button base in the shape of a kaki calyx. The button base is inscribed with four chinese characters “Zhang Yi Zi Sun”. In the outer part of the mirror are eight inward arc patterns. The rim is flat and wide.

Preserved in Zhejiang Museum

華

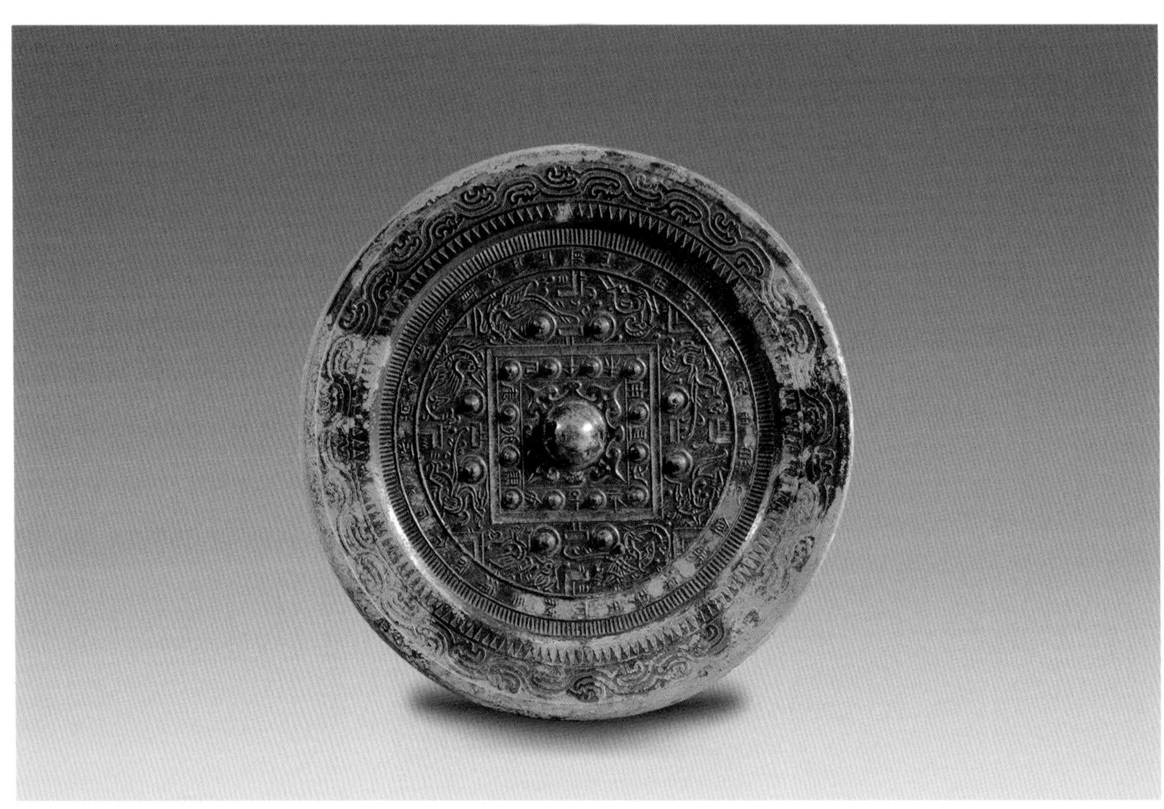

尚方博局纹镜

东汉

青铜质

直径 18 厘米

“Shang Fang” Mirror with Bo-ju Pattern

East Han Dynasty

Bronze

Diameter 18 cm

圆钮，柿蒂钮座。座外围双线方框，内饰乳钉及十二地支。内区饰博局纹与鸟兽纹，外区有铭文一周。因此，研究博局纹镜对探究汉代社会政治、经济、意识形态、思想文化、审美情趣、传统风俗、美术等方面具有极高的参考价值。边缘饰锯齿纹与云纹。浙江绍兴东湖中学出土。

绍兴博物馆藏

The mirror has a circular knob with a button base in the shape of a kaki calyx. The base is circled by a double-line square which are decorated with nipple nails and twelve terrestrial branches inside. The inner area is decorated with Bo Ju pattern and bird-animal pattern. The outer area is a circle of inscription. So the study on the Bo-Ju mirrors could play a key role in the research on the politics, economy, ideology, thoughts, culture, aesthetic tendency, traditional customs, and fine arts in the Han Dynasty. The rim is decorated with sawtooth pattern and cloud pattern. This piece was unearthed in Donghu High School in Shaoxing, Zhejiang.

Preserved in Shaoxing Museum

華

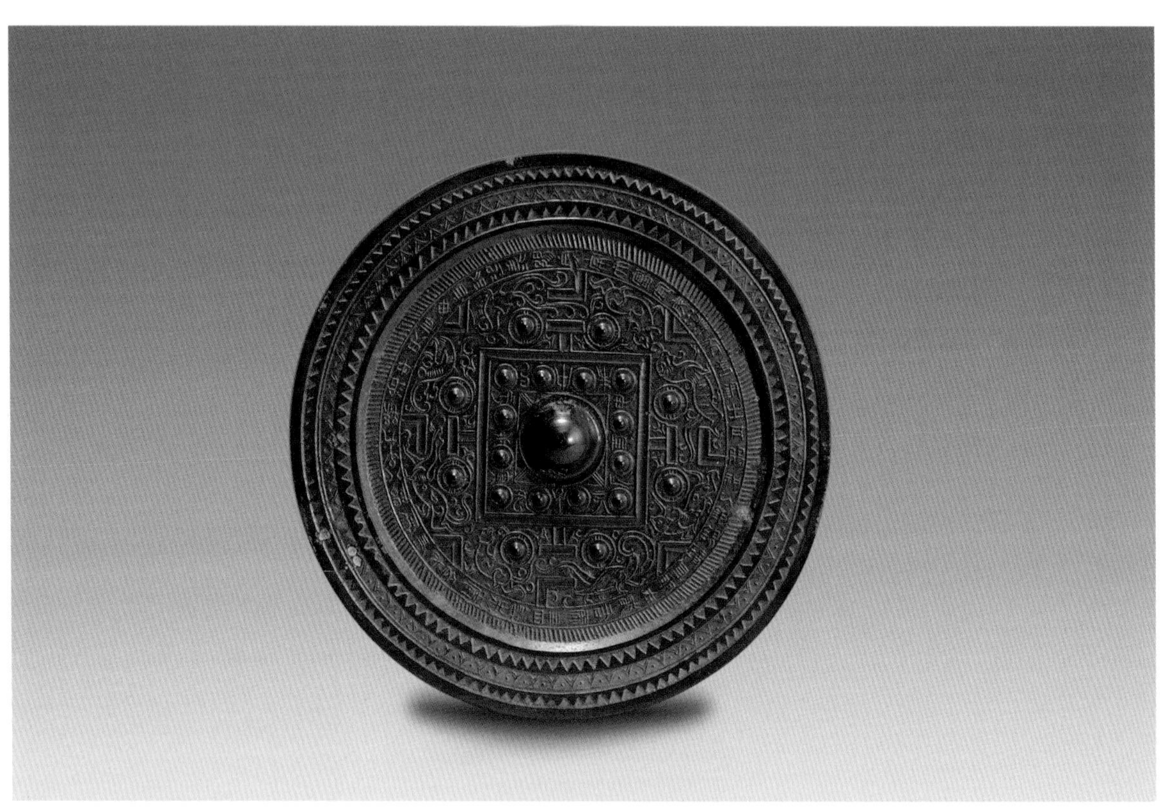

汉有善铜博局纹镜

东汉

青铜质

直径 16.2 厘米

“Han You Shan” Copper Mirror with Bo-ju Pattern

East Han Dynasty

Bronze

Diameter 16.2 cm

圆钮，圆钮座。座外为双线方框，框内排列十二地支铭和十二枚乳钉，框外饰博局纹，配以四灵、瑞兽及八枚乳钉。四灵分别为左龙右虎，上朱雀下玄武。外圈铭文四十八字，镜边饰二周三角锯齿纹。1954年安徽寿县牛尾岗出土。

安徽博物院藏

The mirror has a circular knob with a button base. The base is circled by a double-line square which are decorated with nipple nails and twelve terrestrial branches inside. Outside the square are decorations of Boju patterns matched with four divinities, auspicious beasts, and eight nipple nails. The four divinities are dragon on the left, tiger on the right, rosefinch on the upper and tortoise on the bottom. Forty-eight characters are inscribed on the outer track which is surrounded by two circles of triangle sawtooth patterns. This piece was unearthed in Niu Wei Gang District located in Shou County, Anhui in 1954.

Preserved in Anhui Museum

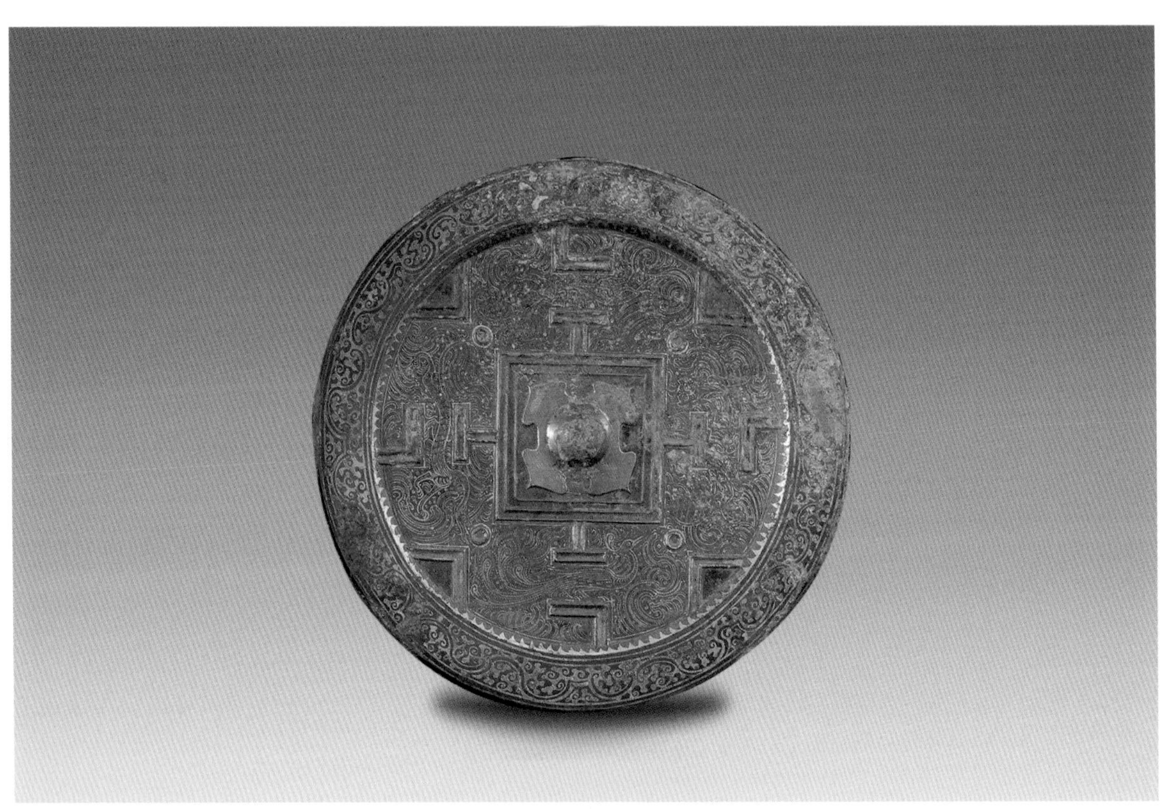

描金四灵博局纹镜

东汉

青铜质

直径 16.4 厘米

Mirror with Bo-ju Pattern and Gold-outlined Four Spirits

East Han Dynasty

Bronze

Diameter 16.4 cm

圆钮，柿形钮座。外围凹形方框两道，纹饰为四神博局纹。青龙作飞腾状，白虎作奔驰状，朱雀作飞翔状，玄武为龟蛇合体并有小蛇缠绕，四灵的空隙处都填以流动的云纹，镜缘饰三角纹和云气纹。此镜特殊之处是四灵纹、博局纹边缘及云气纹、三角纹都用金线绘成，极其精细，这是一种特殊的工艺。

日本千石唯司藏

The mirror has a circular knob with a button base in the shape of a kaki calyx. Surrounding the base is a double concave square framework with four spirits playing Bo-ju patterns. The azure dragon is soaring; the white tiger is galloping; the rosefinch is flying, and the tortoise is the zoarium of turtle and snake twined by little snakes. The spare space among the four spirits is filled with flowing cloud patterns. The rim is decorated with triangle and cloud-qi patterns. The unique of this mirror lies in that all the decoration including four spirits patterns, the margin of Bo-ju patterns, cloud-qi patterns, and triangle patterns are outlined with gold. The decorative patterns are extremely fine and exquisite which belongs to a peculiar technology.

Preserved by Sengoku Tadashi Museum Japan

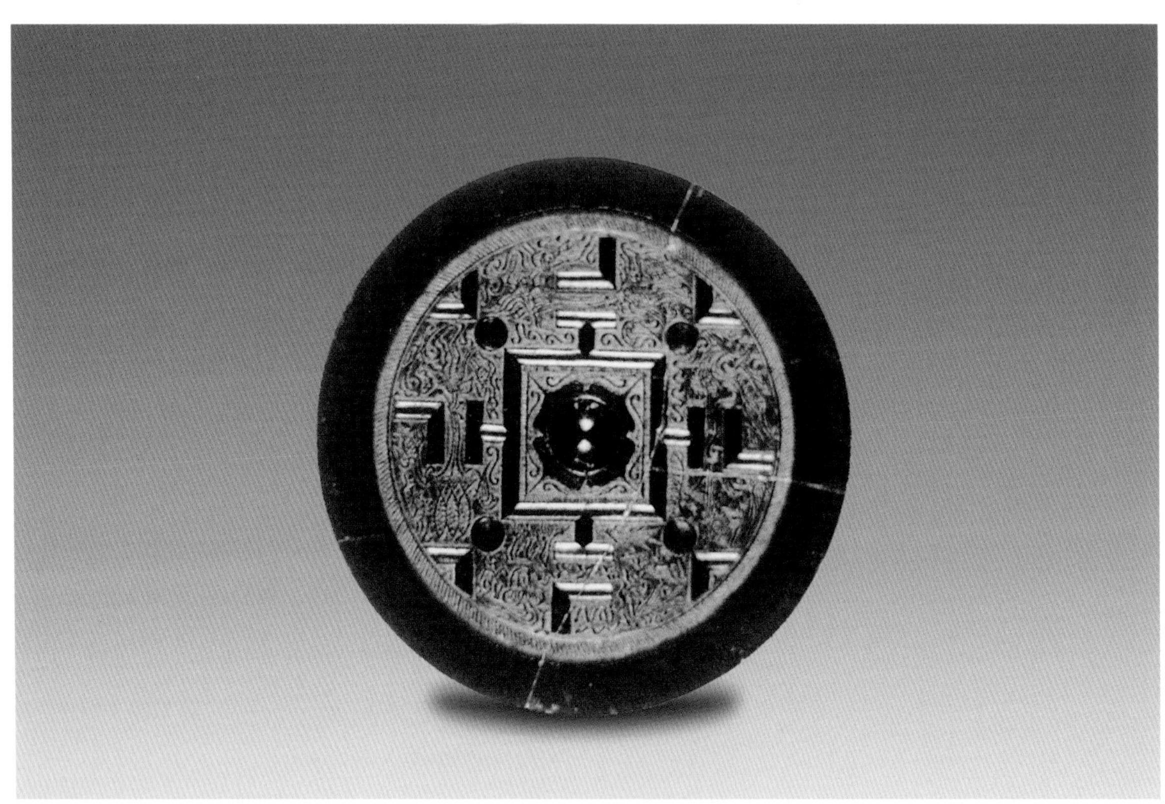

博局纹铜镜

东汉

青铜质

直径 6.5 厘米

Copper Mirror with Bo-ju Pattern

East Han Dynasty

Bronze

Diameter 6.5 cm

镜为圆形，镜背正中呈半球形钮，柿蒂纹座。主纹为宽条组成的博局纹，博局纹内的四角各有凹面圆形纹，在博局间内单线组成鱼、鸟、羽人和虎纹图像。博局纹作为日常用具铜镜的装饰，反映出六博棋在当时的广泛流行。

故宫博物院藏

The circular mirror has a hemispherical knob with a button base in the shape of a kaki calyx. The topical pattern is wide stripe Bo-ju patterns. At the four corners of the Bo-ju patterns are concave circular patterns. Between the Bo-ju patterns are the image of fish, bird, feather man and tiger in a single line. As the decorations of daily utensils, Bo-ju pattern can reflect the popularity of Liu-bo chess at the time.

Preserved in the Palace Museum

華

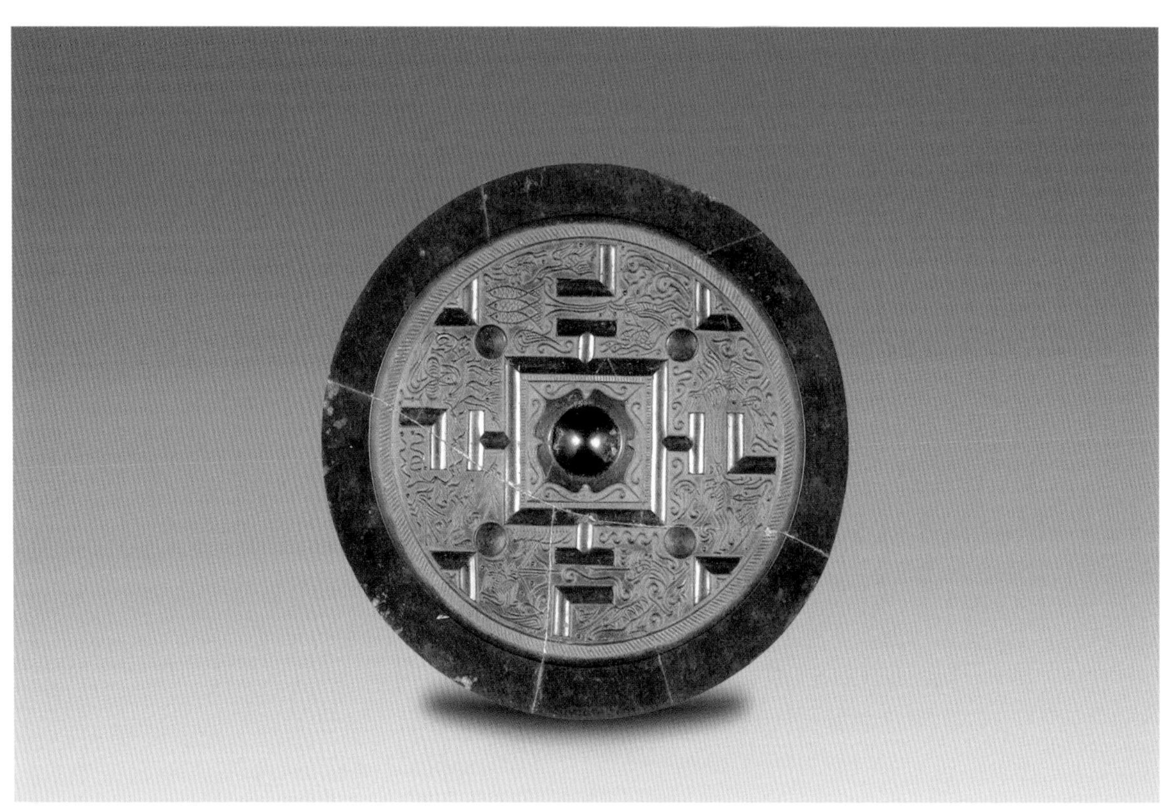

羽人禽兽博局纹镜

东汉

青铜质

直径 16.5 厘米

Mirror with Bo-ju Patterns and Feather Men and Animals

East Han Dynasty

Bronze

Diameter 16.5 cm

圆钮，柿蒂纹钮座。钮座外为浅弧宽条方框。方框四角各有凹面圆形纹。博局纹将纹饰分为八个区域，内饰单线组成的羽人、鱼、鸟、虎等图案。宽平缘。

故宫博物院藏

The mirror has a circular knob with a kaki calyx base. Surrounding the base is a superficial arc and wide stripe square. In the four corners of the square are four concave circular patterns. Bo-ju patterns divide the decorative patterns into eight sections which are decorated with feather men, fish, birds, and tiger in a single line. The rim is wide and flat.

Preserved in the Palace Museum

華

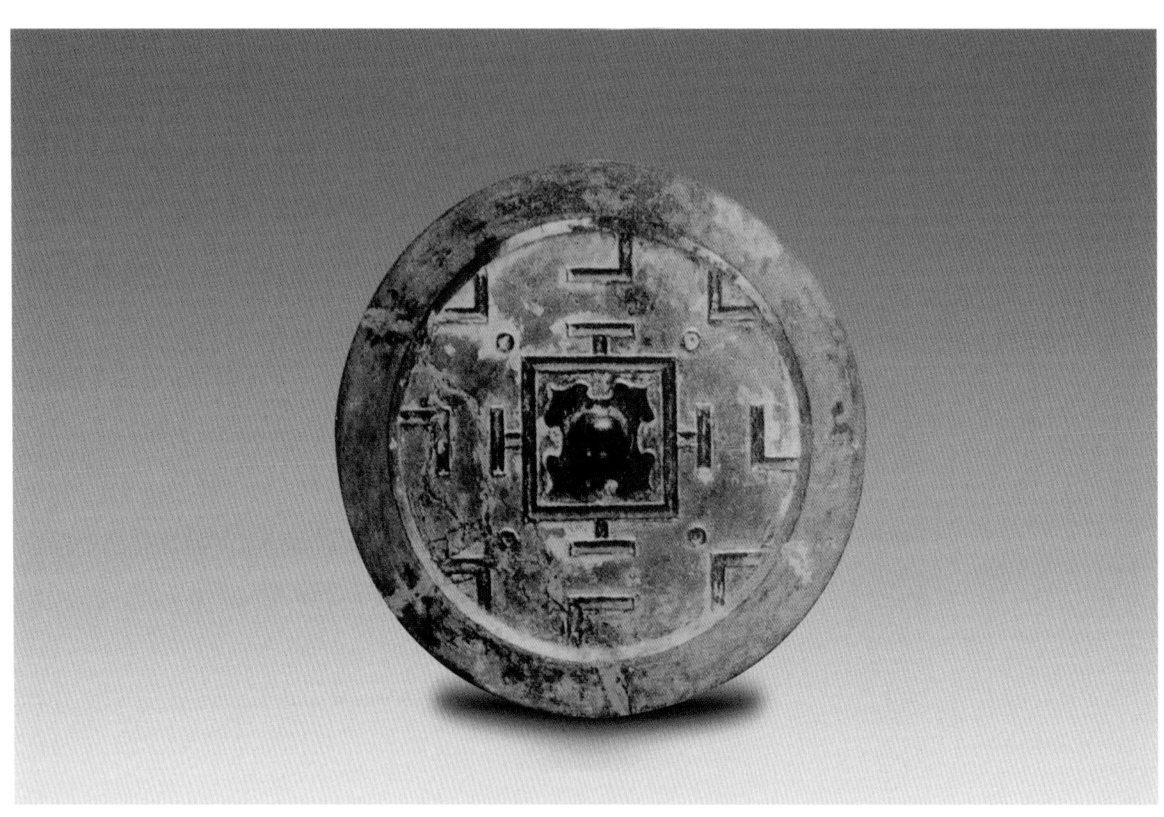

鎏金博局纹铜镜

东汉

鎏金铜质

直径 13.8 厘米

Gilded Mirror with Bo-ju Pattern

East Han Dynasty

Gilded Copper

Diameter 13.8 cm

铜镜为圆形，镜背置半圆形钮，柿蒂钮座。镜背的博局纹饰以“ㄒ”、“ㄱ”、“一”、“口”符号组成了一副六博博局局式，这可以说是汉代六博棋盛行的标志。

湖南省博物馆藏

The circular hemispherical mirror has a circular knob with a kaki calyx button base. The Bo-ju patterns are interphase with the symbols “ㄒ”、“ㄱ”、“一”、“口” which make up a six-bo chessboard. This symbolizes the popularity of Six-bo chess in the Han Dynasty.

Preserved in Hunan Provincial Museum

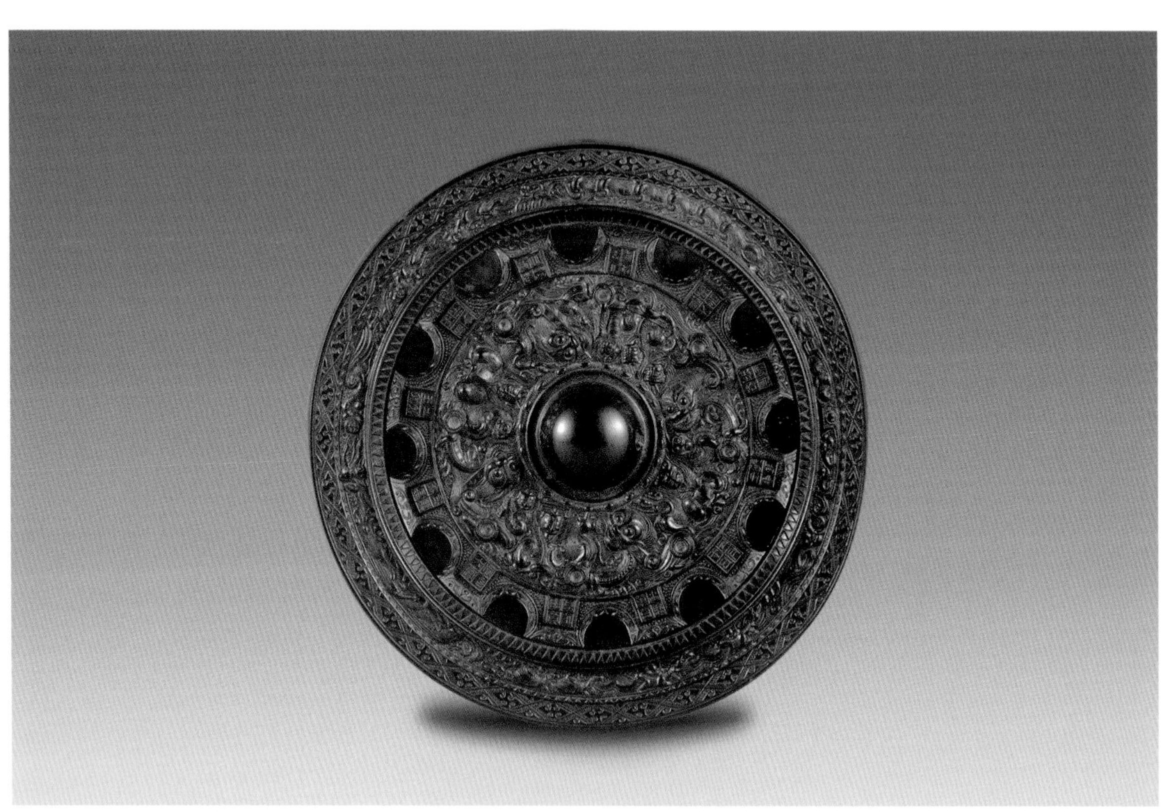

永康元年神兽镜

东汉

青铜质

直径 16.3 厘米

Mirror with Pattern of Sacred Animals in the first Year of Yongkang

East Han Dynasty

Bronze

Diameter 16.3 cm

圆钮，圆钮座。内区饰有四辟邪，下为东王公，上为西王母，左面是黄帝及侍从，右面为伯牙弹琴，一旁似钟子期。外区铭文铸于十二方块内，共四十八字，字多反书。镜缘为二圈纹饰，内圈有两组，一组神人驭龙车，另一组羽人骑独角兽、羽人骑鼋乘鸟。两组纹饰间以神人捧日捧月。外圈是菱形纹连续图案。

上海博物馆藏

The mirror has a circular knob with a circular button base. The inner area is decorated with four Bixie (sacred animals for avoiding evils): Tung Wang Kung (God of the Immortals) is on the bottom, Xi Wang Mu (Queen Mother of the West) is on the top, yellow Emperor and his servants are on the left, the image of Boya playing the lyre is on the right with Zhong Ziqi standing aside. On the outer area, forty eight characters are engraved reversely in twelve squares. The rim is decorated with two circles of patterns. The inner circular pattern consists of two groups: one group is immortals riding dragon carriages; the other is feather men riding unicorn, pelochely bibroni and birds. Between the two circles is the picture of the immortals holding the sun and the moon. The outer circle is decorated with continuous diamond patterns.

Preserved in Anhui Museum

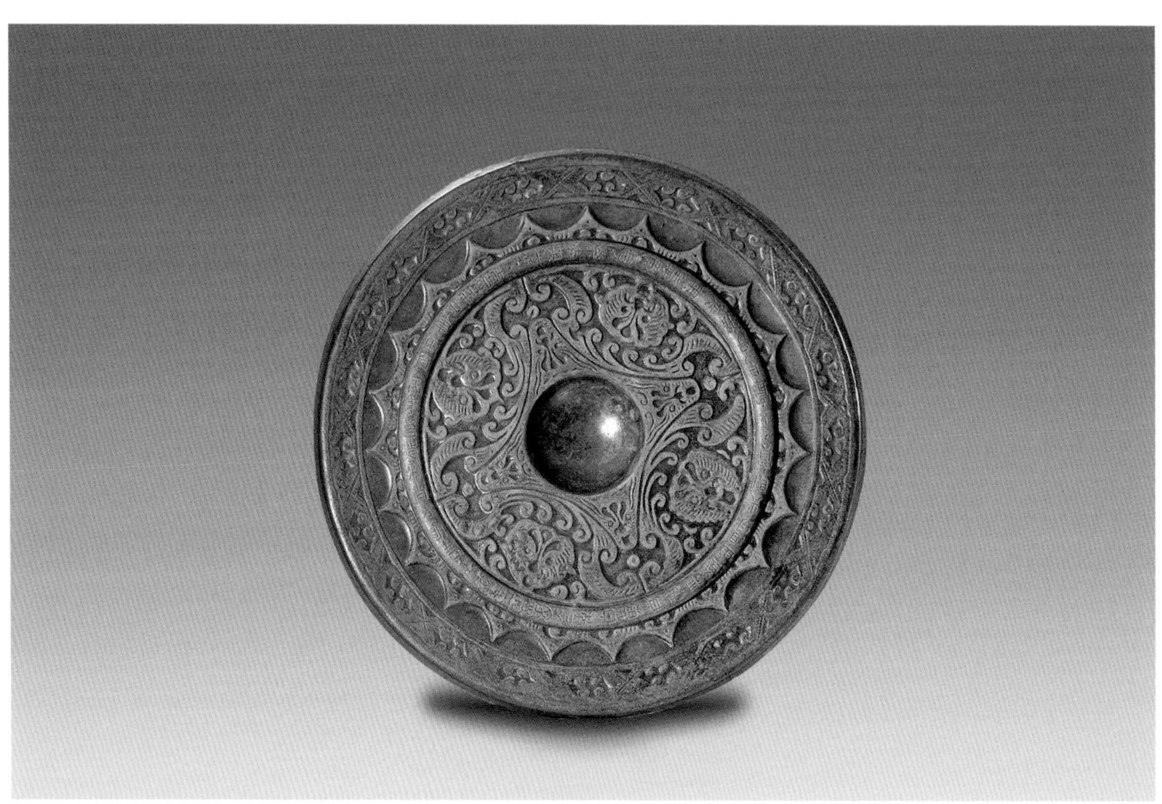

熹平三年狮纹镜

东汉

青铜质

直径 17.8 厘米

Mirror with Lion Pattern in the Third Year of Xiping

East Han Dynasty

Bronze

Diameter 17.8 cm

圆钮，菱形钮座。内区饰四个正视狮面纹，狮怒目吐舌。其外镌“熹平三年正月丙午吾造作尚方明镜……”铭文一周。外区饰连弧纹一周。边缘饰一周菱纹，内饰卷云纹。1951 年卫聚贤捐献。

重庆市博物馆藏

The mirror has a circular knob with a diamond button base. The inner area is decorated with four positive lions with glaring eyes and protruding tongues. Outside is a circle of inscriptions which show the production time of the mirror. The outer area is decorated with a circle of arc patterns. The rim is decorated with a circle of diamond patterns with the rolling-cloud patterns inside. This piece was contributed by Wei Juxian in 1951.

Preserved in Chongqing Museum

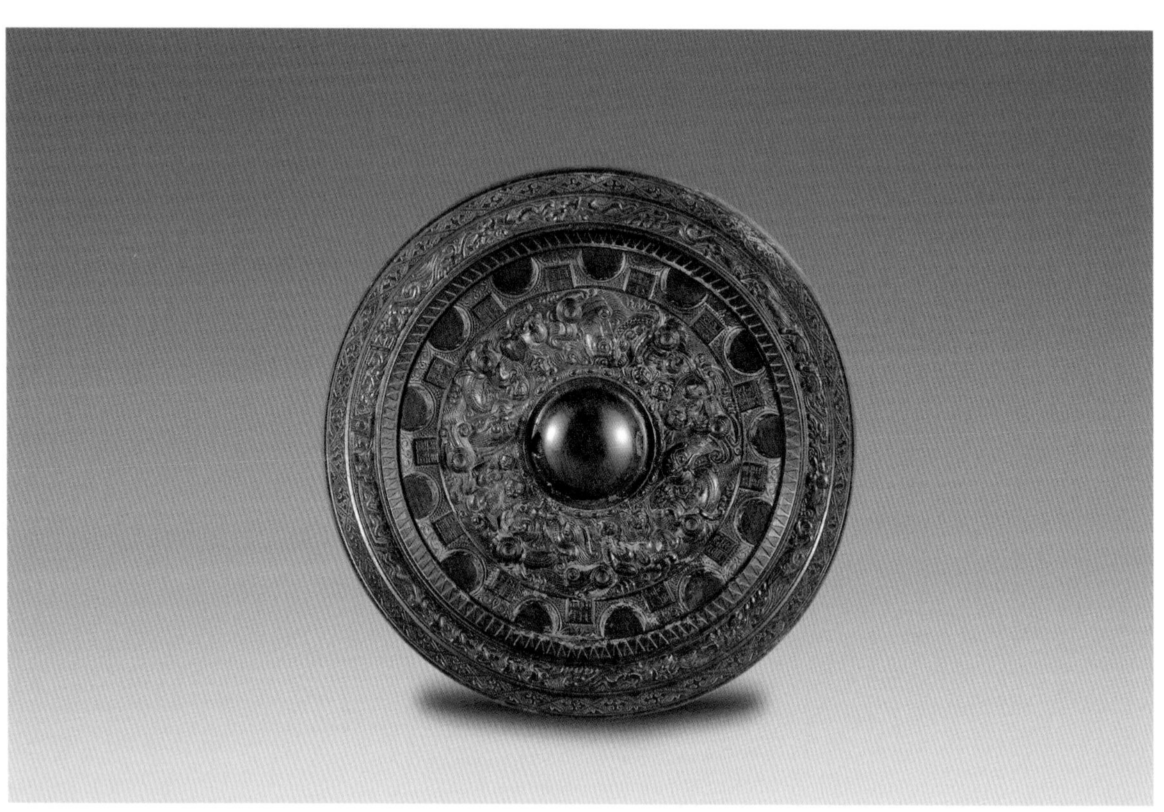

中平四年神兽镜

东汉

青铜质

直径 19.2 厘米

Mirror with Pattern of Sacred Animals in the Fourth Year of Zhongping

East Han Dynasty

Bronze

Diameter 19.2 cm

圆钮，连珠纹钮座。内区为浮雕纹饰，由四神兽将纹饰分为四组，一组为东王公、玉女、神兽，一组为西王母、青鸟、神兽，一组为黄帝、侍者，一组为伯牙奏琴。外区铭文铸于十三方块内，每块四字，共五十二字："中平四年五月午日，幽湅白铜早作明镜……"。铭文外为锯齿纹。中平四年，为公元一八七年。

上海博物馆藏

The mirror has a circular knob with a button base ornamented with a string of beads. The inner relief patterns area are divided by four sacred animals into four groups. The first group is decorated with Tung Wang Kung (God of the Immortals), jade women, and sacred animals; the second group is decorated with Hsi Wang Mu (Queen Mother of the West), bird messenger of Fairy God-Mother, and sacred animals; the third group is decorated with Huangdi and his servants; the fourth group is decorated with the image of Boya playing the lyre. On the outer area, the inscription is engraved in 13 squares with 4 characters in each square. Totally, there are 52 characters which foretell good wishes. The rim is decorated with saw tooth patterns. The fourth year of Zhongping was in the year of 187 A.D.

Preserved in Shanghai Museum

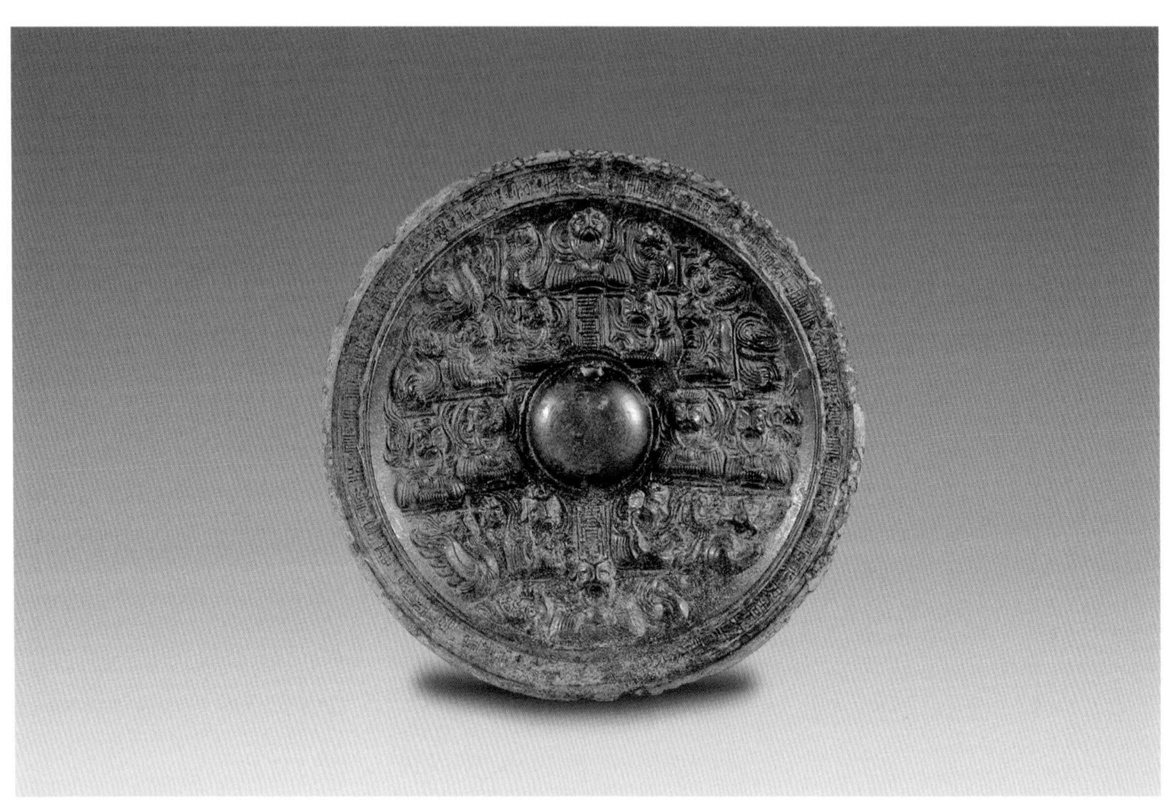

建安七年神兽镜

东汉

青铜质

直径 13.2 厘米

Mirror with Pattern of Sacred Animals in the Seventh Year of Jianan

East Han Dynasty

Bronze

Diameter 13.2 cm

圆钮。主纹共置十三神人、十二神兽，横列成五排。第二、四排中为“君宜官”三字。外缘有铭文一周“建安七年朱氏造大吉祥……”，共五十字。建安七年，为公元 202 年。

上海博物馆藏

The mirror has a circular button. The topical patterns consist of 13 immortals and 12 sacred animals horizontally arranged in 5 rows. The second and forth rows are decorated with “Jun Yi Guan”, three characters which means that it is suitable for the owner to be officer. The rim is circled by 52-character inscription which means the production time of the mirror and its goodness. The 7th year of Jian’an was in the year of 202 A.D.

Preserved in Shanghai Museum

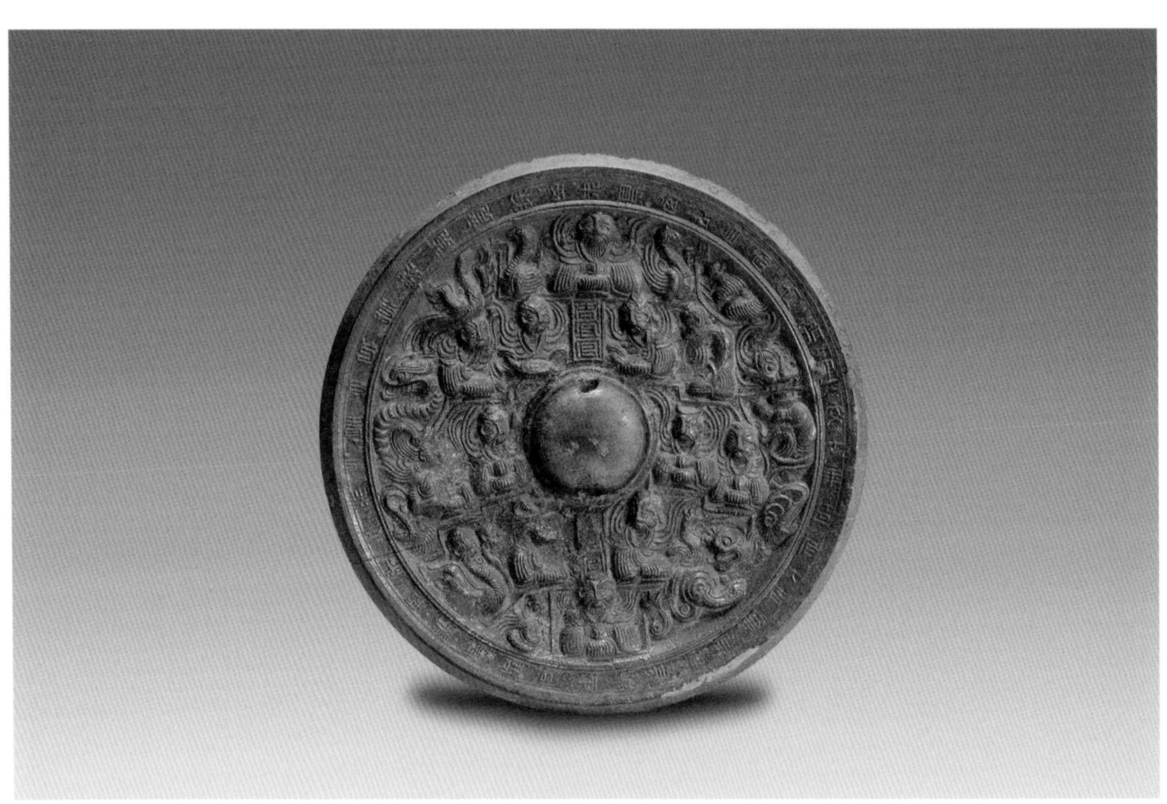

建安十年神兽镜

东汉

青铜质

直径 13.5 厘米

Mirror with Pattern of Sacred Animals in the 10th Year of Jianan

East Han Dynasty

Bronze

Diameter 13.5 cm

圆钮，圆钮座。纹饰为高浮雕神人神兽，作重列式，共五层。钮上下各直列铭文“君宜官”。镜缘处铭文一周四十字：“吾作明竟，幽湅宫商，周罗客象，五帝三皇，白牙单琴，黄竟除凶，朱鸟玄武，白虎青龙，建安十年，造作大吉”。建安十年，为公元 205 年。1954 年安徽芜湖赭山 2 号墓出土。

安徽博物院藏

The mirror has a circular knob with a circular button base. The decorative patterns are high relief immortals and sacred animals rearranged in 5 layers. On the top and the bottom of the base, the inscription “Jun Yi Guan” is engraved respectively which means that it is suitable for the owner to be an officer. The rim is circled by forty character inscription which tell the good reason to produce the mirror. The 10th year of Jianan was in the year of 205 A.D. This piece was unearthed in the No.2 tomb in Zhe Mountain located in Wuhu, Anhui in 1954.

Preserved in Anhui Museum

華

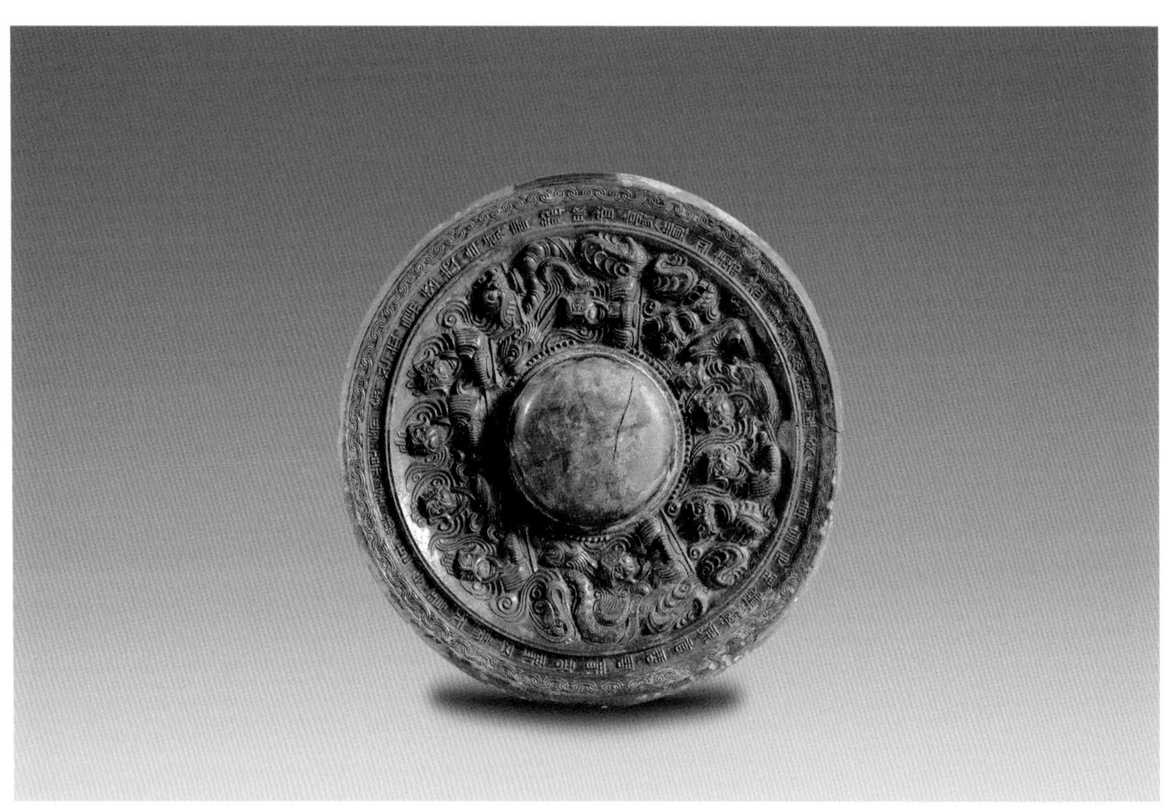

建安十年神兽镜

东汉

青铜质

直径 14.7 厘米

Mirror with Pattern of Sacred Animals in the Tenth Year of Jianan

East Han Dynasty

Bronze

Diameter 14.7 cm

圆钮，连珠座。钮外圈饰神人、青龙、白虎及瑞兽，外缘饰铭文一周及链纹带。浙江绍兴出土。

绍兴博物馆藏

The mirror has a circular knob with a button base patterned with a string of beads. Outside the base is decorated with the image of the immortals, azure dragons, white tigers, and auspicious animals. The rim is decorated with a circle of inscriptions and chain patterns. This piece was unearthed in Shaoxing, Zhejiang.

Preserved in Shaoxing Museum

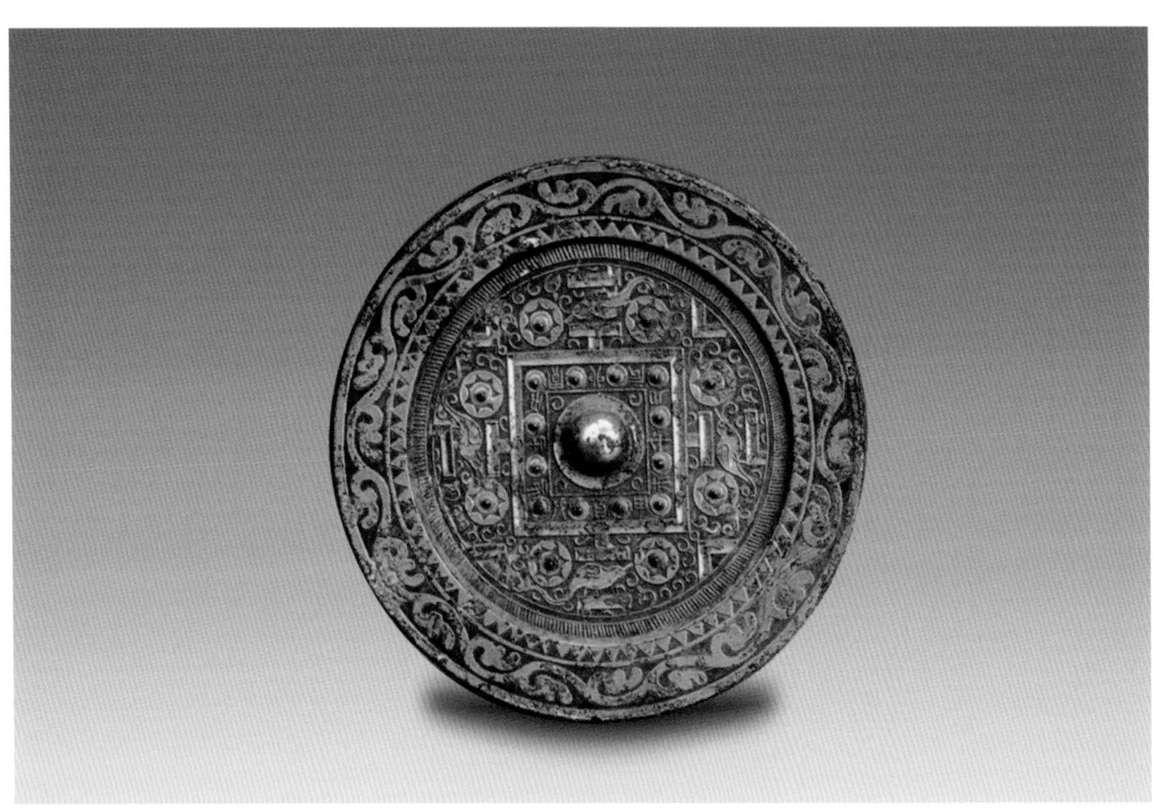

地支铭文镜

汉

青铜质

直径 16.2 厘米

Mirror with Inscription of Terrestrial Branches

Han Dynasty

Bronze

Diameter 16.2 cm

圆形。半圆钮，圆钮座，座外大方格中环列十二生肖及地支铭。主区博局纹间四朱雀环绕，其外短斜线纹和锯齿纹带各一周，云纹外缘。

山西博物院藏

The circular mirror has a semicircular knob with a button base. Outside the base are the twelve Chinese zodiac signs and terrestrial branches. Four rosefinches ornament the topical Bo-ju pattern. Outside are two circles of short slash patterns and sawtooth patterns respectively. The rim is decorated with cloud patterns.

Preserved in Shanxi Museum

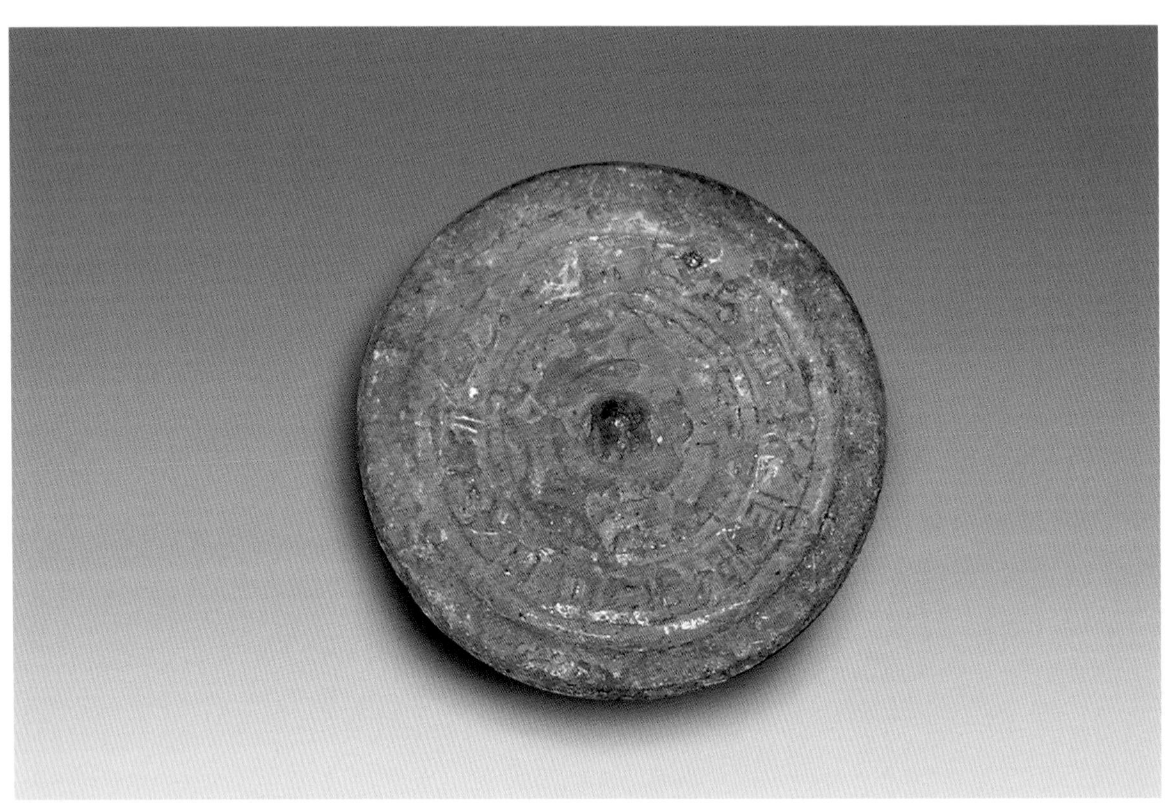

铜镜

汉

铜质

直径 8 厘米，厚 0.3 厘米，重 100 克

Bronze Mirror

Han Dynasty

Copper

Diameter 8 cm/ Thickenss 0.3 cm/ Weight 100g

圆形，镜中间有一圆钮，边沿扁平，有铭文。生活用器。完整无损。陕西省咸阳市征集。

陕西医史博物馆藏

The circular mirror has a circular knob in the center and a flat rim. It also has inscriptions and is still intact. It was collected in Xianyang, Shaanxi Province.

Preserved in Shaanxi Museum of Medical History

華

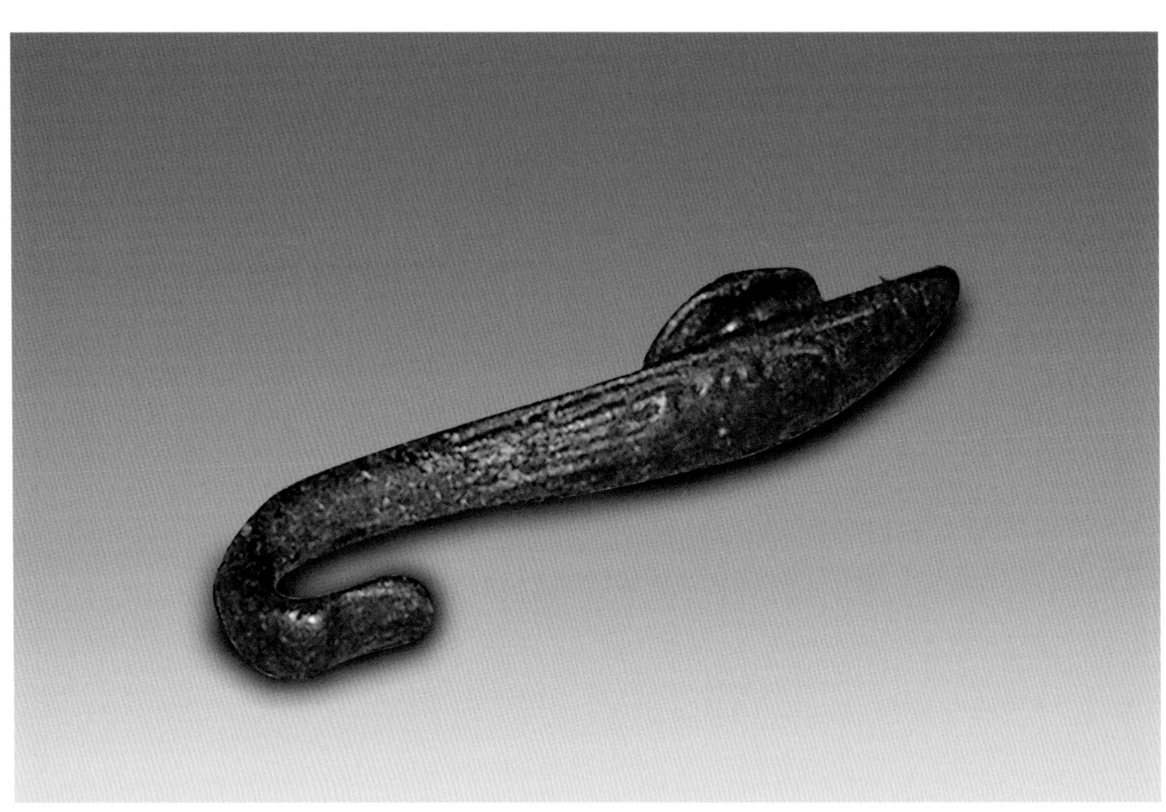

铜衣钩

汉

铜质

长 4.7 厘米，宽 0.7 厘米，重 1 克

Copper Clothes Hook

Han Dynasty

Copper

Length 4.7 cm/ Width 0.7 cm/ Weight 1g

“S” 形，底部中心有一圆钮，面部有纹饰。生活器具。完整无损。内蒙古自治区成陵征集。

陕西医史博物馆藏

There is a circular knob in the center of the base of the S-shaped hook. The surface is decorated with patterns. The clothes hook is an article for daily use and is still intact. It was collected in Chengling, Inner Mongolia Autonomous Region.

Preserved in Shaanxi Museum of Medical History

華

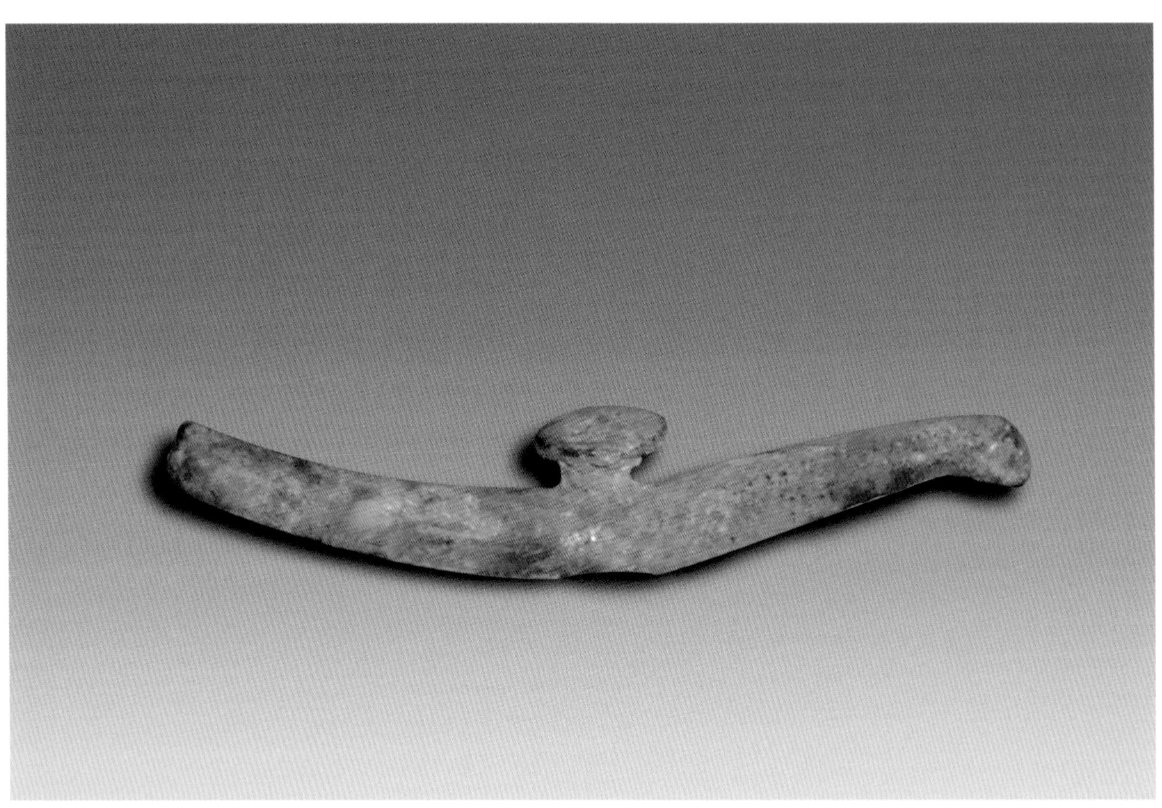

铜衣袋勾

汉

铜质

长 11.5 厘米，宽 0.7 厘米，底径 0.5 厘米，重 100 克

Copper Pouch-like Hook

Han Dynasty

Copper

Length 11.5 cm/ Width 0.7 cm,/ Bottom Diameter 0.5 cm/ Weight 100 g

“S”形，中有一圆钮。生活用器。完整无损。陕西省咸阳市征集。

陕西医史博物馆藏

The S-shaped hook has a circular knob in the center. It is used as a household item and is preserved intact. It was collected from Xianyang, Shaanxi Province.

Preserved in Shaanxi Museum of Medical History

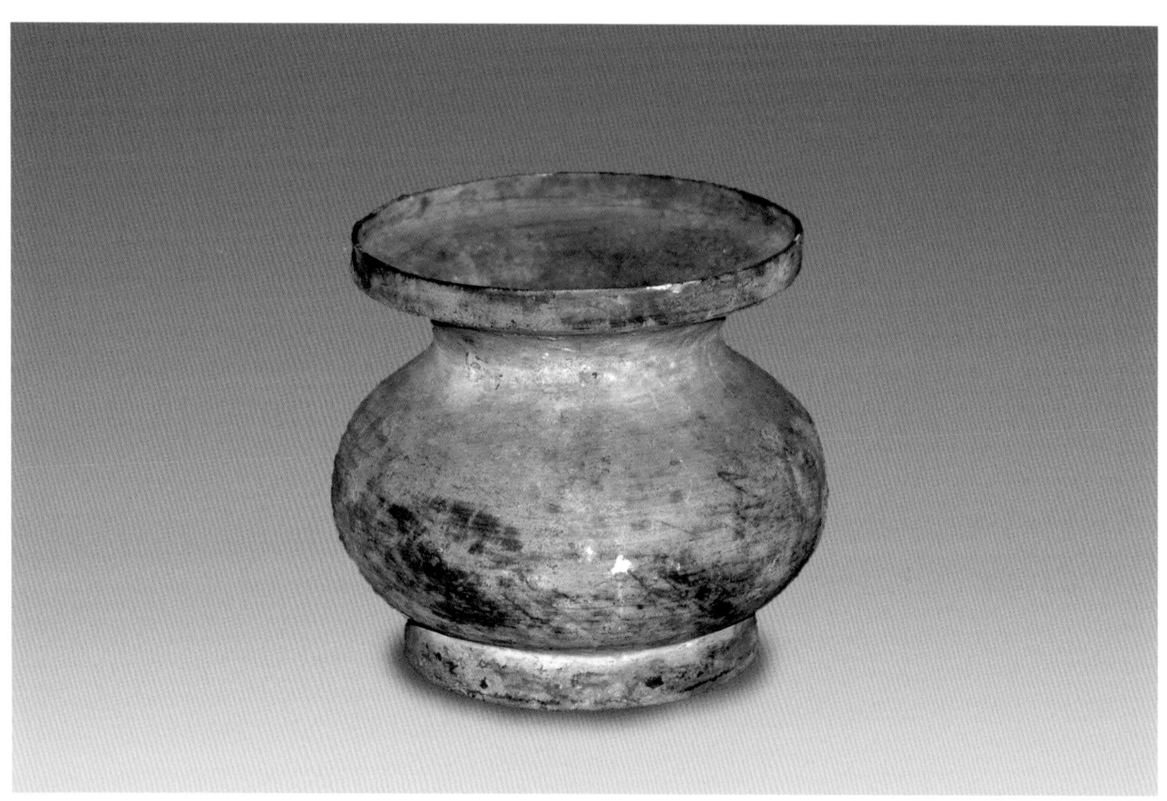

铜痰盂

汉

铜质

口径 12.4 厘米，底径 10 厘米，通高 12 厘米，重 700 克

Copper Cuspidor

Han Dynasty

Copper

Caliber 12.4 cm/ Bottom Diameter 10 cm/ Height 12 cm/ Weight 700g

盘口，鼓腹，圈足。生活器具。完整无损。陕西省西安市征集。

陕西医史博物馆藏

The cuspidor has a discoid mouth, a swelling belly, and a circular-like foot. This article for daily use is still intact and was collected in Xi'an, Shaanxi Province.

Preserved in Shaanxi Museum of Medical History

華

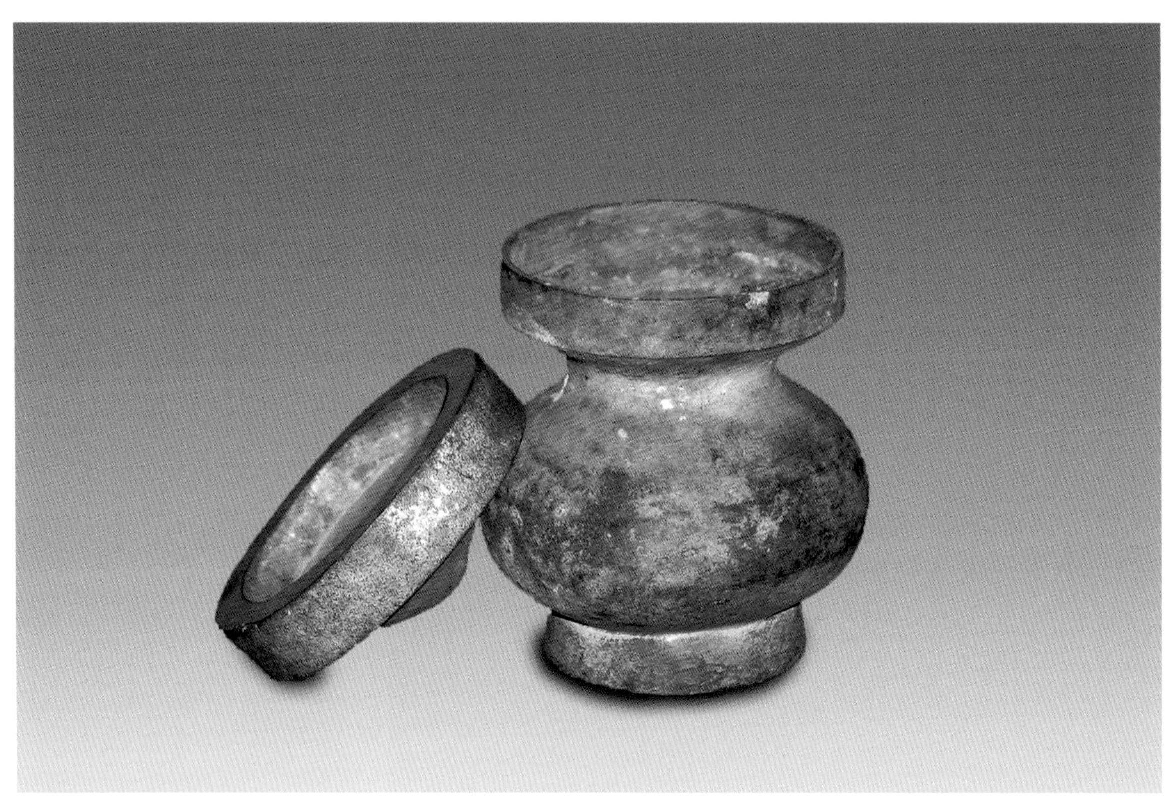

铜痰盂

汉

铜质

口径 8 厘米，底径 5.6 厘米，通高 9.2 厘米，重 1050 克

Copper Cuspidor

Han Dynasty

Copper

Caliber 8 cm/ Bottom Diameter 5.6 cm/ Height 9.2 cm/ Weight 1,050g

盘口，鼓腹，圈足，口上有一漏斗。生活器具。完整无损。陕西省咸阳市征集。

陕西医史博物馆藏

The cuspidor has a ring foot, a swelling belly, and a discoid mouth. It is covered with a funnel-shaped lid. This article for daily use is still intact. It was collected in Xianyang, Shaanxi Province.

Preserved in Shaanxi Museum of Medical History

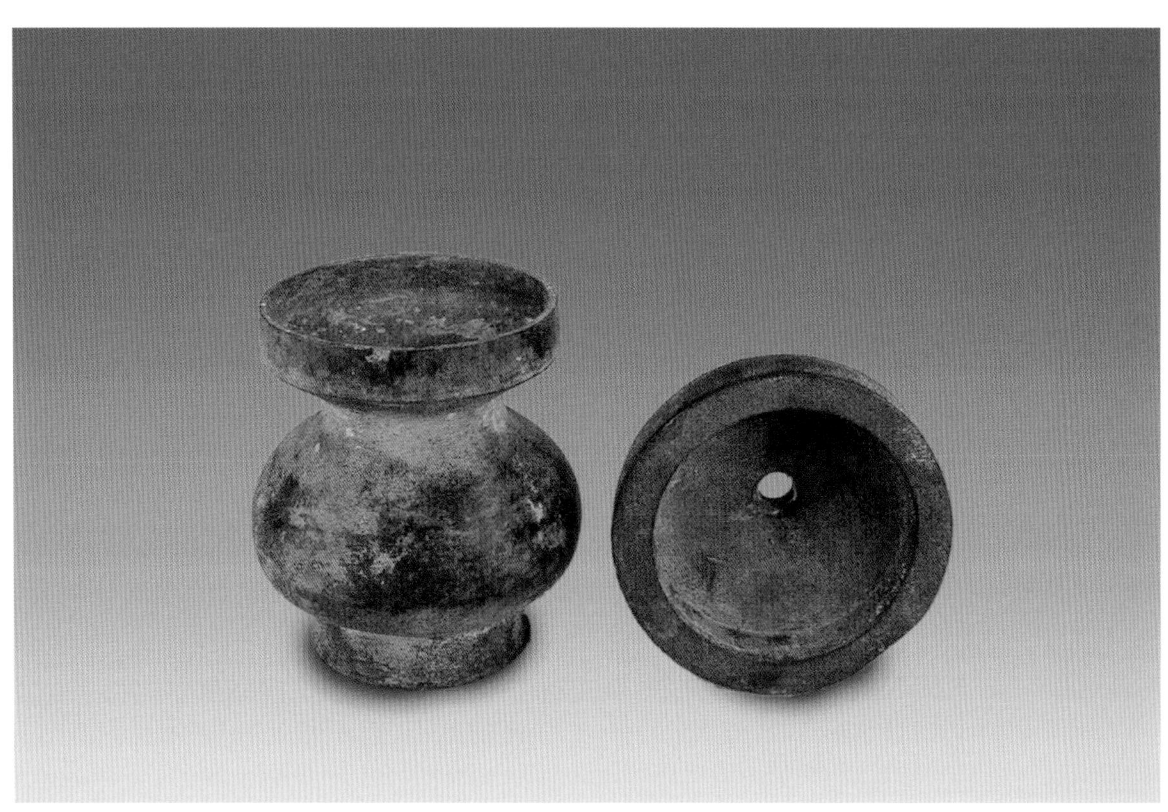

唾盂

西汉

铜质

盖盘口径 7.9 厘米，通高 9.5 厘米

Cuspidor

Western Han Dynasty

Copper

Lid Caliber 7.9 cm/ Total Height 9.5 cm

分盂盖与盂体两部分。盖中有漏孔，盖可取下，便于清洗。陕西咸阳出土。

陕西医史博物馆藏

The cuspidor consists of two parts, lid and body. There is a leak hole in the center of the lid. The lid is detachable and easy to clean. The cuspidor was unearthed from Xianyang, Shaanxi Province.

Preserved in Shaanxi Museum of Medical History

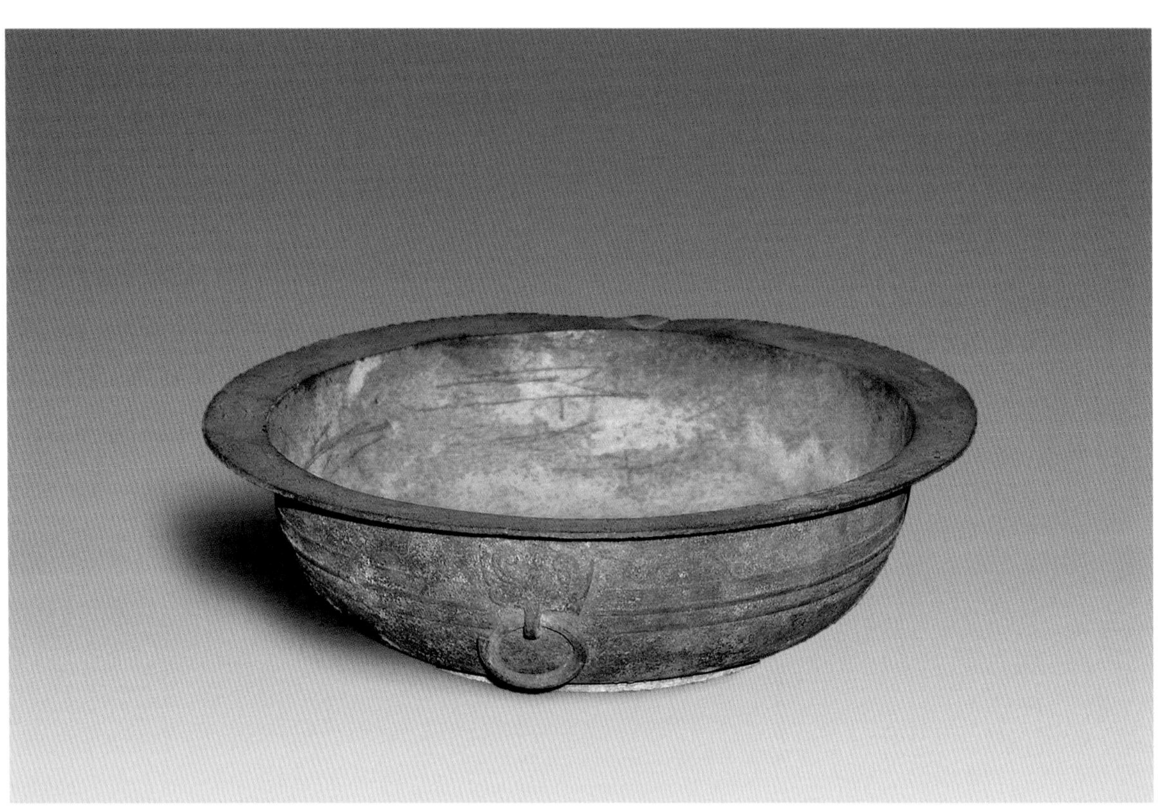

铜便盆

汉

铜质

口径 16.2 厘米，底径 8.5 厘米，通高 4.5 厘米，重 400 克

Copper Bedpan

Han Dynasty

Copper

Caliber 16.2 cm/ Bottom Diameter 8.5 cm/ Height 4.5 cm/ Weight 400g

平口沿，圆腹，圈足，腹上有三道弦纹，双兽头耳环。生活用器。完整无损。陕西省西安市征集。

陕西医史博物馆藏

The bedpan has a flat mouth edge, a circular foot, a swelling belly engraved with three string patterns, and double animal head holding rings. This article for daily use is still intact. It was collected from Xi'an, Shaanxi Province.

Preserved in Shaanxi Museum of Medical History

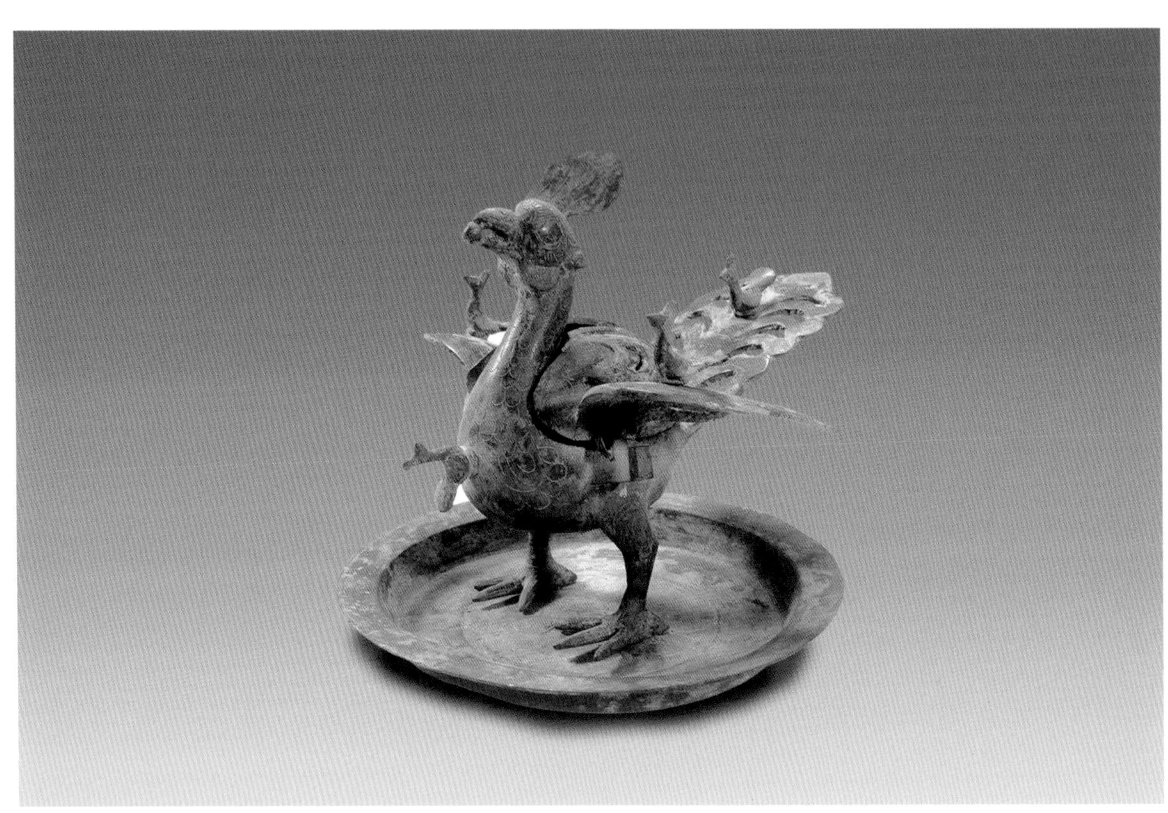

五凤熏炉

西汉

铜质

直径 21.5 厘米，通高 20 厘米

Aromatherapy Censer with Five Phoenix Pattern

Western Han Dynasty

Copper

Diameter 21.5 cm/ Height 20 cm

盘为平底，三只小乳足。大凤双爪铆在盘上，昂首引颈，口衔圆球，振翅挺胸，阔尾上翘，胸前与双翅上均有阴刻羽状纹饰。翅、腹连接处用穿钉连接，可自由张合。尾翅上均有弧形与长方形小镂孔。胸前、双翅和尾部另饰四只雏凤。熏炉是古时用来熏香和取暖的炉子。1989 年河南省焦作嘉禾屯窖藏出土。

河南博物院藏

The censer has a plate-shaped pedestal and three little feet. The big phoenix raises his head and cranes his neck with its two claws riveting to the pedestal. Biting a ball, the big phoenix flutters and thrust the chest out while tailing up. The chest and the wing are decorated with feather-like patterns in intaglio. Connected with the belly by driftbolts, two wings are free to fold and spread. Some arc and rectangle holes are engraved along the tail and wing. Four young phoenixes stand on the chest, the two wings, and the tail respectively. Aromatherapy censer is a furnace used to incense and keep warm. This piece was unearthed from the cellar in Jiahetun, Jiaozuo City, Henan Province in 1989.

Preserved in Henan Museum

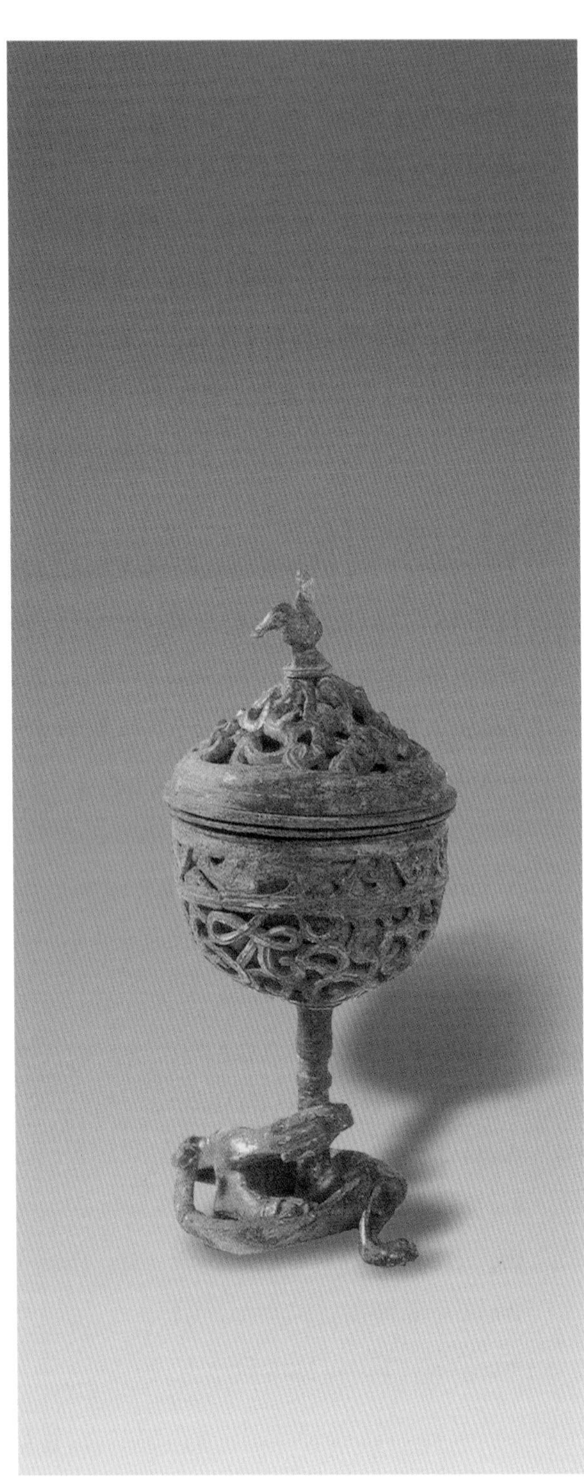

鎏金透雕蟠龙熏炉

西汉

鎏铜质

通高 19.4 厘米

Gilded Aromatherapy Censer with Openwork Engraved Curled-up Dragon

Western Han Dynasty

Gilded Copper

Height 19.4 cm

器座作蟠龙形，三爪外伸着地，一爪压住龙尾。蟠龙张口咬住一柱，柱上呈熏炉。熏炉深腹透雕，口沿饰两虎两羊，各具神态。腹部及盖均饰不规则的云纹。整个容器另有一层内套，可容燃烧的香料。盖作双层透雕，以散发香气。炉顶立一朱雀。

上海博物馆藏

The pedestal of the article takes the shape of curled-up dragon with three claws down to the ground and the last one stepping on the tail. He bites the pillar firmly which supports the aromatherapy censer. The censer has a deep openwork belly. The mouth edge is decorated with two lifelike tigers and sheep. The belly and the lid are decorated with irregular cloud patterns. There is an inner container for storing the fragrance. The double-layered openwork lid facilitates the distribution of the fragrance. On the top of the heater stands a rosefinch.

Preserved in Shanghai Museum

華

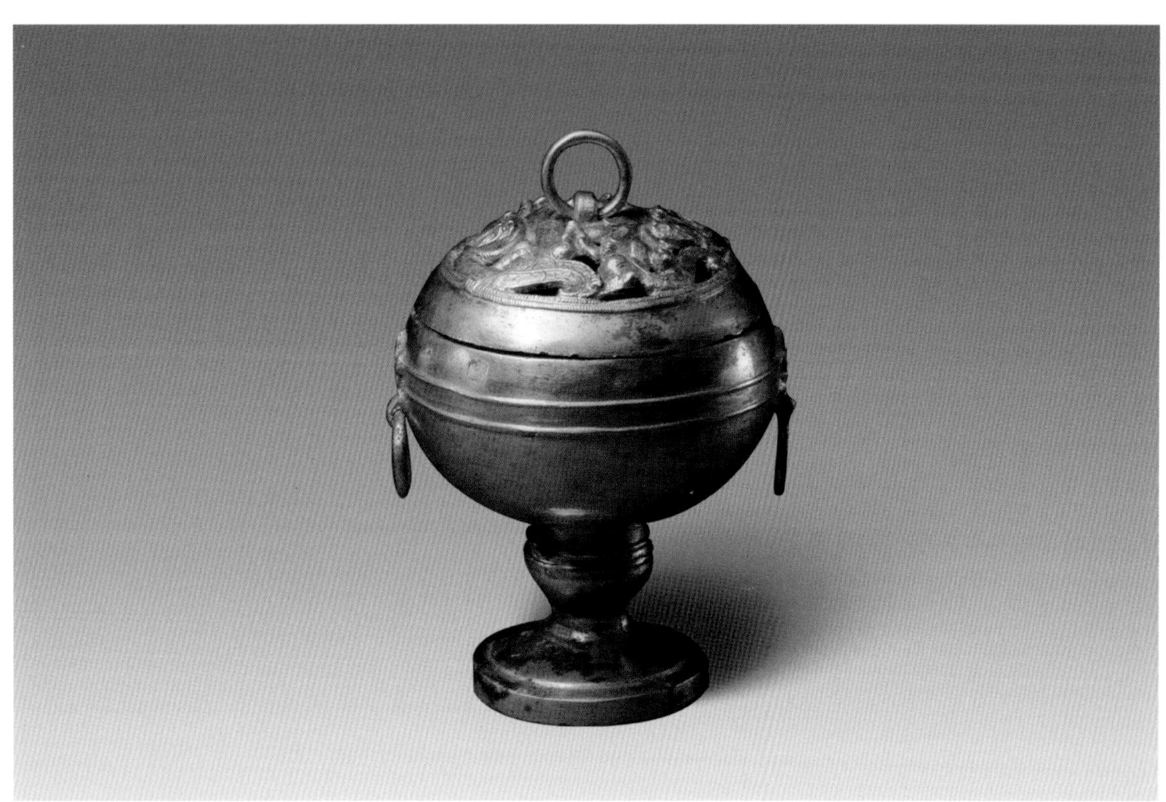

鎏金铜熏炉

西汉

鎏金铜质

口径 9.3 厘米，通高 14.4 厘米

Gilded Copper Aromatherapy Censer

Western Han Dynasty

Gilded Copper

Caliber 9.3 cm/ Total Height 14.4 cm

腹部刻“左重三斤六两”,“今三斤十一两”。通体鎏金。弧形盖，顶饰一环钮，周围透雕盘龙两条，首尾相接。字母口，圆腹。

山东省临淄区齐国故城博物馆藏

The belly is inscribed with characters which tell the weight of the article. The entire body is gilded. It has an arc-like lid with a circular knob, two matching mouths, and a swelling belly. The body is engraved with two intertwined dragons with their heads and tails connected.

Preserved in Museum of Gucheng of Qi State in Linzi district, Shandong Province

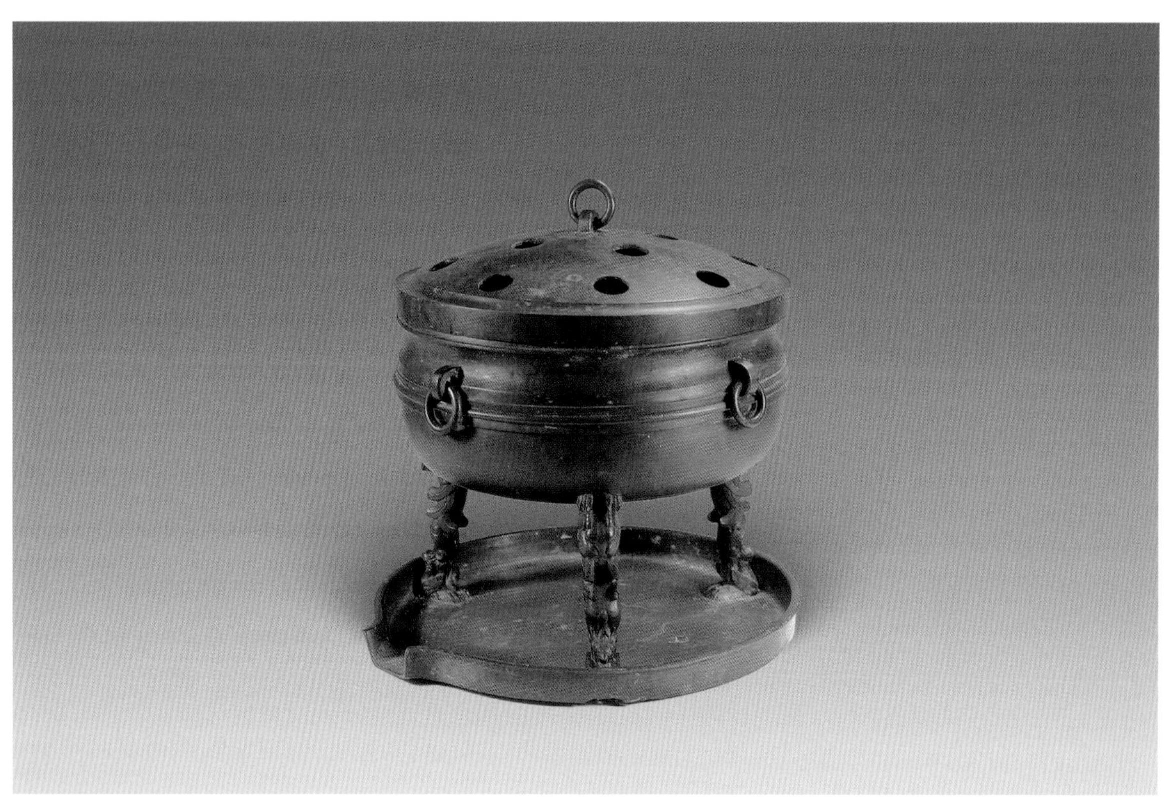

龙凤足带盘熏炉

西汉

青铜质

口径 26 厘米，承盘径 30 厘米，盖高 5.1 厘米，通高 28.5 厘米

Aromatherapy Censer with Tray and Feet Decorated with a Dragon Treading on a Phoenix

Western Han Dynasty

Bronze

Caliber 26 cm/ Tray Diameter 30 cm/ Thickness of Lid 5.1 cm/ Total Height 28.5 cm

炉身敞口，腹微鼓，大平底，三高足，足作龙踩凤状。腹部有对称四环钮，钮下饰宽带凸弦纹一周。平底中心镂一小圆孔，周围有 12 个长方形孔。盖作半球形，上有一环钮，盖面有镂圆形孔 12 个。炉下有一直壁平底的圆形承盘，盘壁开一流状缺口，炉体内灰烬落入承盘时，可从缺口处加以清除。

河北博物院藏

The censer has an open mouth, a swelling belly, a big flat base, and three long feet decorated with a dragon treading on a phoenix. Four symmetrical rings are placed around the belly. Below the rings is a circle of broad convex string pattern. In the center of the base is a small circular hole surrounded by twelve rectangular holes. With a circular knob, the hemispherical lid is carved with 12 circular holes. The circular tray has a straight wall, a flat base, and a breach for ashes cleaning.

Preserved in Hebei Museum

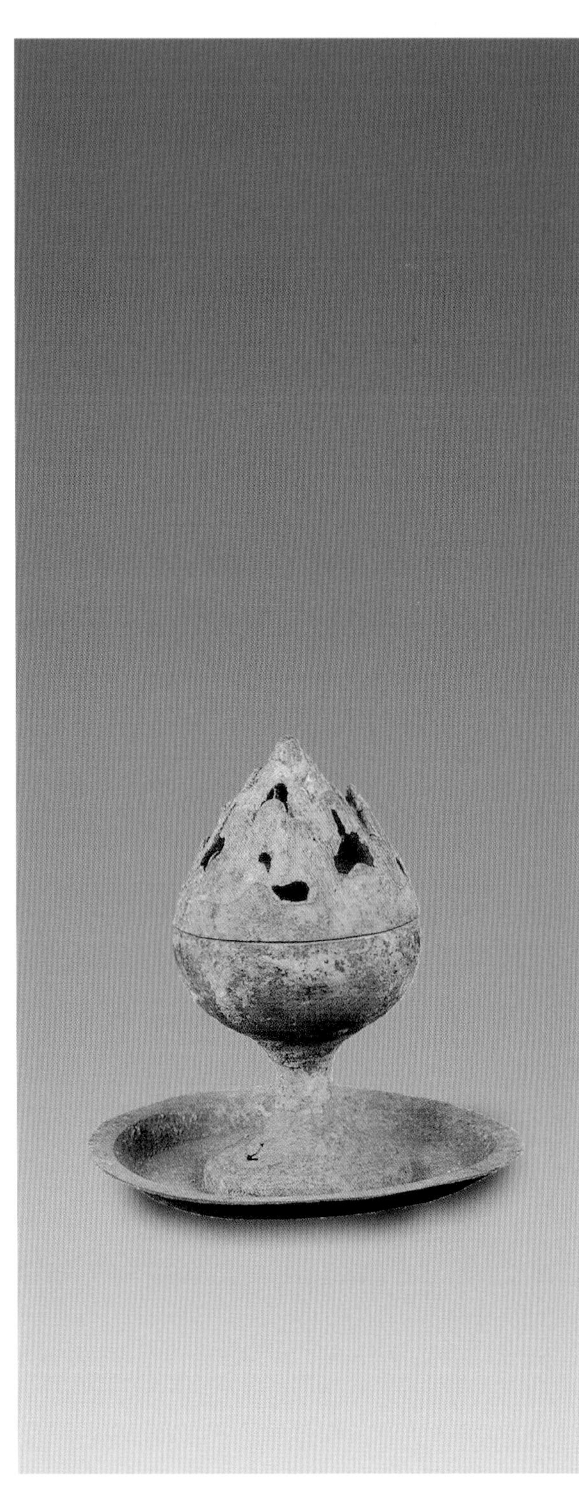

博山炉

西汉

铜质

盘口径 10 厘米，通高 11 厘米

炉盖镂空。用于熏香。陕西西安出土。

上海中医药博物馆藏

Boshan Censer

Western Han Dynasty

Copper

Tray Caliber 10 cm/ Censer Total Height 11 cm

The lid of the censer is hollowed for aroma releasing. The censer was unearthed from Xi'an, Shaanxi Province.

Preserved in Shanghai Museum of Traditional Chinese Medicine

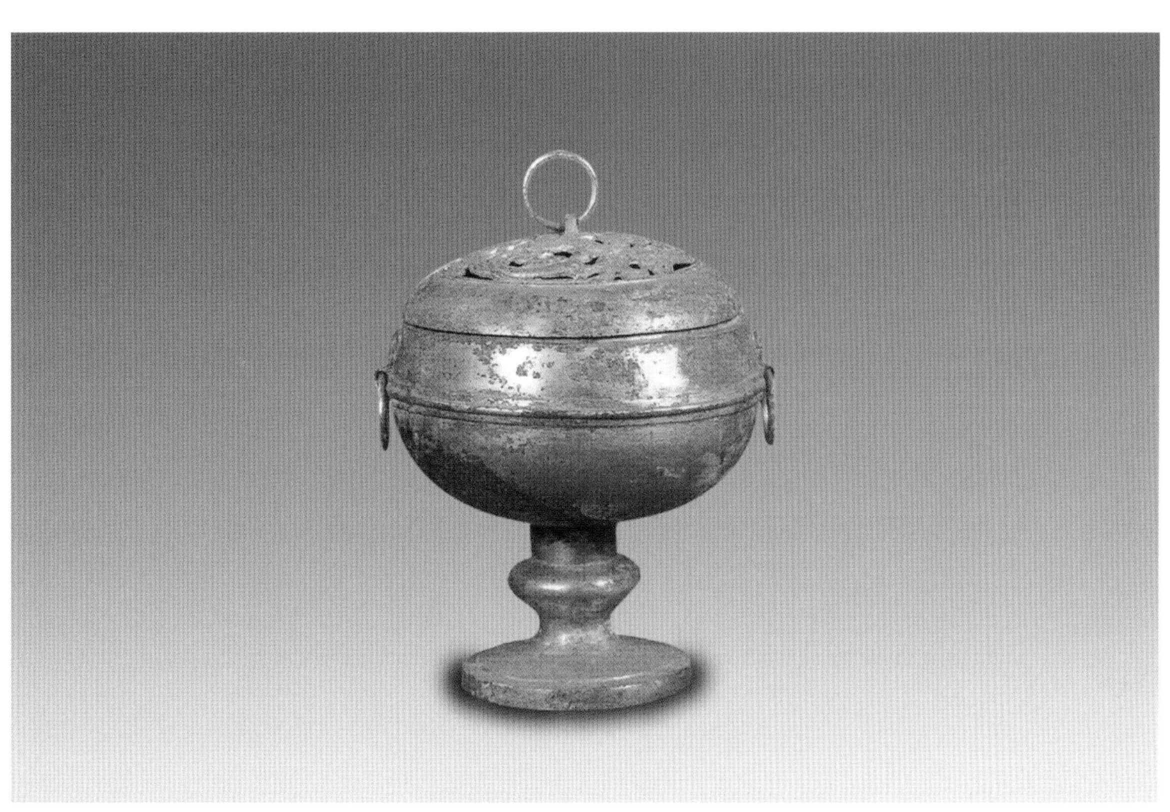

鎏金透雕香熏

西汉

鎏金铜质

底径 6 厘米，高 18 厘米

盖上透雕。

上海中医药博物馆藏

Gilded Censer with Openwork Engravings

Western Han Dynasty

Gilded Copper

Base Diameter 6 cm/ Height 18 cm

There are openwork engravings on the lid.

Preserved in Shanghai Museum of Traditional Chinese Medicine

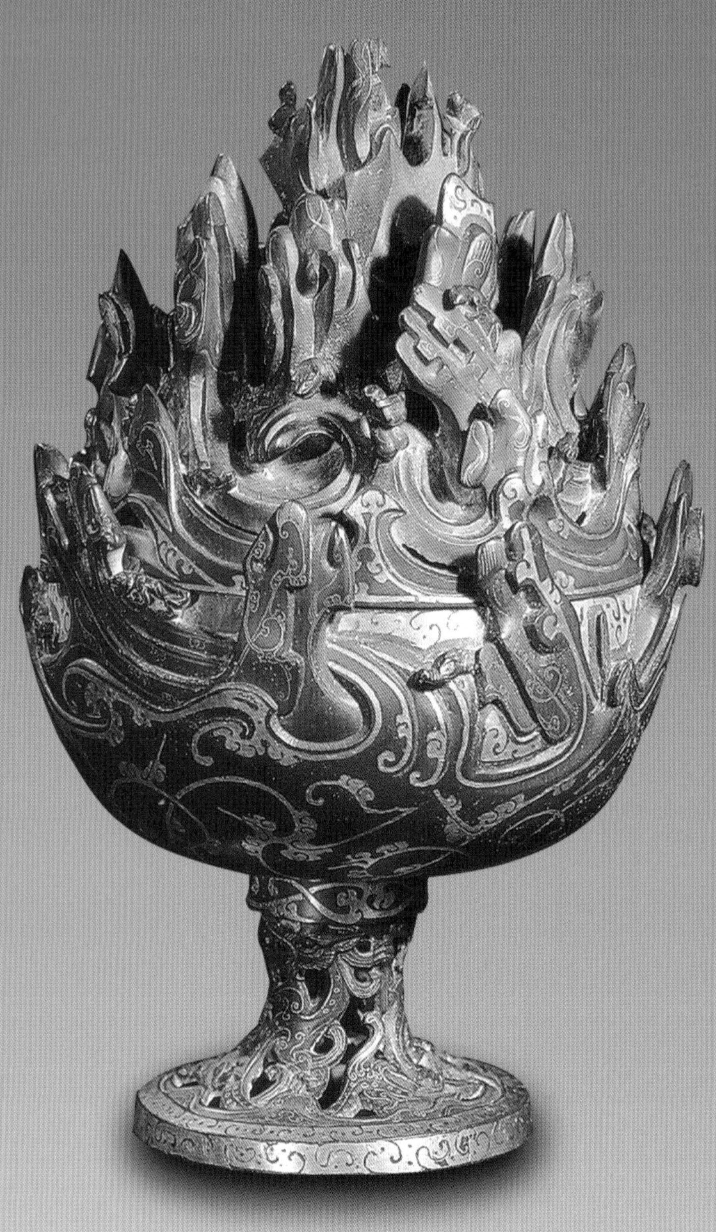

错金博山炉

西汉

金质

通高 26 厘米

炉身似豆形，通体用金丝和金片错出舒展的云气纹。炉盘上部和炉盖铸出高低起伏的山峦。炉盖上因山势镂孔，雕塑出生动的山间景色。山间神兽出没，虎豹奔走，轻捷的小猴或蹲踞在峦峰高处，或骑坐在兽背上嬉戏玩耍，猎人手持弓箭巡猎山间。座把透雕成三龙出水状，以龙头擎托炉盘。1968 年河北满城陵山中山靖王刘胜墓出土。

河北博物院藏

Gold-inlaid Boshan Censer

Western Han Dynasty

Gold

Total Height 26 cm

The body of censer takes the shape of bean with the decoration of floating cloud design interlaced by the golden threads and flakes. Undulating mountain range is carved on the upper part of the tray and the lid according to the ups and downs of the mountains, vividly portraying the beautiful scenery. Among the mountain range are walking mythical creatures, tigers, and leopards. The naughty monkeys have fun while squatting on peak or sitting on the back of the beast. With bow and arrow in hand, hunters are patrolling in the woods. The pedestal is engraved with three dragons rising out of the water with the dragons' head upholding the tray. The piece was unearthed from the mausoleum of King Jing-Liu Sheng in Man County of Hebei Province in 1980.

Preserved in Hebei Museum

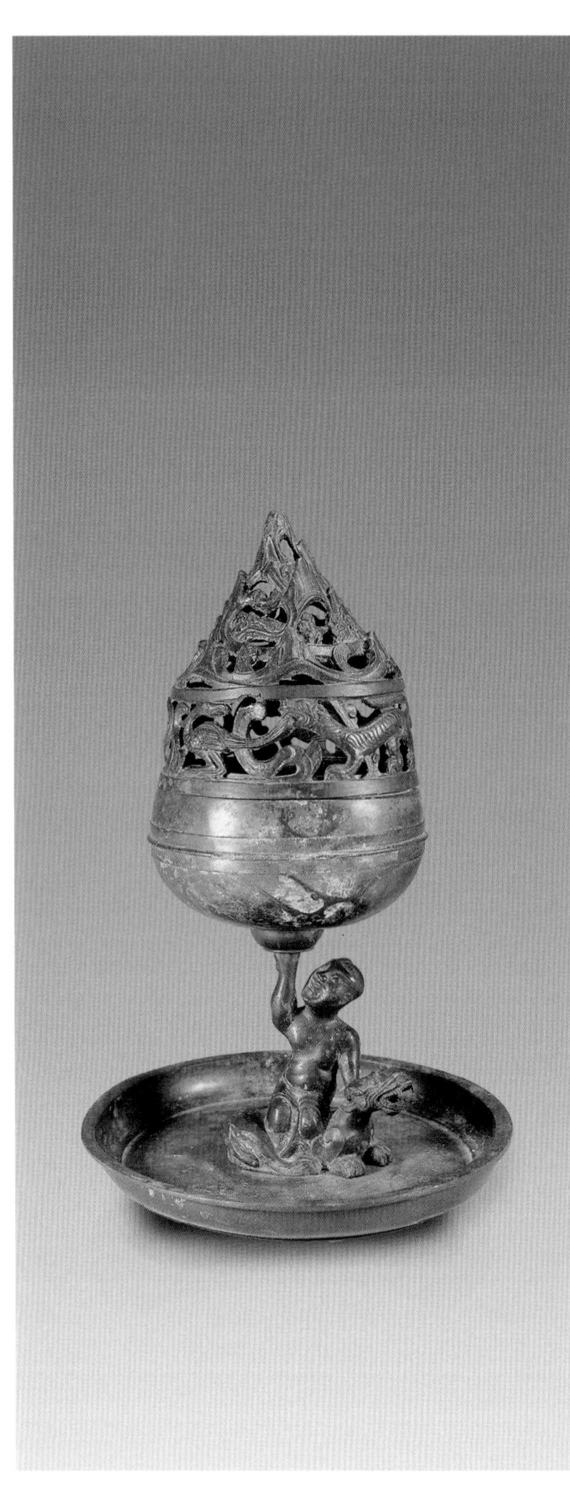

鎏银骑兽人物博山炉

西汉

鎏银铜质

底盘径 22.3 厘米，通高 32.3 厘米

Silver-gilded Boshan Censer with Decoration of a Man Riding Beast

Western Han Dynasty

Silver-gilded

Tray Caliber 22.3 cm/ Total Height 32.3 cm

由底盘、炉身、炉盖三部分组成。底盘内卧一海兽，昂首，张口欲噬，颈部前伸作挣扎状。兽背上跪坐一力士，上身裸露，左手按住兽颈，右手高擎炉身。炉盖铸上下两层：上层群山叠翠，流云四绕，云山间虎熊出没，人兽搏斗和人物驱赶牛车的场面。下层铸龙虎、朱雀、骆驼以及草木云气等纹饰。1968 年河北满城陵山中山靖王刘胜墓出土。

河北博物院藏

The censer includes three parts: the tray, the body, and the lid. On the tray crouches a struggling marine beast with its head rising, its mouth open, and its neck craning. A strong man is sitting on the back of the beast with his upper body naked while his left hand grips the beast's neck and his right hand holds the censer's body. The censer is casted into two layers. The upper layer shows the following scene: tigers and bears come and go among the clouding mountain range; people fight against beast or drive bullock cart. The lower layer is casted with pattern of dragon, tiger, rosefinch, flowers, and floating clouds.

Preserved in Hebei Museum

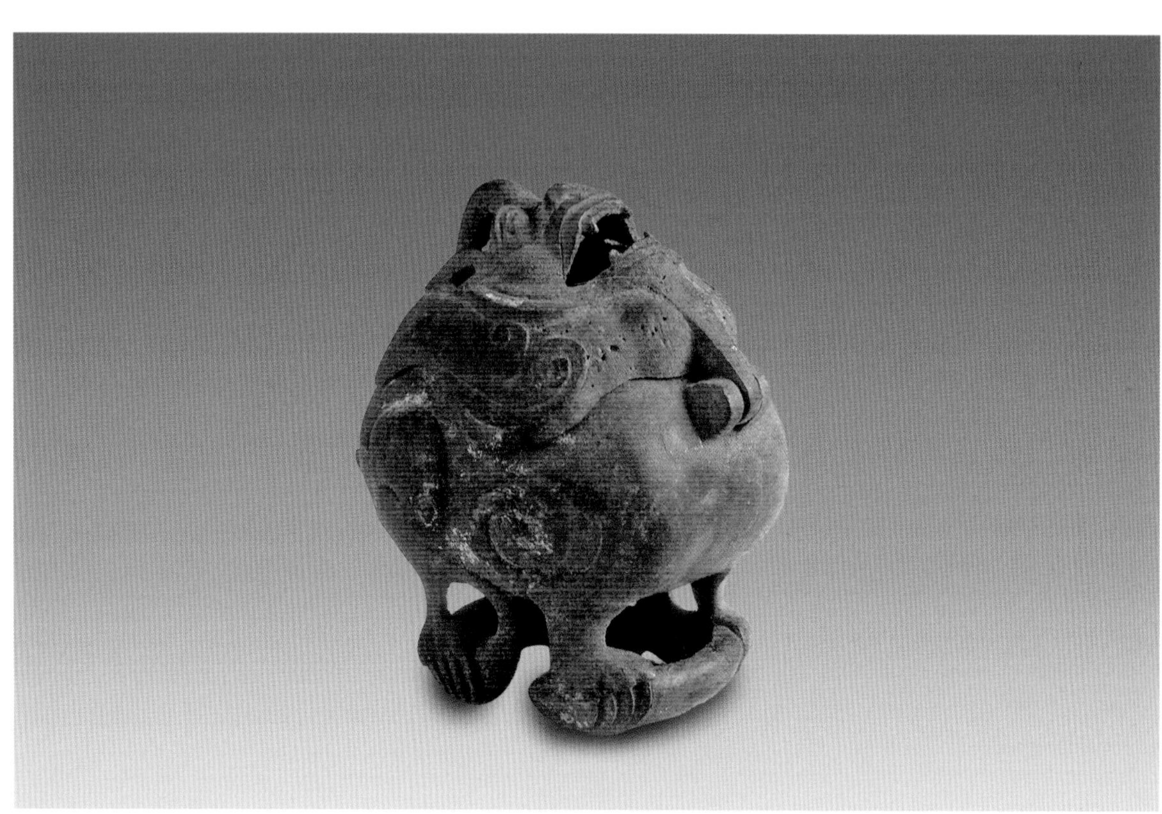

辟邪踏蛇铜薰

西汉

铜质

通高 9.5 厘米

Copper Censer with Bixie (a mythical creature) Treading Snake

Western Han Dynasty

Copper

Total Height 9.5 cm

器体雕铸成一站立的辟邪状，身体作薰身，头、肩部作盖，与身铰链于胸部，辟邪体浑圆，强壮有力，昂首向天，大鼻、突目、独角、口大张露齿，口、角、额部镂空作薰孔。体饰双翼，翼上饰卷云纹，四足爪形，抓踏一条盘成“S”形的蛇，蛇之头、尾卷至辟邪腹部。1989 年扬州市郊西湖胡场 7 号墓出土。

扬州博物馆藏

The censer is casted into a standing Bixie. Bixie's body is casted into the censer's body. Its head and shoulders are casted into lid which is hinged to the chest. Bixie looks strong and powerful with a chubby body. With his mouth open wide and his teeth exposed, he is raising his head to the sky with a huge nose, a single horn, and protruding eyes. The mouth, horn and forehead of Bixie are hollowed out for aroma releasing. With two scrolled-cloud-patterned wings, Bixie grips the S-shaped snake in his four claws. The snake's head and tail curl down to Bixie's belly. The censer was unearthed in No. 1 tomb in Huchang country, Xihu Town, Yangzhou City in 1989.

Preserved in Yangzhou Museum

華

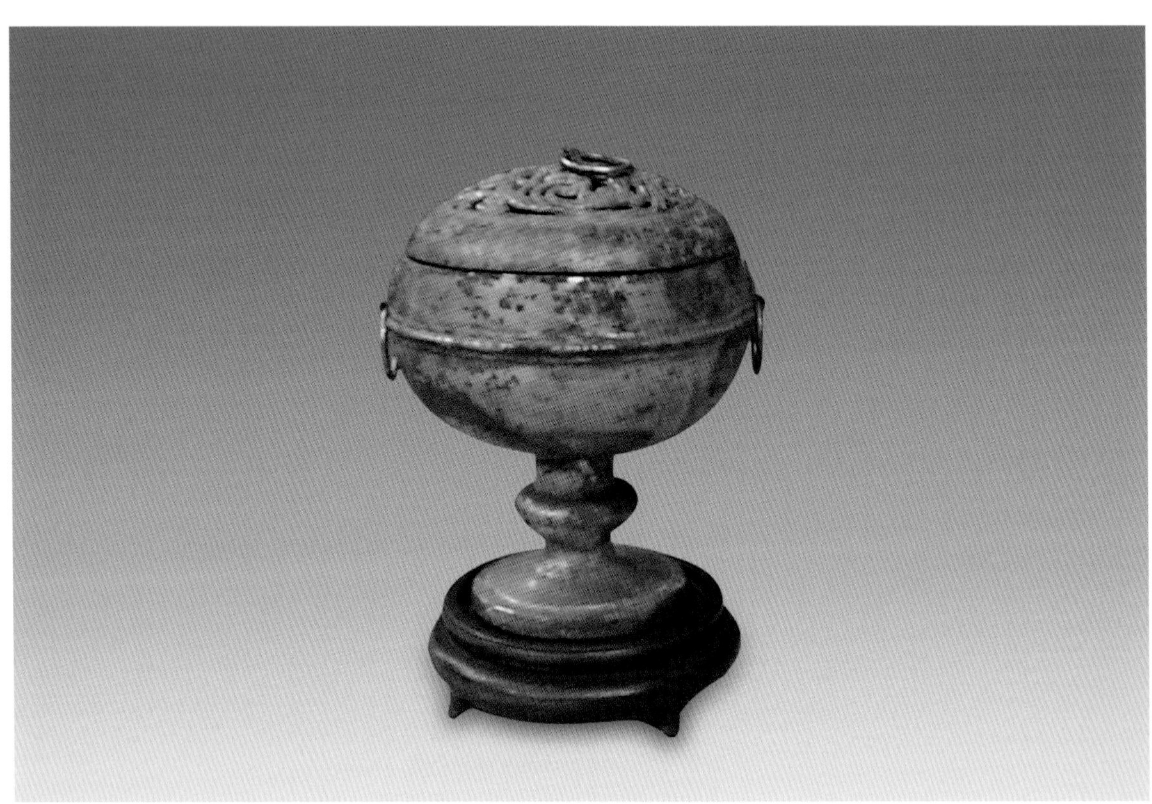

鎏金铜熏炉

汉

鎏金铜质

口径 10.6 厘米 , 胸径 13.2 厘米，腰径 3.2 厘米，底径 8.2 厘米 , 通高 16.2 厘米，盖高 2.6 厘米

Gilded Copper Censer

Han Dynasty

Gilded Copper

Caliber 10.6 cm/ Chest Diameter 13.2 cm/ Waist Diameter 3.2 cm/ Base Diameter 8.2 cm/ Total Height 16.2 cm/ Thickness of Lid 2.6 cm

熏炉形，为香熏。该藏表面鎏金，两侧有环状耳，上部有镂空盖，工艺精湛。鎏金局部脱落。1983年入藏。

中华医学会/上海中医药大学医史博物馆藏

The censer is an aroma furnace with a gilded surface. The censer is decorated with two rings on each side and a hollowed-out lid. It was exquisitely casted. It was collected in 1983,

Preserved in Chinese Medical Association/Museum of Chinese Medicine History, Shanghai University of Traditional Chinese Medicine

華

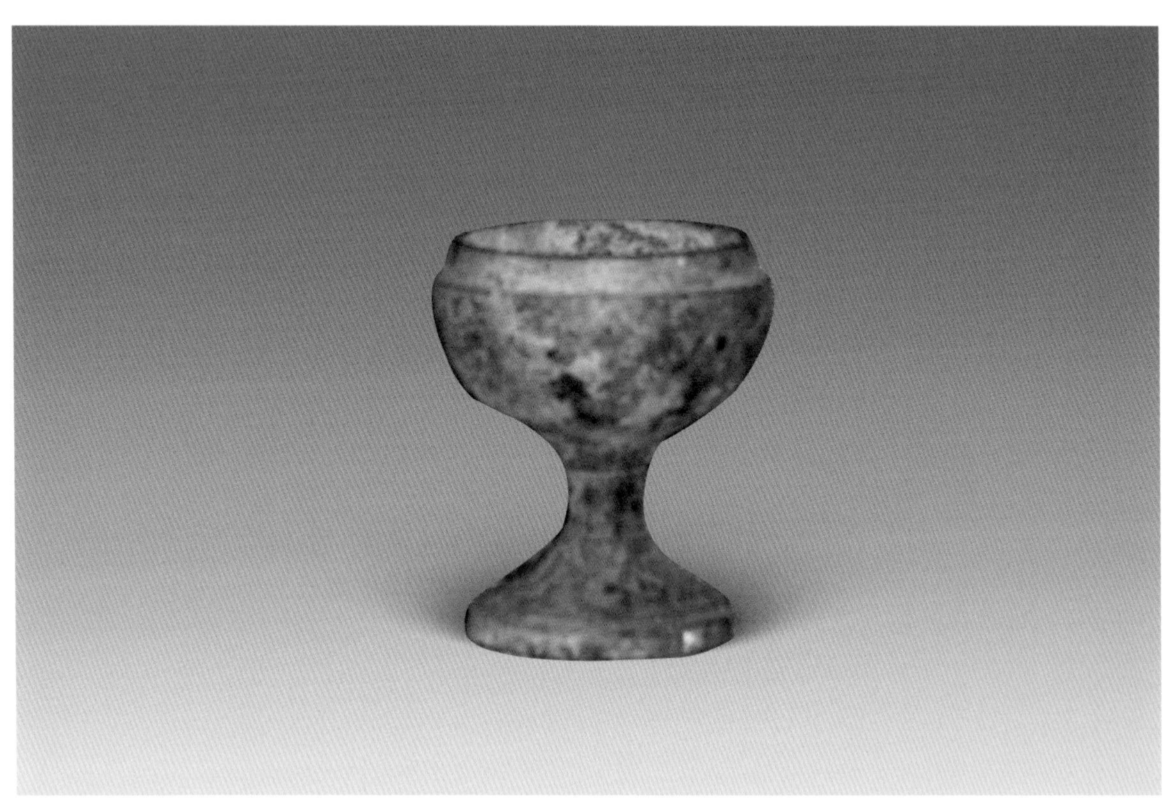

铜薰器

汉

铜质

口径 5.5 厘米，底径 4.8 厘米，通高 7 厘米，重 100 克

Copper Aromatherapy Utensil

Han Dynasty

Copper

Caliber 5.5 cm/ Base Diameter 4.8 cm/ Height 7 cm/ Weight 100g

子母口，中为高脚杯状，无底座。卫生器具。无盖，无底座。陕西省咸阳市废品站征集。

陕西医史博物馆藏

The utensil has a matched mouth and takes the shape of goblet without pedestal and cover. It is a sanitary ware and was collected from a salvage station of Xianyang, Shaanxi Province.

Preserved in Shaanxi Museum of Medical History

華

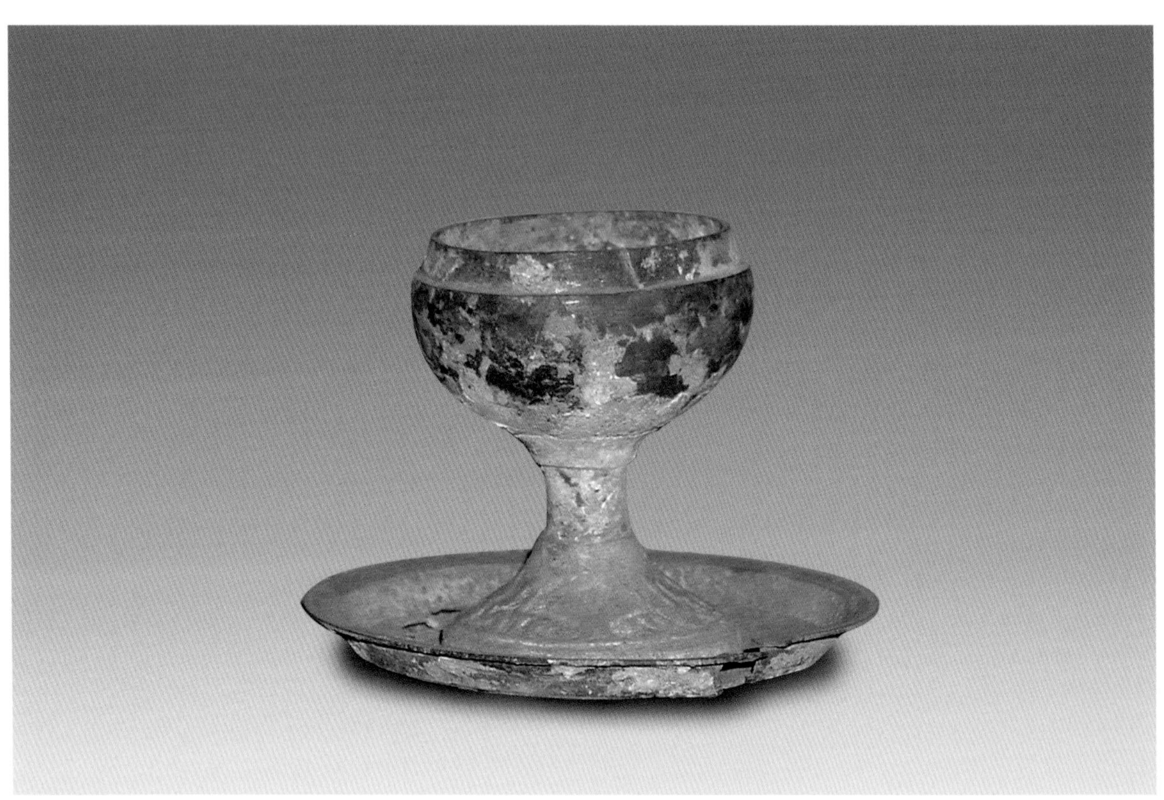

铜薰器

汉

铜质

口径 5 厘米，底径 10.5 厘米，通高 8 厘米，重 200 克

Copper Aromatherapy Utensil

Han Dynasty

Copper

Caliber 5 cm/ Base Diameter 10.5 cm/ Height 8 cm/ Weight 200g

子母口，中为高脚杯状，下为一圆盘。卫生器具。无盖，底残。陕西省咸阳市废品站征集。

陕西医史博物馆藏

The utensil has a matched mouth, a tray, and no cover. It takes the shape of goblet and is a kind of sanitary ware. The base is damaged. It was collected from a salvage station of Xianyang, Shaanxi Province.

Preserved in Shaanxi Museum of Medical History

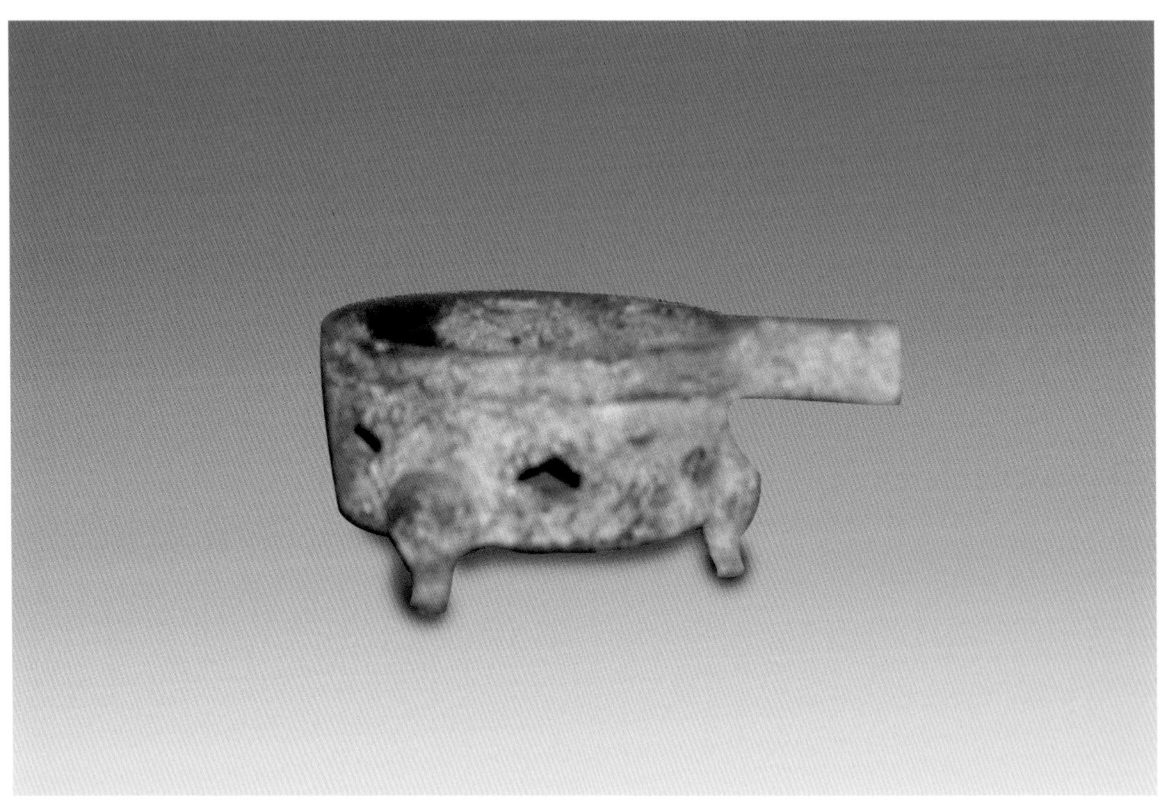

铜薰器

汉

铜质

口径 9.2 厘米，底径 8.1 厘米，通高 5.5 厘米，重 450 克

Copper Aromatherapy Utensil

Han Dynasty

Copper

Caliber 9.2 cm/ Base Diameter 8.1 cm/ Total Height 5.5 cm/ Weight 450 g

直口直腹，平底三兽足，上腹有一把，下腹有六个棱形孔。卫生器具。完整无损。陕西省西安市南郊边家村征集。

陕西医史博物馆藏

The utensil has an upright mouth, an upright belly, a flat base, and three animal-shaped feet. A handle is attached to the upper belly and six prismatic holes are in the lower belly. It is a sanitary ware and is still in good condition. The utensil was collected from Bian Village in the southern suburbs of Xi'an, Shaanxi Province.

Preserved in Shaanxi Museum of Medical History

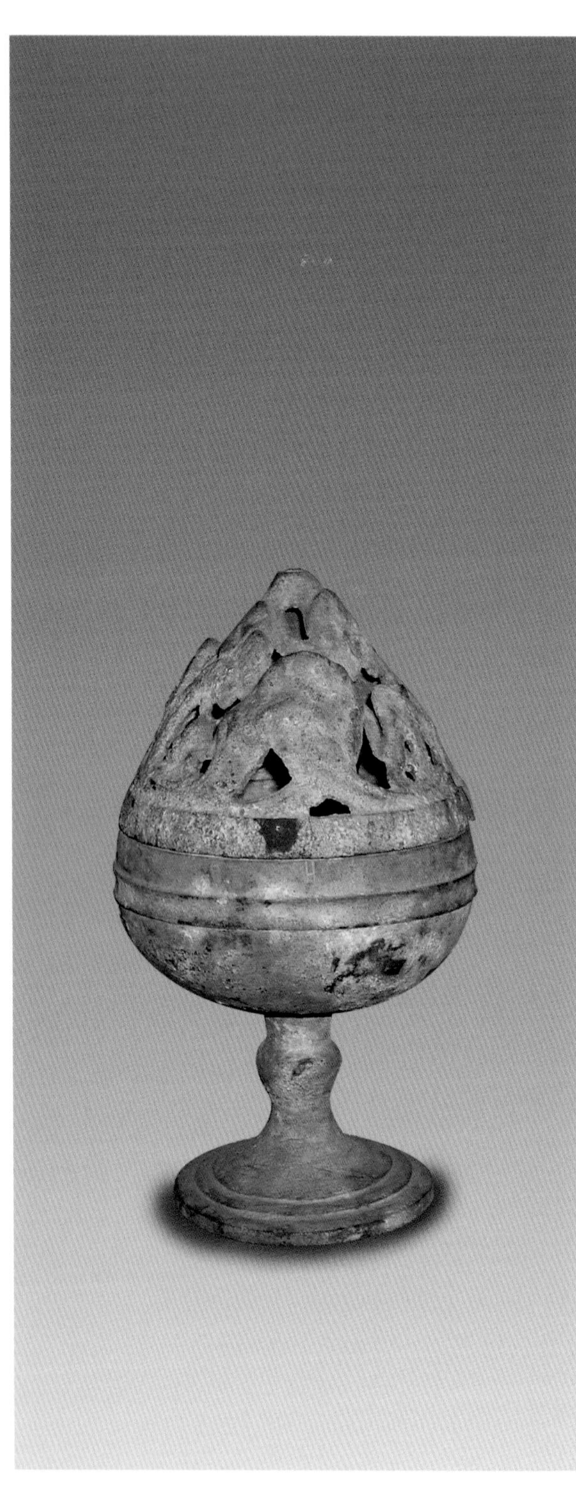

铜薰器

汉

铜质

口径 7 厘米，底径 6.2 厘米，通高 15.5 厘米，重 450 克

Copper Aromatherapy Utensil

Han Dynasty

Copper

Caliber 7 cm/ Base Diameter 6.2 cm/ Total Height 15.5 cm/ Weight 450 g

博山炉盖，子母口，圆腹，倒喇叭底座。卫生器具。有残。陕西省咸阳市征集。

陕西医史博物馆藏

The utensil has a Boshan cover, a matched mouth, a belly belly, and an inverted trumpet-shaped pedestal. It is a sanitary ware with some damages. The utensil was collected from Xianyang, Shaanxi Province.

Preserved in Shaanxi Museum of Medical History

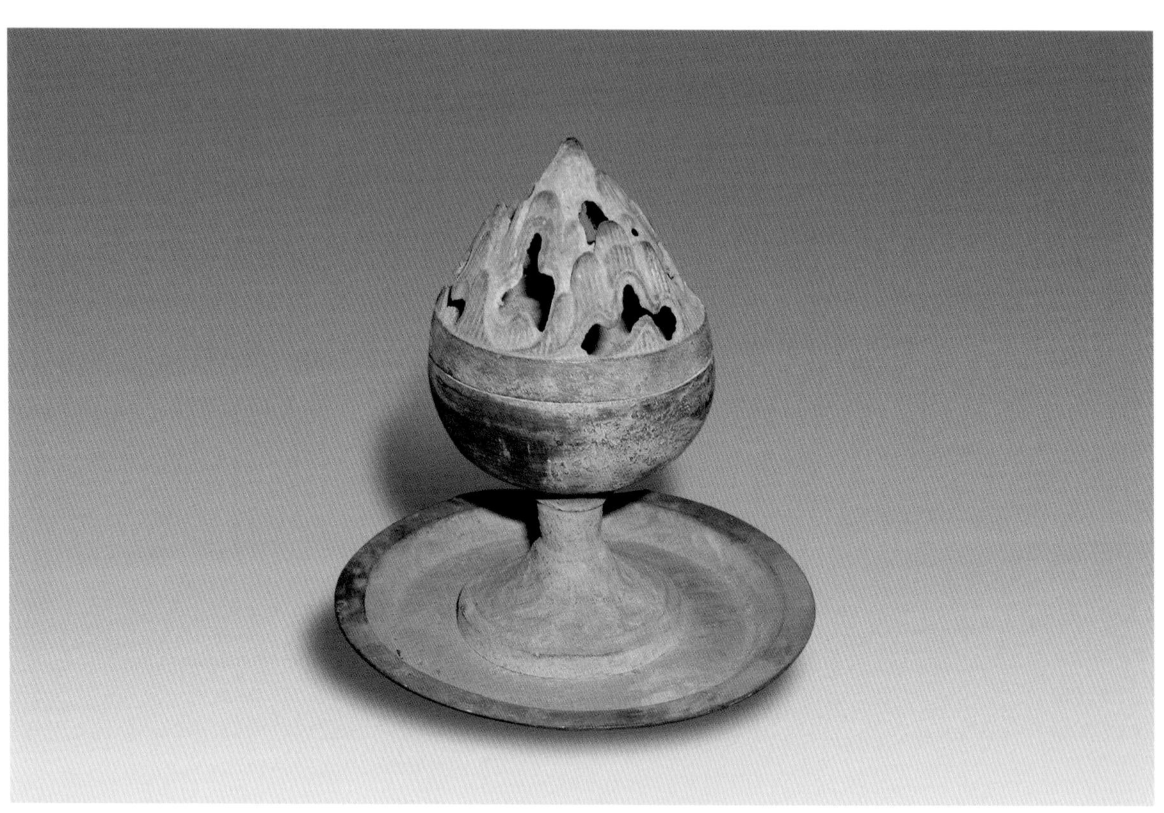

铜薰器

汉

铜质

口径 3 厘米，底径 10.5 厘米，通高 11 厘米，重 200 克

Copper Aromatherapy Utensil

Han Dynasty

Copper

Caliber 3 cm/ Base Diameter 10.5 cm/ Total Height 11 cm/ Weight 200 g

上为火焰状罩盖，中为一高脚杯状，下为一圆盘。卫生器具。完整无损。陕西省绥德县征集。

陕西医史博物馆藏

The utensil takes the shape of goblet with a flamboyant cover and a circular tray. It is still in good condition. This sanitary ware was collected from Suide County, Shaanxi Province.

Preserved in Shaanxi Museum of Medical History

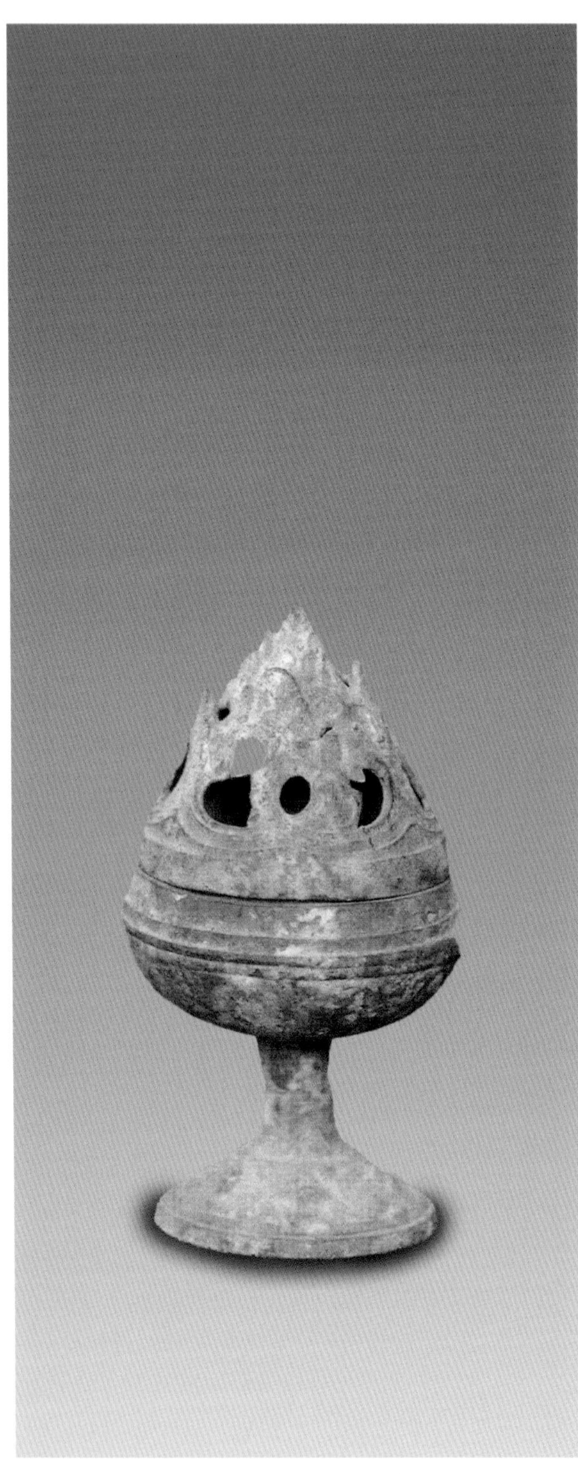

博山炉

西汉

铜质

高 17 厘米

Boshan Censer

Western Han Dynasty

Copper

Height 17 cm

炉盖呈山峰状，底为喇叭状。系西汉时期常见的熏香器具。

陕西医史博物馆藏

The censer has a mountain range cover and a trumpet-shaped base. It was a common utensil for aroma releasing in the Western Han Dynasty.

Preserved in Shaanxi Museum of Medical History

華

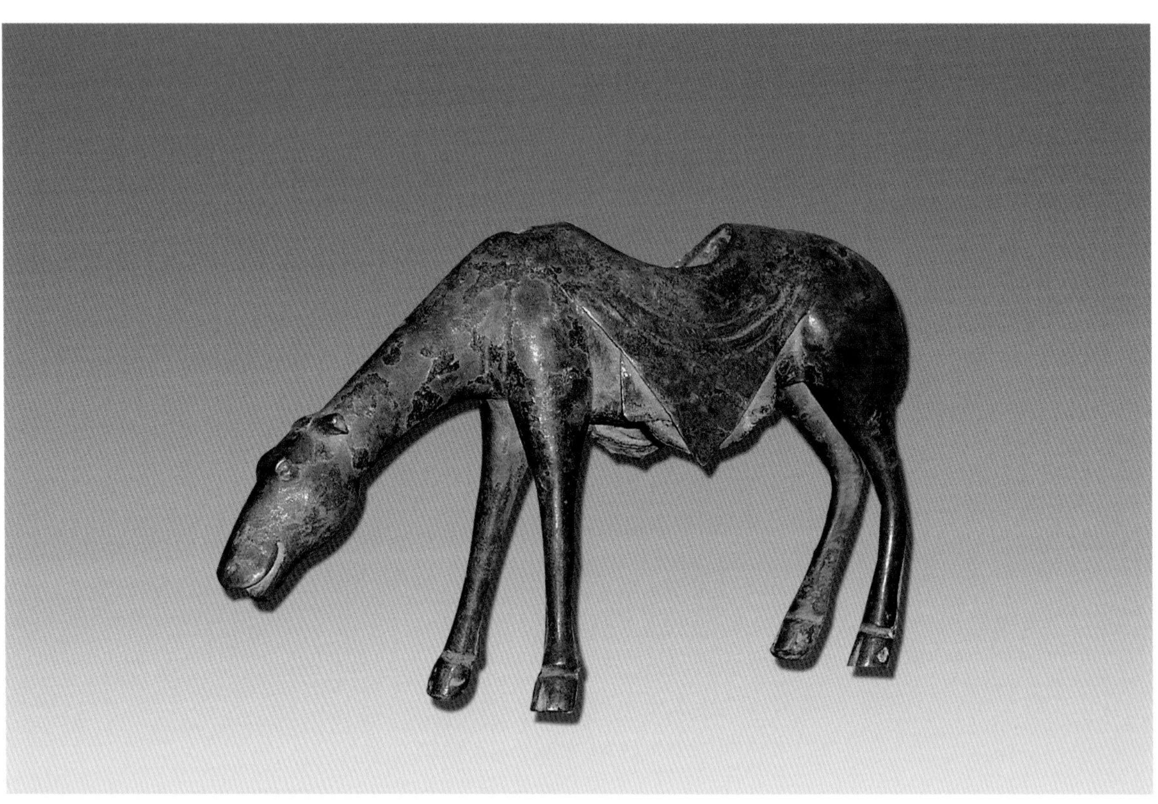

铜薰炉

汉

铜质

口径 23 厘米，底径 11 厘米，通高 11 厘米，重 550 克

Copper Aromatherapy Censer

Han Dynasty

Copper

Caliber 23 cm/ Base Diameter 11 cm/ Total Height 11 cm/ Weight 550 g

走马状，马鞍处有一椭圆孔，两边各有一小孔。生活器具。无盖。

陕西医史博物馆藏

The censer takes the shape of a walking horse but has no lid. The saddle has an oval hole on it and two small holes on each side.

Preserved in Shaanxi Museum of Medical History

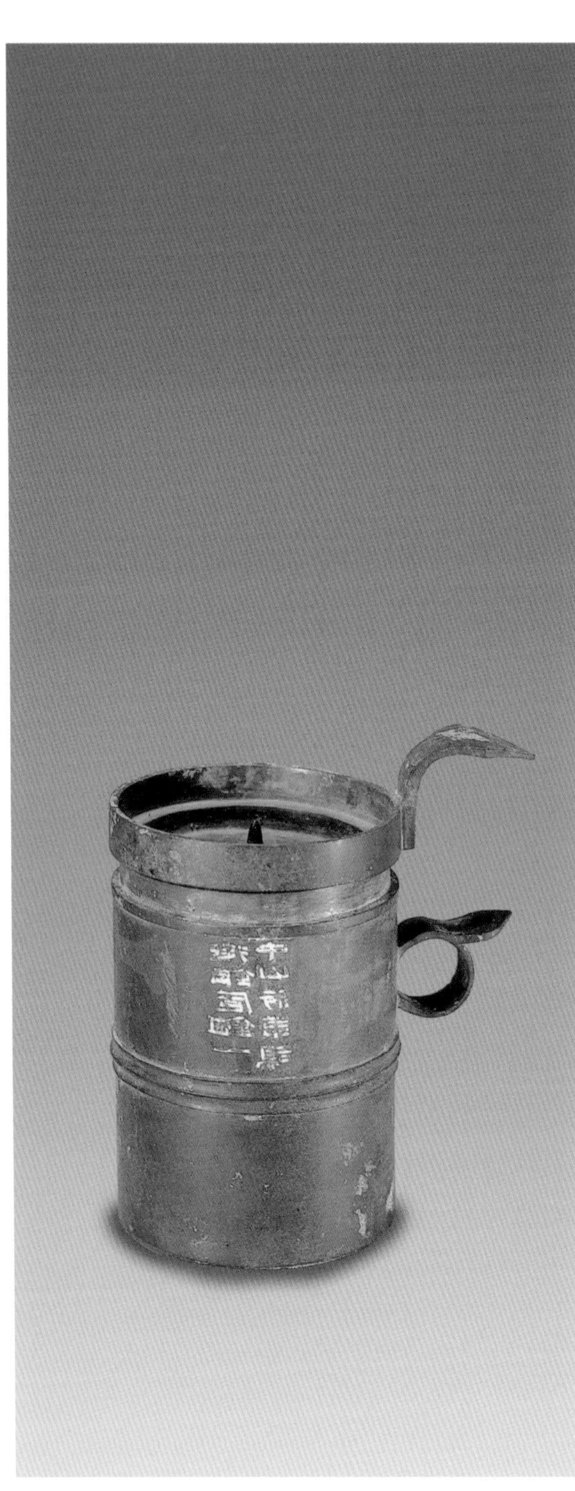

带铭铜卮灯

西汉

铜质

通宽 10.7 厘米，高 12.2 厘米

Copper Zhi-shaped Lamp with Inscription

Western Han Dynasty

Copper

Total Width 10.7 cm/ Height 12.2 cm

灯为带盖直筒杯形。杯作子口，平底，上腹有菱形带环鋬，腹中部隆起宽带瓦纹两周。盖似覆盘，使用时翻转即为灯盘。灯盘直口，假圈足。壁一侧伸出菱形鋬，鋬面有可与杯身菱形鋬扣合的凹槽。假圈足恰好纳入杯口中。盘心有烛扦。杯身及盖外侧均有铭文。杯名“御铜卮锭一，中山内府，第鸪”；盖铭“卮锭，第鹊”。

河北博物院藏

The cup-shaped lamp has a matched mouth, a flat base, and a circular handle attached to the upper belly. Around the middle part of the belly are two circles of relief pattern of tiles. The inverted plate-shaped lid can be used as lamp tray when turned over. With an upright mouth and a fake circular foot, the tray extends a diamond-shaped handle, of which the indentation can interlock with the handle on the cup-shaped body. Thus the fake foot can be embedded in the mouth of body. On the center of tray stands a candle stick. There are inscriptions on the surface of the lid and the body which record that this lamp was once used in the imperial palace.

Preserved in Hebei Museum

華

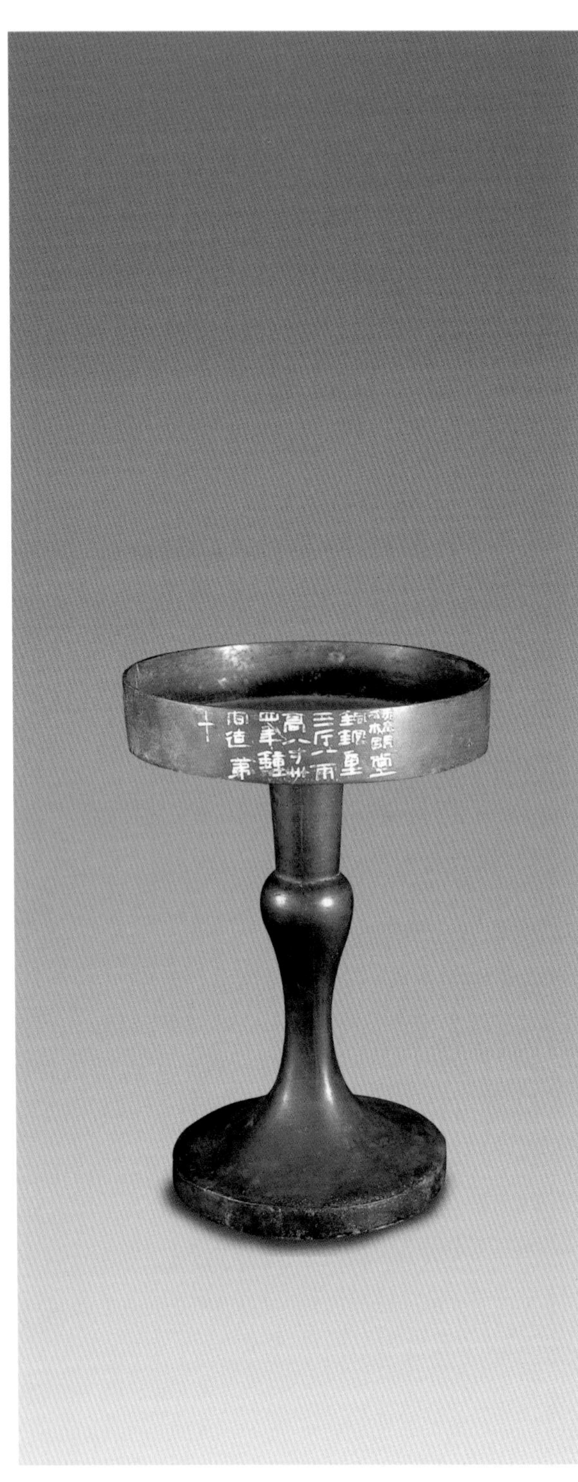

椒林明堂豆形铜灯

西汉

铜质

灯盘径 12.3 厘米，通高 18 厘米，重 850 克

Jiaolin Bean-shaped Copper Lamp

Western Han Dynasty

Copper

Tray Diameter 12.3 cm/ Total Height 18 cm/ Weight 850 g

灯盘直壁，平底。细座把上部呈圆柱形，中部隆起，向下渐细。喇叭形底座，圈足。盘和座把分铸，盘下有小柱插入把腔内，用铜钉铆合。盘壁外侧刻有铭文“椒林明堂铜锭，重三斤八两，高八寸，卅四年，锺官造，第十”。

河北博物院藏

The tray has an upright wall and a flat base. The lamp has a trumpet-shaped pedestal and a circular-like foot. The narrow post takes the shape of cylinder in the upper part, while it grows wide in the middle part and tapers at the base. Casted respectively, the lamp tray and the post are riveted together by the bronze nails, with the small pillar plugged into the cavity of post. On the outer wall of the tray is the inscription which records that this eight-cun-high lamp weighed three Jin and eight Liang and was casted by the court artisan in the 34th year of the Western Han Dynasty.

Preserved in Hebei Museum

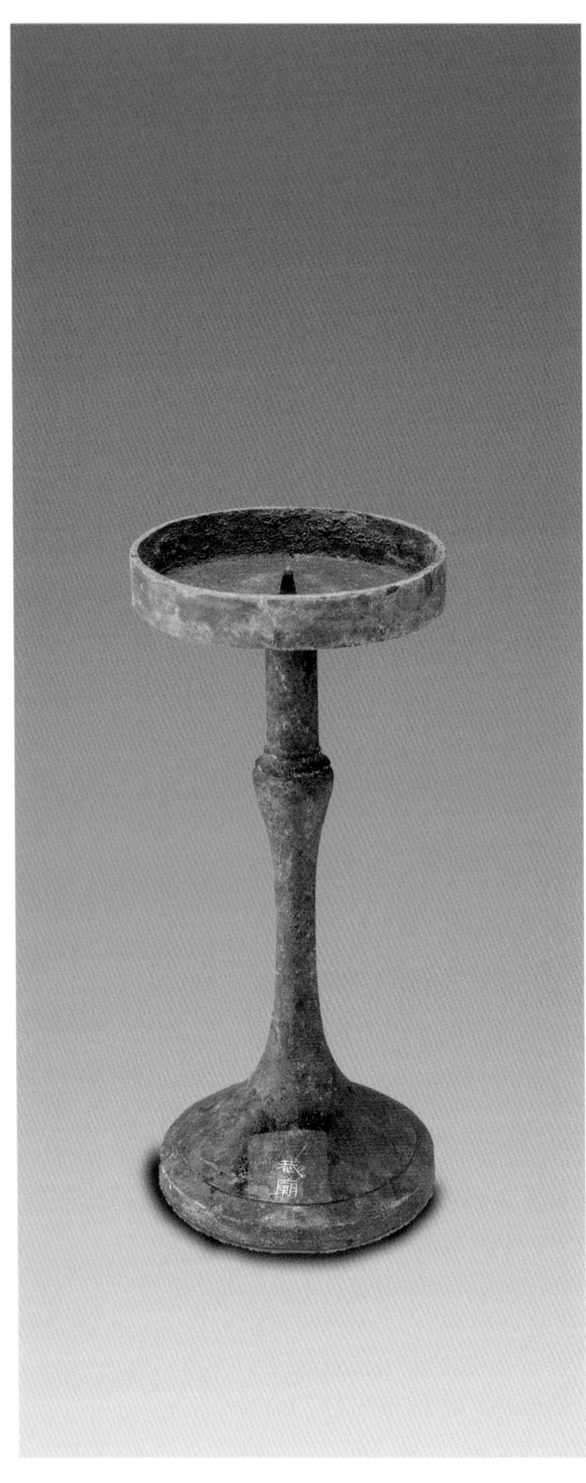

“恭庙”铜灯

西汉

铜质

灯盘直径 15.9 厘米，圈足直径 15.6 厘米，高 34.6 厘米

Gongmiao Copper Lamp

Western Han Dynasty

Copper

Tray Diameter 15.9 cm/ Diameter of the circular foot 15.6 cm/ Height 34.6 cm

灯盘直盘口，盘中心有一支钉。细高蒜头形柄，喇叭形圈足座。足面阴刻隶书“恭庙”二字，字体规整。该灯系广陵国祖庙内的祭祀用器。1985 年邗江杨寿镇李岗村宝女墩汉墓出土。

邗江区文物管理委员会藏

The lamp has a long bulb-like post, a trumpet-shaped pedestal with a circular foot and a tray with an upright mouth. There is a nail in the center of the tray. On the surface of the foot are two neatly-lettered characters "Gong Temple " cut in intaglio. The lamp is the ritual object used in ancestral temple in Guangling (today named Yangzhou). It was unearthed from Baonvdun Tomb (Han) in Ligang Village, Yangshou Town ship, Hanjiang District.

Preserved in Hanjiang District Administration Committee of Cultural Relics

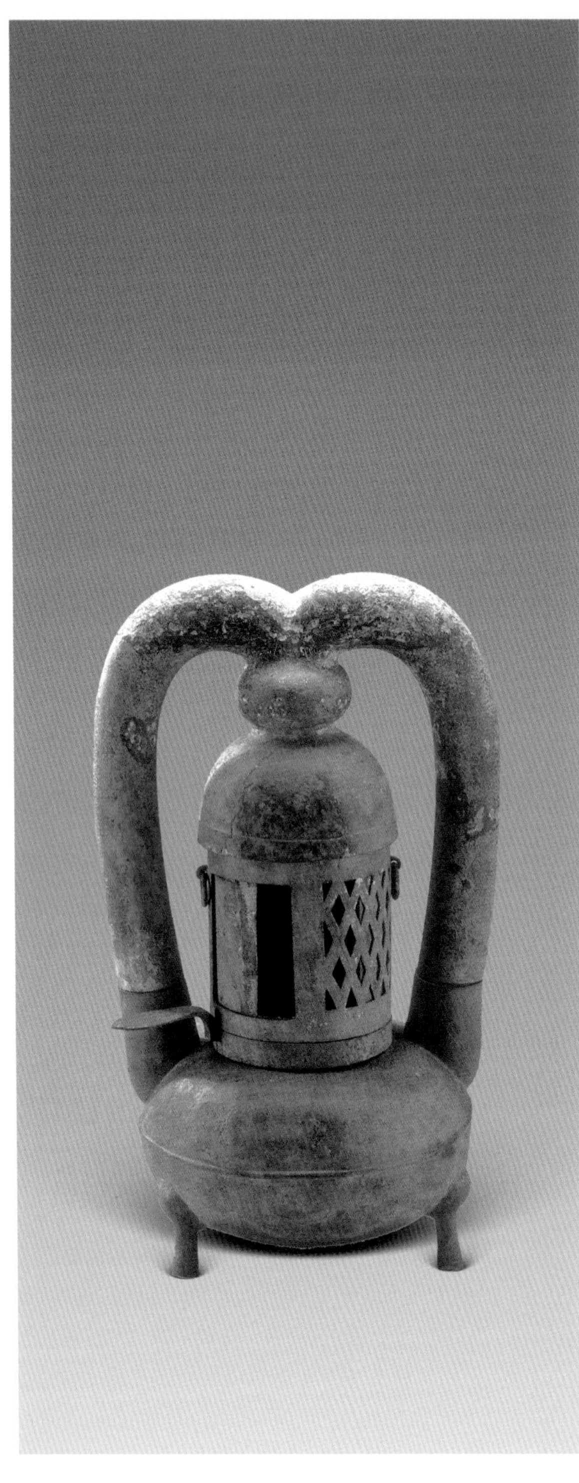

铜釭灯

西汉

铜质

宽 35 厘米，通高 58 厘米

Copper Oil Lamp

Western Han Dynasty

Copper

Width 35 cm/ Total Height 58 cm

此灯造型属鼎形釭灯类。全器由灯盘、双层灯罩、左右双导烟管和兼有底座与贮水消烟双重功能的三足釜形器四部分组成。在导烟管的两面各以阴线刻饰一条昂首爬升的蛟龙纹样。转动灯盘手柄，可使卡扣其上的内层灯罩的窗口在约150° 的范围内随意移位，以此增减通光量。导烟管可使灯汕芯或烛炬燃烧时的废气消融于釜形器内的水中，减轻了室内的污染。1991 年出土于邗江县甘泉乡姚湾村之巴家墩的一座木椁墓中，墓主当为西汉昭宣时期广陵国内有很高身份的贵族。

扬州博物馆藏

This tripod-shaped oil lamp consists of four parts, a tray, a double-layered lamp chimney, two smoke conduit pipes on both sides, and three-foot cauldron which could serve as the pedestal as well as the water reservoir for smoke abatement. Both sides of the conduit pipes are engraved with two strong climbing dragons in intaglio. The window on the inside layer of the lamp chimney could shift in the range of 150° to adjust the amount of light when the handle of the tray is moved. The conduit pipes help the water in the cauldron absorb the burnt gas, which could reduce the indoor pollution. The lamp was unearthed in a big wooden tomb in Bajiadun, Yanwan Village, Ganquan Township, Hanjiang County, which shows that the tomb owner was a noble with high status in Guangling during the period of the reign of Emperor Xuan and Zhao in the Western Han Dynasty.

Preserved in Yangzhou Museum

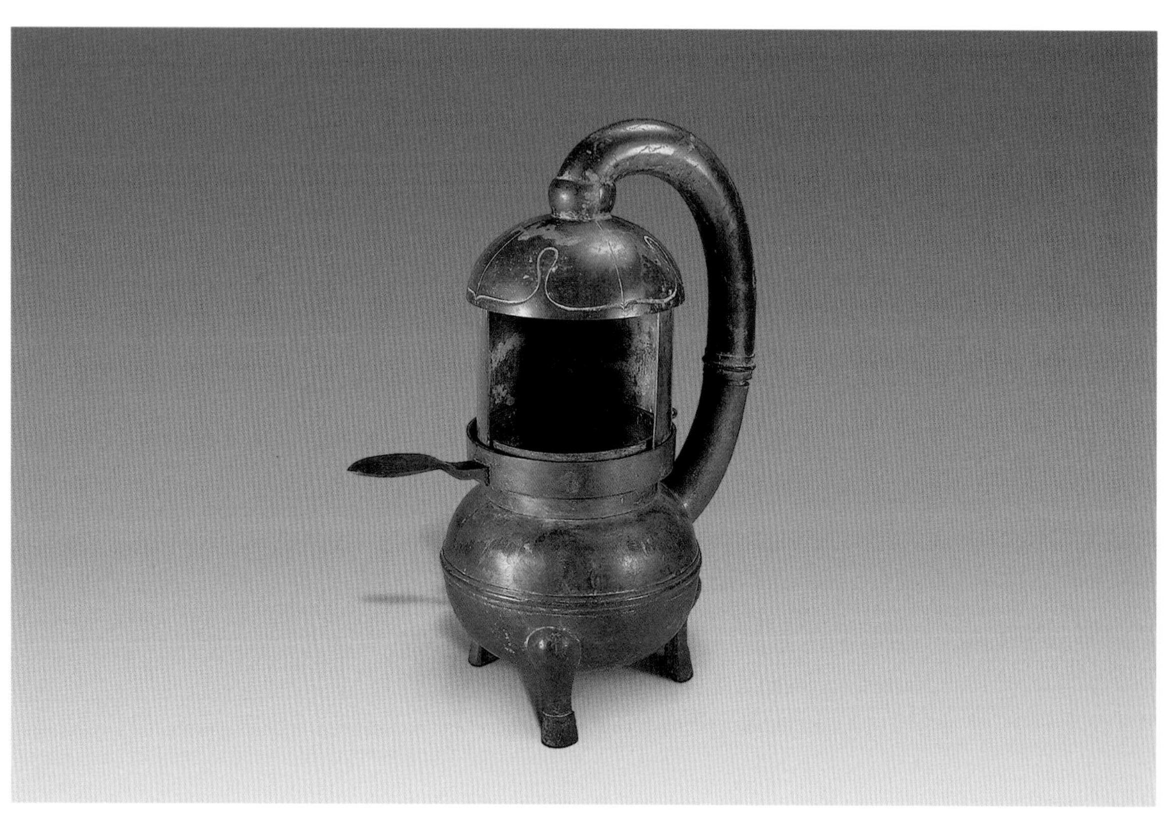

带罩铜灯

西汉

铜质

通高 33 厘米

Copper Lamp with Cover

Western Han Dynasty

Copper

Total Height 33 cm

器由三足空心炉、灯盘、灯罩、灯盖、烟道等部分构成。灯盘圈足套置于炉上。盘壁双重，灯罩屏板插于其间。灯盘外壁平伸叶形长鋬，用以移动灯盘。灯罩为弧形屏板，对称的两下角均有小钮，用来推移屏板。灯盘、灯罩的转动可随意调节灯光的亮度和方向。灯盖形如覆钵，置于灯罩屏板之上。盖顶伸出管形烟道，弯曲向下和三足炉身伸出之烟道扣合，整个烟道作灯把。灯的各部分均可拆卸。

河北博物院藏

The lamp constitutes a hollow censer with three feet, a tray, a chimney, a cover, and a pipe. The circular foot of the tray is harnessed to the censer. The screen board of the chimney plugs between two layers of tray wall. Stretching from the outer wall of the tray, the long leaf-shaped handle could control the movement of tray. In the symmetrical inferior angles of the arc chimney are small holes which are used to push the screen board. The brightness and the direction of light can be modulated by the rotation of the tray and the chimney. Standing on the screen board, the inverted-bowl-shaped cover extends a tube-like smoke pipe, which curls down and connects with pipes on the censer. The whole smoke pipes act as the handle and every part of the lamp is detachable.

Preserved in Hebei Museum

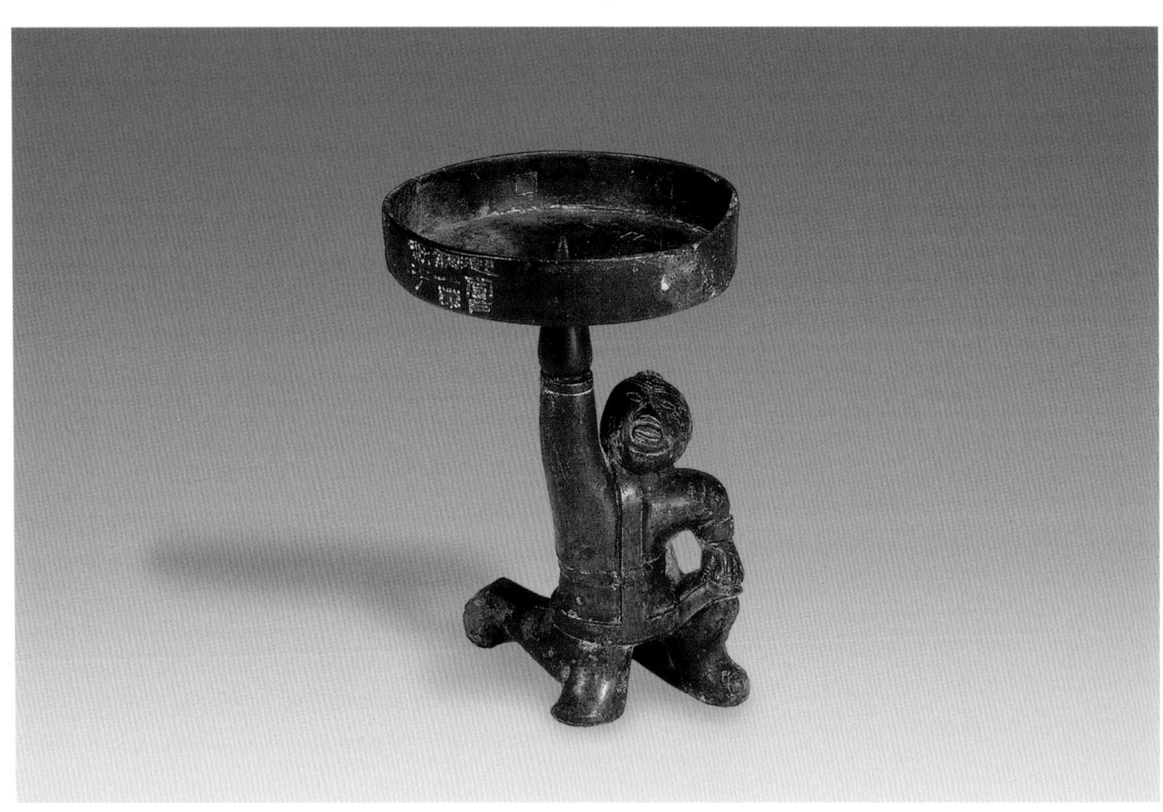

铜当户灯

西汉

铜质

灯盘径 8.5 厘米，通高 12 厘米

Copper Danghu Lamp

Western Han Dynasty

Copper

Tray Diameter 8.5 cm/ Total Height 12 cm

作铜俑半跪托灯状。俑昂首，右腿跪地，左手按左膝，右手上举承托灯盘。灯盘直口，直壁，平底，盘心有烛扦。盘、俑分铸，在俑右臂上用铜钉铆合。铜俑身着胡服，短衣直襟左袒，衣后部束成长尾状拖曳于地，以支持灯座不致倾倒。手有臂褠，脚着长靴。为匈奴官吏形象。灯盘壁刻有铭文“御当户锭一，第然于”八字。

河北博物院藏

The lamp tray has an upright mouth, a vertical wall, a flat base, and a candle stick standing in the center. Holding up the lamp, the bronze warrior kneels down on his right foot and raises his head with his left hand on the left knee. Casted respectively, the figurine and the tray are riveted together by the bronze nail at the right arm of the figurine. The bronze warrior wears Hu clothes with short tops and a straight front garment and naked left shoulder. The clothes are bundled up at the rear of the bronze warrior and tail down to the ground to balance the lamp. His hands wear arm cover and his feet puts on thigh boots. The figurine was an image of governmental official in Hu (an ancient nationality in China). The inscription engraved on the tray records that this lamp is an imperial souvenir for the peace between Han and Hua.

Preserved in Hebei Museum

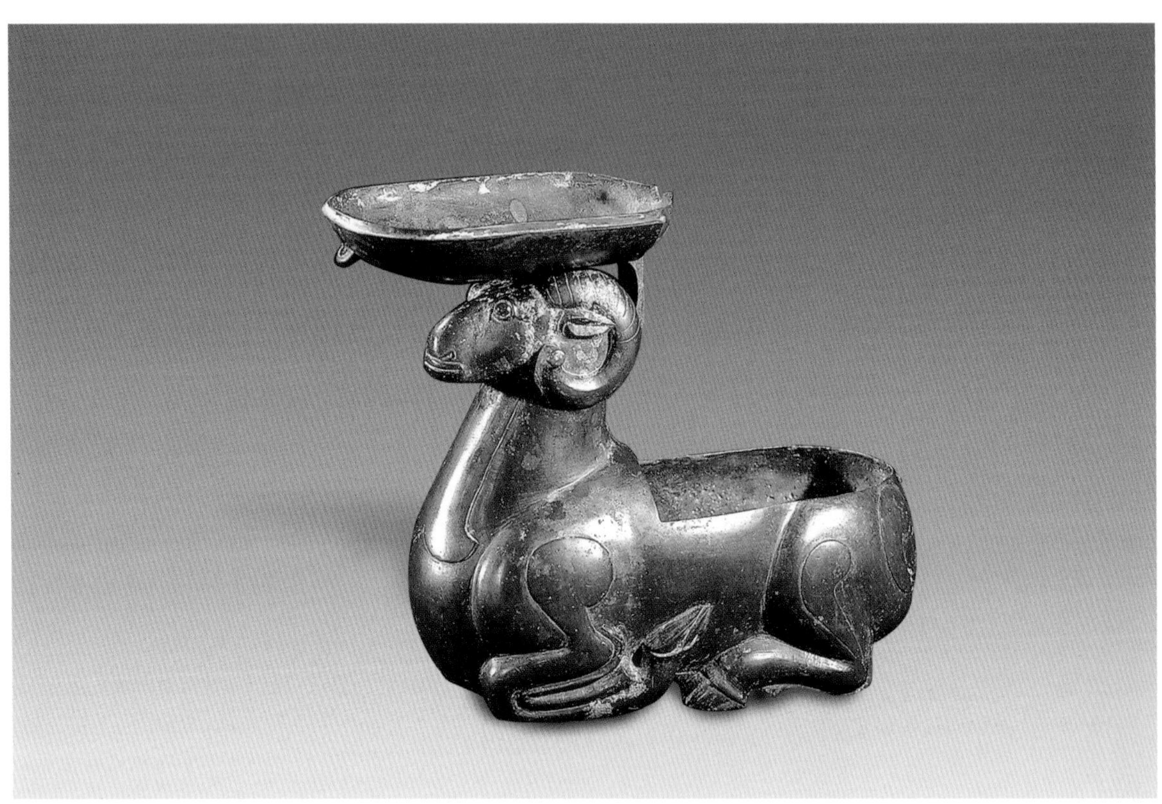

铜羊尊灯

西汉

铜质

长 23 厘米，通高 18.6 厘米

Copper Sheep-shaped Square Lamp

Western Han Dynasty

Copper

Length 23 cm/ Total Height 18.6 cm

灯作卧羊形。羊昂首，双角卷曲，身躯浑圆，短尾。羊背和身躯分铸，颈后置活钮，可将羊背向上翻开，平放于羊头上作为灯盘。灯盘为椭圆形，子口，一端有小流嘴。羊腹中空，用以储油，出土时腹腔内残留有含油脂成分的白色沉积物。

河北博物院藏

The lamp takes the shape of a crouched sheep with rising head, curled horns, a chubby belly, and a short tail. The back and the body are casted respectively. The back could be lifted upside down when the knob on the neck is moved. The oval-shaped tray has a matching mouth with a small spout. The sheep belly is hollowed out for storing the oil. The lamp was unearthed with some white deposit left in the abdominal cavity which may contain fat or oil.

Preserved in Hebei Museum

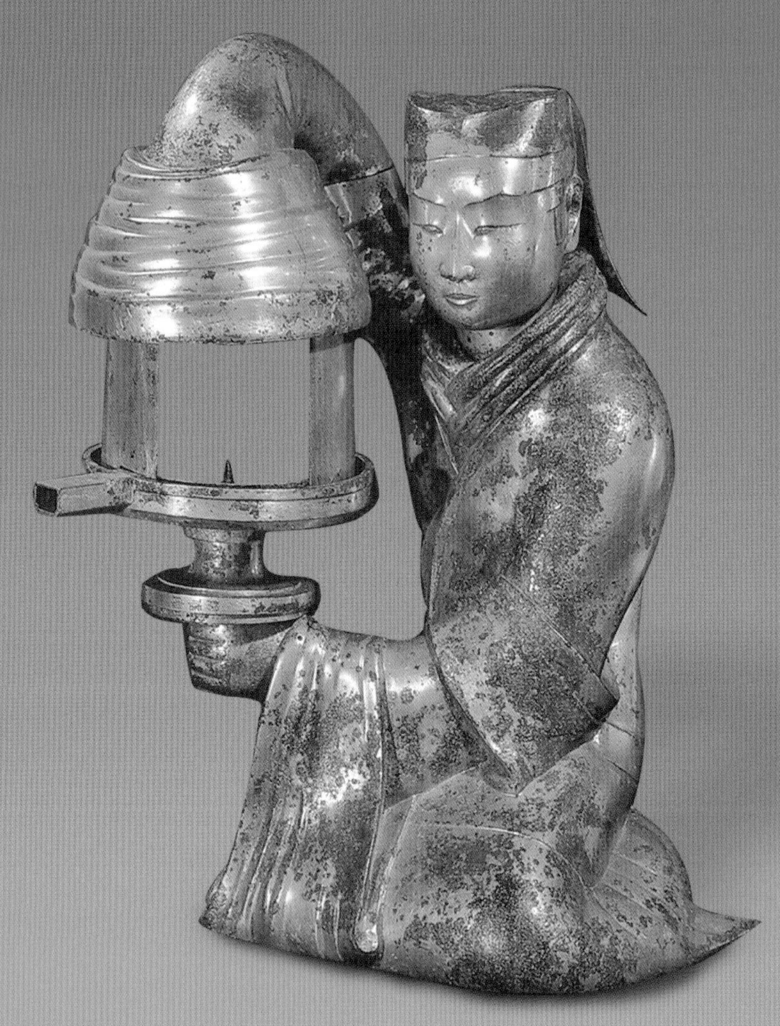

长信宫灯

西汉

铜质

通高 48 厘米

Changxin Palace Lamp

Western Han Dynasty

Copper

Total Height 48 cm

通体鎏金，作宫女跪坐执灯形象。宫女梳髻覆帼，着深衣，跣足。由头部、身躯、右臂、灯座、灯盘、灯罩等部分组成。各部分可拆卸，灯盘可转动，灯罩可开合。宫女体臂中空，右臂为烟道，可将灯烟导入器内，以保持室内清洁。灯上刻铭文九处，内容包括灯的重量、容量、铸造时间和所有者等。因刻有“长信尚浴”字样，故名长信宫灯。

河北博物院藏

The gilded lamp takes the shape of a kneeling court maid who holds a lamp. The barefooted maid wears a suit of dark clothes with hair covered with a kerchief. The lamp consists of a head, a body, a right arm, a pedestal, a tray, and a chimney. Every part is detachable: the tray is movable and the chimney is free to open or close. The hollowed arm of the maid is the conduit pipe which can lead the smoke to the body cavity, thus keeping interior clean. There are inscriptions engraved on nine places of the lamp, which record the weight, the volume, the casting time, and the owner of the lamp. According to the inscription, the lamp was used in Changxin Palace and thus named Changxin.

Preserve in Hebei Museum

華

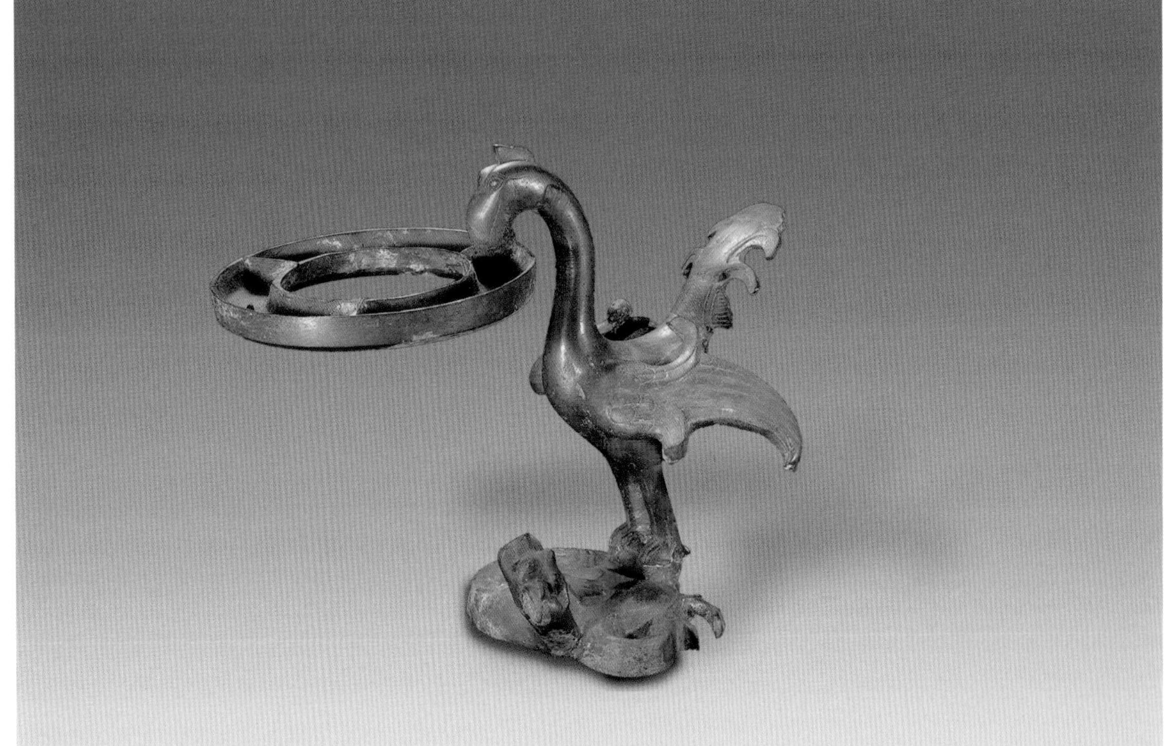

朱雀灯

西汉

铜质

盘径 19 厘米，通高 30 厘米

Rosefinch Lamp

Western Han Dynasty

Copper

Tray Diameter 19 cm/ Total Height 30 cm

朱雀昂首翘尾，脚踏蟠龙，口衔灯盘，做展翅欲飞状。灯盘为环状凹槽，内分三格，各有烛扦一个。灯座为一蟠龙，龙首昂起。

河北博物院藏

Biting the tray, the rosefinch, with its head and tail extending upwards. treads on the curled dragon and spread its wings to fly. The indented circular tray is divided into three cells with a candle stick in each one. The pedestal takes the shape of a curled dragon who is holding up its head.

Preserved in Hebei Museum

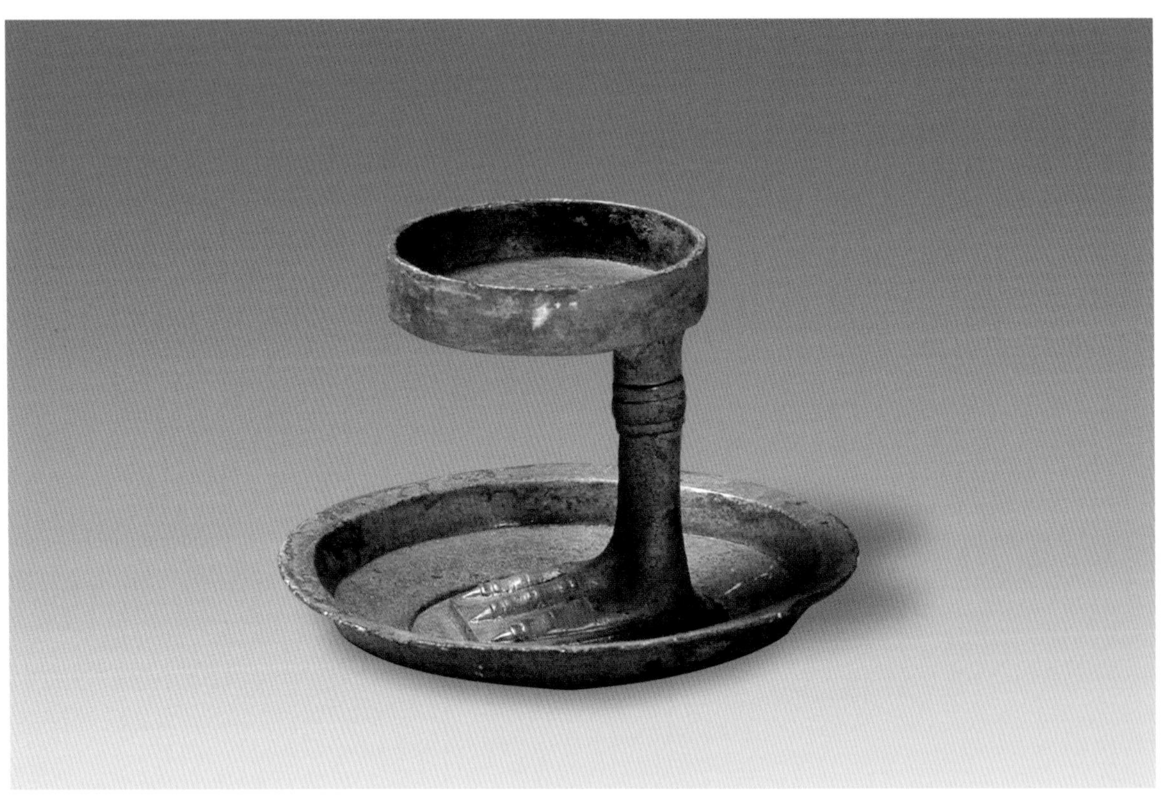

青铜雁足灯

东汉

青铜质

通高 10.2 厘米

Bronze Lamp with Wild Goose's feet

Eastern Han Dynasty

Bronze

Total Height 10.2 cm

圆盘形底座内立一雁足支撑，其上承托小盘的底，雁足承柱与盏盘为一次浇铸，底座下用铜铆钉与承柱连成一体。

高淳区文物保管所藏

Taking the shape of the feet of a wild goose, the post stands in the plate-shaped pedestal and holds the base of the little tray. The post and the tray were both casted at a time. The pedestal was riveted to the post with the bronze nail.

Preserved in Cultural Relics Preservation of Gaochun

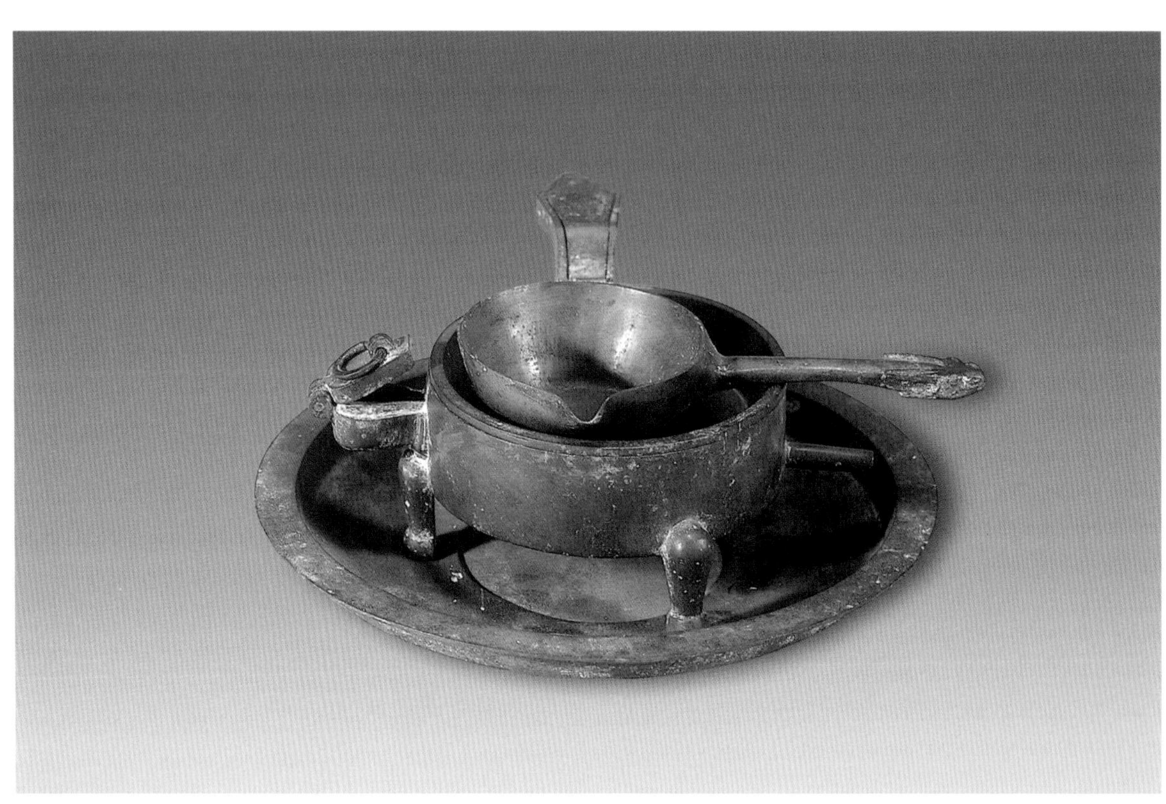

青铜组合灯

西汉

青铜质

灯身径 9.6 厘米，通高 7 厘米

承盘口径 18.6 厘米，高 2.4 厘米

小勺口径 6.6 厘米，把长 7.1 厘米，高 2.7 厘米

Bronze Combined Lamp

Western Han Dynasty

Bronze

Lamp: Body Diameter 9.6 cm/ Total Height 7 cm

Tray: Diameter 18.6 cm/ Height 2.4 cm

Spoon: Caliber 6.6 cm/ Handle Length 7.1 cm/ Height 2.7 cm

由灯、承盘、小勺三器组成。灯为直壁，浅腹，平底，三蹄形足，器壁一侧有一小嘴，作子口，嘴上有带环纽的小盖；另一侧下方有一管状流。在嘴、流间的器壁上方伸出一菱形长鋬，鋬上有槽。盖呈盘形，口侧伸出一较小的菱形鋬，恰好纳入灯身长鋬的凹槽中。灯下有敞口折腹承盘。小勺为大口，小平底，一侧有小流嘴，龙首形长把。

河北博物院藏

The relic constitutes three parts: a lamp, a tray, and a small spoon. The lamp has a vertical wall, a shallow belly, a flat base, and three horseshoe-shaped feet. A small spout (which has a lid with a ring knob) is on one side of the wall and a tubular spout on the other side. On the wall between the mouth and spout is a long diamond-shaped handle with indentation, which fit the smaller handle stretching from the mouth of the plate-shaped lid. The tray under the lamp has an open mouth and a folded belly. The spoon has a big mouth, a small flat base, a small spout on one side, and a long handle in the form of dragon head.

Preserved in Hebei Museum

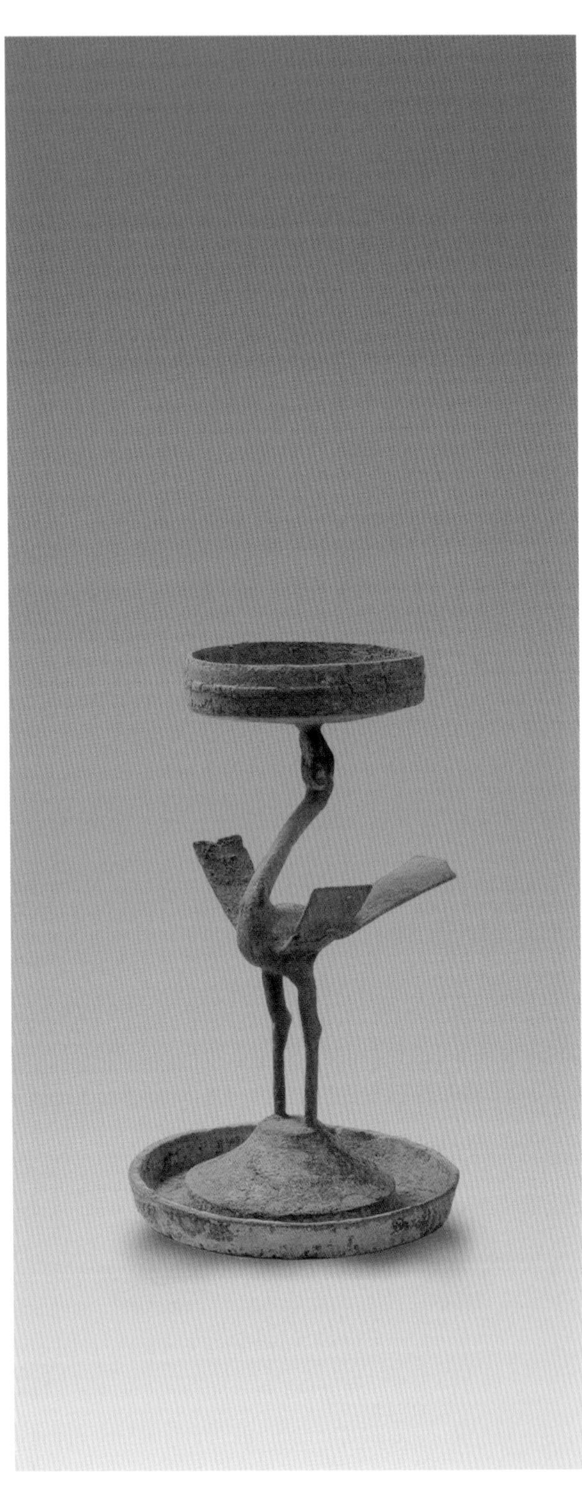

青铜朱雀灯

东汉

青铜质

底盘径 9.3 厘米，灯盏径 6.7 厘米，通高 16 厘米

Bronze Rosefinch Lamp

Eastern Han Dynasty

Bronze

Base Diameter 9.3 cm/ Tray Diameter 6.7 cm/ Total Height 16 cm

圆盘形底座，朱雀双足分开，立于盘心的圆锥形台座上。通体光素无纹，两翅伸展，尾翼翘起。朱雀引颈上扬，喙顶置一圆盘状灯盏，盏外沿饰弦纹一道。该青铜朱雀灯造型简洁生动，反映了汉代工匠高超的抽象思维和丰富的想象能力。

南京博物院藏

With two feet apart, the rosefinch stands on the center of the conical pedestal on the plate-shaped base. Spreading its wings, raising its tail, and craning its neck, the sacred bird holds a plate-shaped tray at the top of its beak. The edge of the plate is ornamented with a circle of string pattern. The concise and lively portrayal demonstrates the abstract thinking and imagination of the craftsman.

Preserved in Nanjing Museum

華

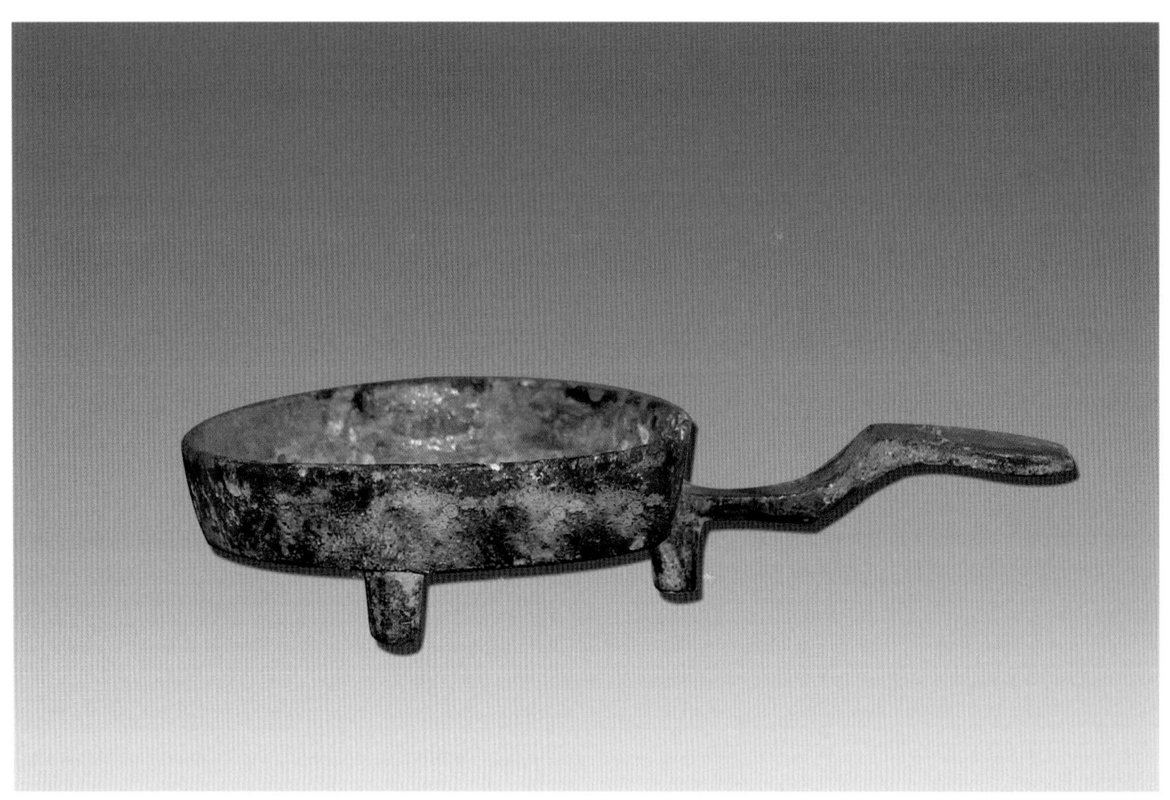

铜灯

汉

铜质

口径 9 厘米，底径 8.5 厘米，通高 3 厘米，重 200 克

Copper Lamp

Han Dynasty

Copper

Caliber 9 cm/ Base Diameter 8.5 cm/ Total Height 3 cm/ Weight 200 g

直口直腹，平底三足，有一勺形把，盘内有灯眼。生活用器。完整无损。陕西省咸阳市征集。

陕西医史博物馆藏

The lamp has an upright mouth, an upright belly, a flat base, three feet, and a spoon-shaped handle. There is a wick in the tray. This household article is intact. It was collected from Xianyang, Shaanxi Province.

Preserved in Shaanxi Museum of Medical History

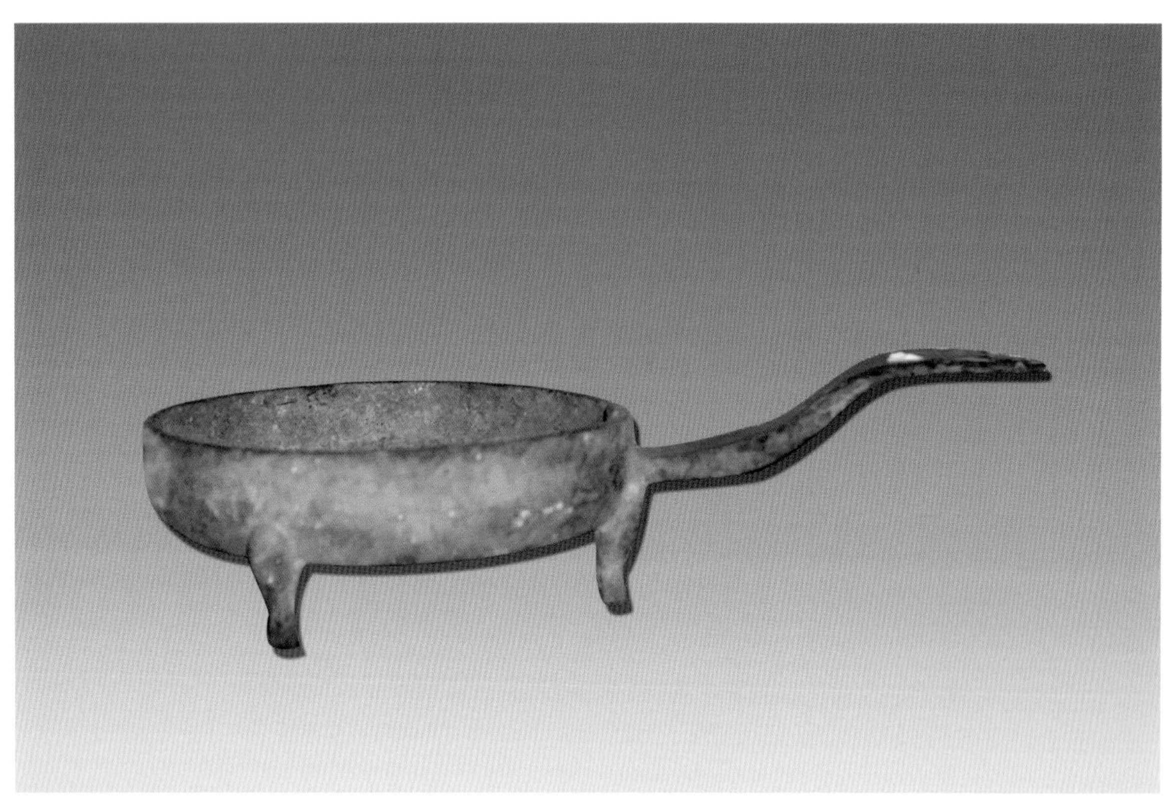

铜灯

汉

铜质

口径 14 厘米，底径 13 厘米，通高 5.5 厘米，重 900 克

Copper Lamp

Han Dynasty

Copper

Caliber 14 cm/ Base Diameter 13 cm/ Total Height 5.5 cm/ Weight 900 g

直口直腹，平底三兽足，腹上有勺形把。生活用器。完整无损。陕西省咸阳市征集。

陕西医史博物馆藏

The lamp has an upright mouth, an upright belly, a flat base, three animal-shaped feet, and a spoon-shaped handle attached to the belly. This household article is intact. It was collected in Xianyang, Shaanxi Province.

Preserved in Shaanxi Museum of Medical History

華

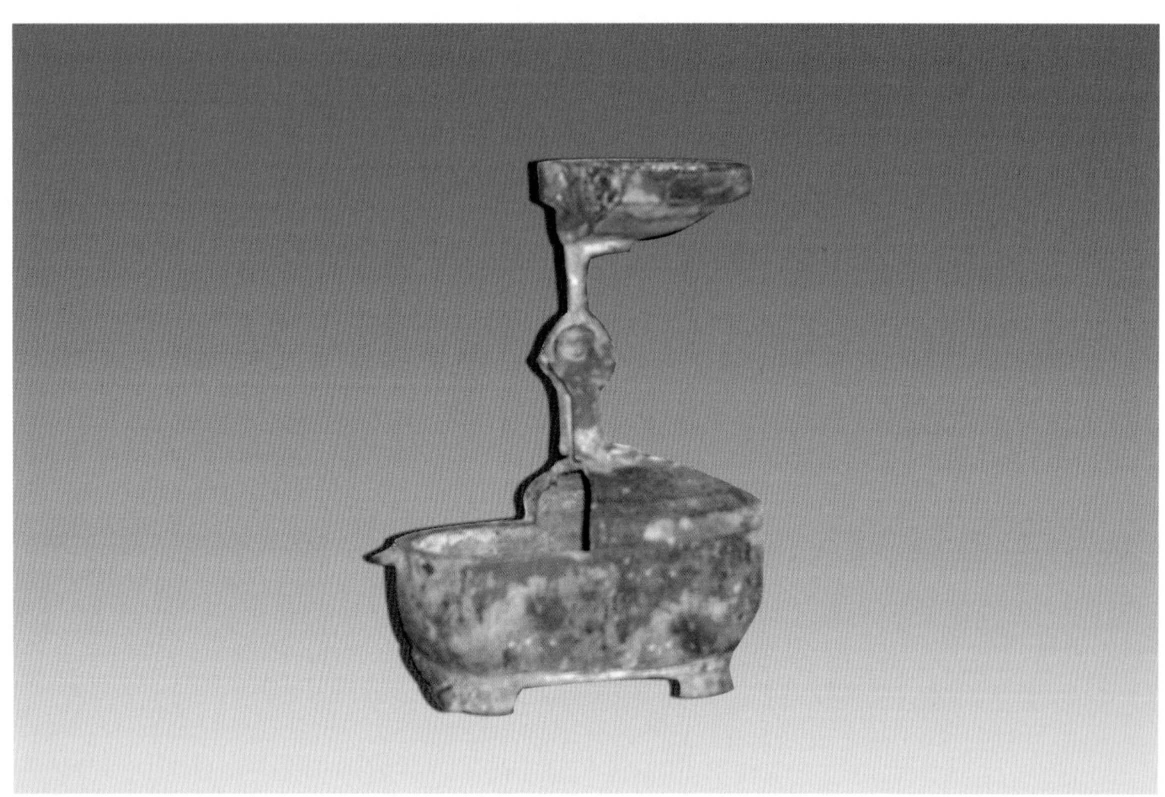

铜盒子灯

汉

铜质

口径 13 厘米，底径 7.2 厘米，通高 16 厘米，重 500 克

Copper Box-shaped Lamp

Han Dynasty

Copper

Caliber 13 cm/ Base Diameter 7.2 cm/ Total Height 16 cm/ Weight 500 g

椭圆盒状，腹为长形，圆腹，两个马蹄形座有三乳丁。生活用器。三级。完整无损。1965年入藏。陕西省历史博物馆调拨。

陕西医史博物馆藏

Taking the shape of an oval box, the lamp has a circular rectangular belly and two horseshoe-shaped pedestals with three nipple nails. This household article is still in good condition. It was collected in 1965 and allocated by Shaanxi History Museum.

Preserved in Shaanxi Museum of Medical History

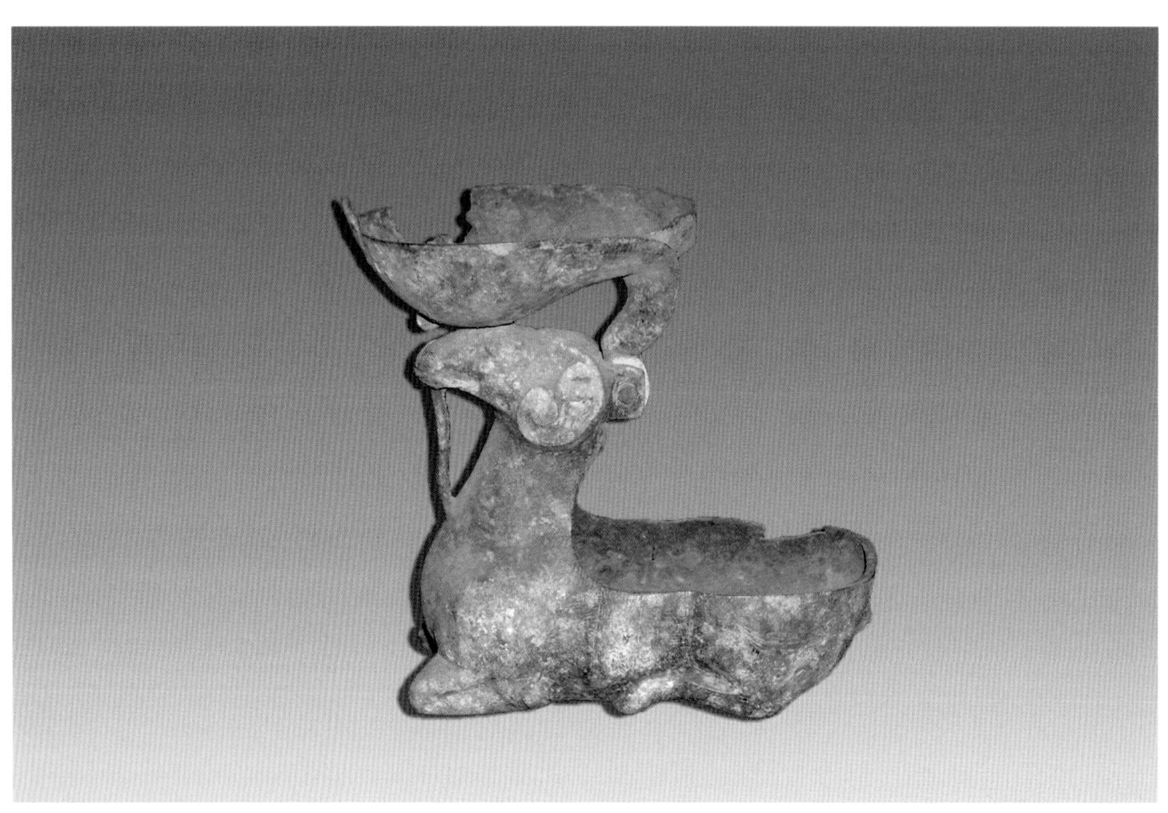

铜羊灯

汉

铜质

长 13.8 厘米，通高 13 厘米，重 300 克

Copper Sheep-shaped Lamp

Han Dynasty

Copper

Length 13.8 cm/ Height 13 cm/ Weight 300 g

一卧羊状，羊背有一盖，翻上为一灯盘。生活用器。三级。完整无损。陕西省西安市征集。

陕西医史博物馆藏

The lamp takes the shape of a crouched sheep. The lid on the back of sheep can be turned over as the lamp tray. This household article is intact and was collected from Xi'an, Shaanxi Province.

Preserved in Shaanxi Museum of Medical History

華

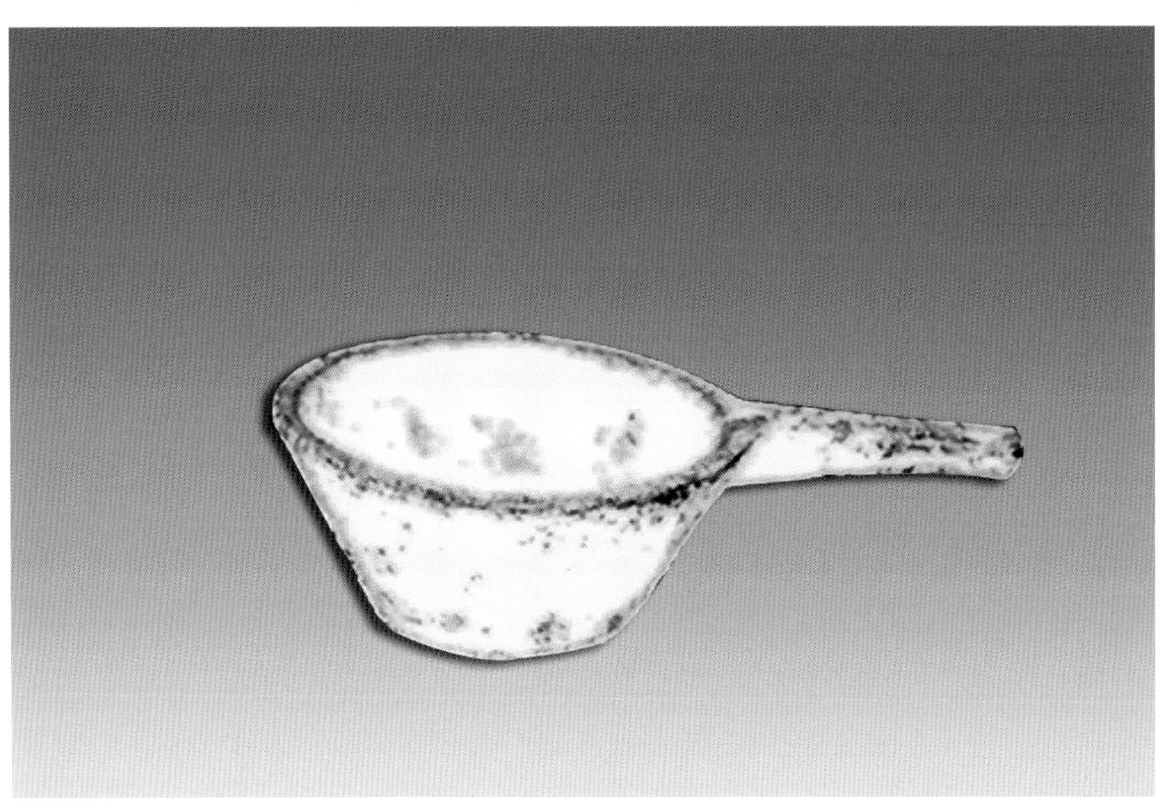

铜量

汉

铜质

口径 2.7 厘米，底径 1.5 厘米，通长 4.2 厘米，通高 1.1 厘米，重 9.5 克

Copper Measuring Tool

Han Dynasty

Copper

Caliber 2.7 cm/ Base Diameter 1.5 cm/ Length 4.2 cm/ Total Height 1.1 cm/ Weight 9.5 g

侈口，平底，斜腹，口沿处连接一把。量器。完整无损。陕西省咸阳市征集。

陕西医史博物馆藏

The measuring tool has a big mouth, a flat base, an oblique belly, and a handle attached to the mouth edge. This measuring tool was collected from Xianyang, Shaanxi Province and is still in good condition.

Preserved in Shaanxi Museum of Medical History

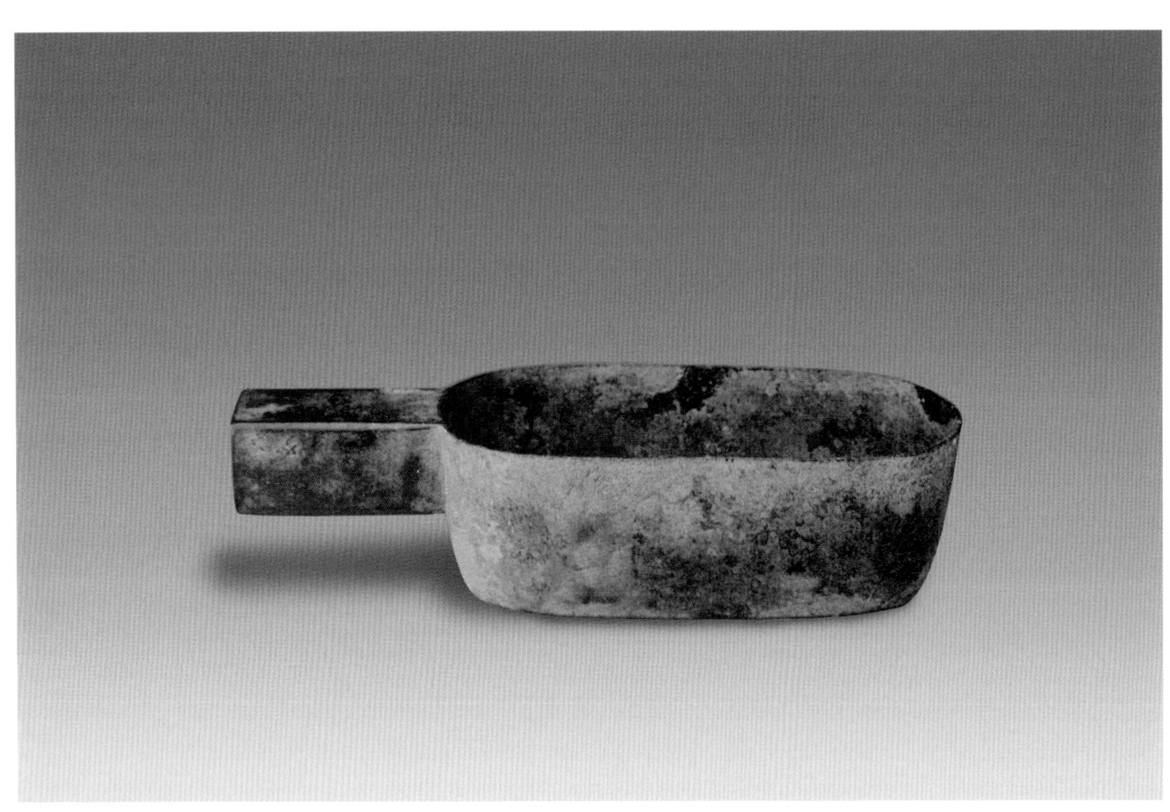

常方半椭量

汉

铜质

通长 20 厘米，宽 10 厘米，高 6.6 厘米

Oval-shaped Measuring Tool

Han Dynasty

Copper

Length 20 cm/ Width 10 cm/ Height 6.6 cm

量呈椭圆形，直口深腹，平底，口略大于底，一端有柄，柄作上平下弧的筒形。

山西博物院藏

This oval-shaped measuring tool has an upright mouth, a deep belly, a flat base, and a handle attached to the mouth edge. The mouth is a little larger than the base and the cylindrical handle is flat at the top but arc-like at the base.

Preserved in Shanxi Museum

華

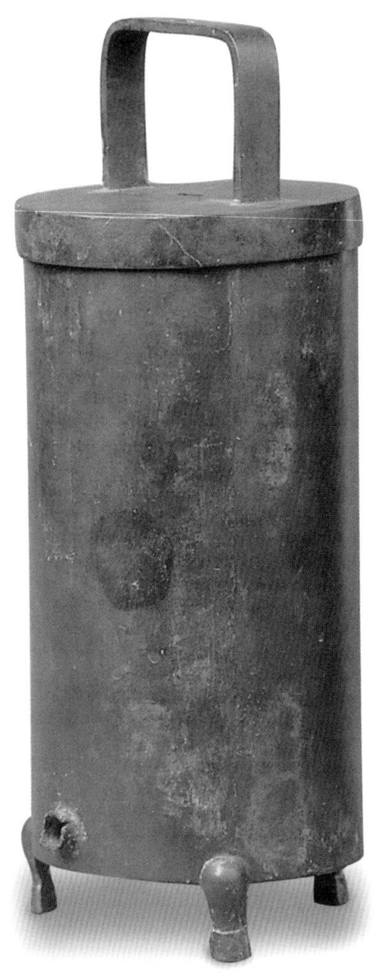

铜漏壶

西汉

铜质

腹径 8.6 厘米、通高 22.5 厘米，腹深 15.6 厘米

Copper Water Clock

Western Han Dynasty

Copper

Belly Diameter 8.6 cm/ Total Height 22.5 cm/ Belly Depth 15.6 cm

圆筒形，平底，三蹄足，近底部伸出细管状流口。壶身与盖紧密扣合。盖面平，中央有个 1 厘米 ×0.4 厘米的长方孔，盖上作长方形提梁，提梁中段也开有与盖孔相对，大小相同的孔。两孔可能是用于插置刻箭的，刻箭应属木质或竹质，立于壶中的舟上，随壶内盛水盈减而浮降，从而指示时辰。

河北博物院藏

This cylindrical water clock has a flat base, three horseshoe-shaped feet, and a tube-like spout extended from the base. The mouth is firmly buttoned with a flat lid. In the middle of the rectangular hoop handle is a 1×0.4 oblong-shaped hole which is the same size as the one in the center of the lid. Passing through two holes, the mark arrow made of wooden or bamboo can stand on the boat in the vessel. The arrow floats up or down according to the water level in the vessel and thus to indicate the time.

Preserved in Hebei Museum

華

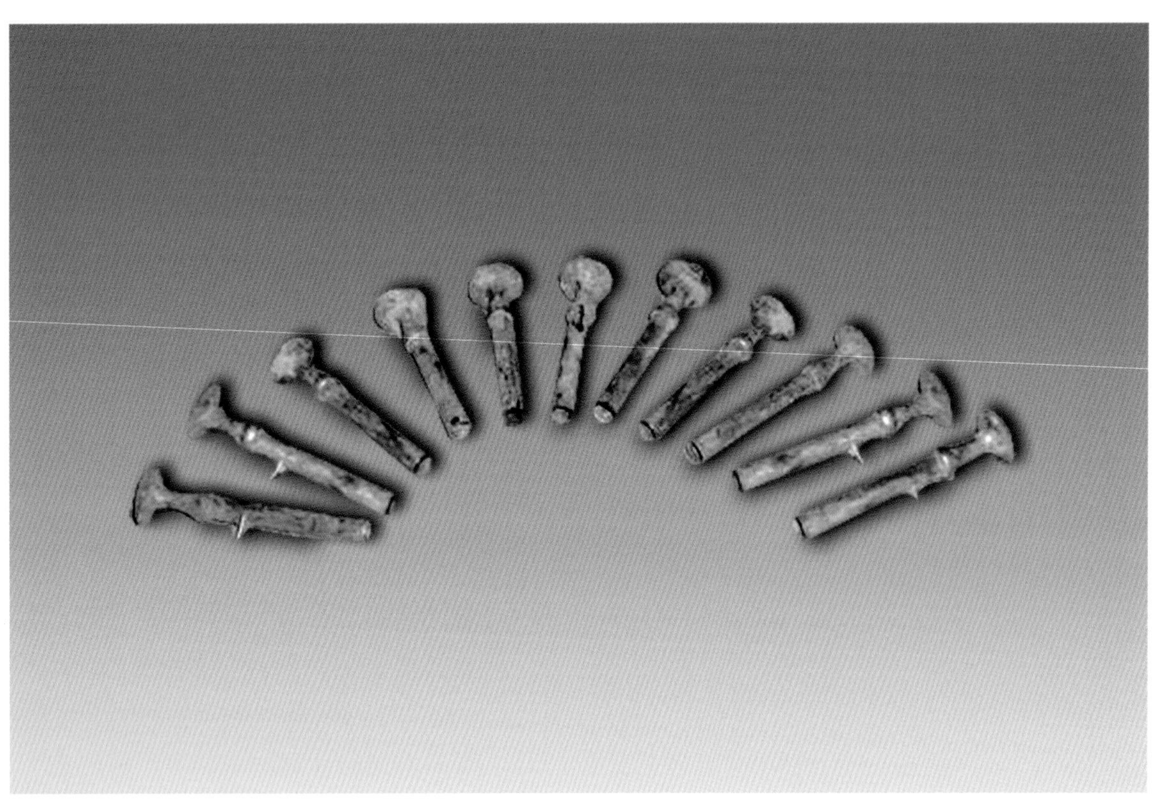

铜器插座

汉

铜质

高 7 厘米，底径 1.8 厘米，重 14 克

Copper Sockets

Han Dynasty

Copper

Height 7 cm/ Bottom diameter 1.8 cm/ Weight 14g

直口中腹下有一钩，底座呈喇叭状。车饰部件。完整无损。陕西省咸阳市废品站征集。

陕西医史博物馆藏

The sockets, intact and undamaged, are decoration parts for carriage. They have a hook in the middle and a trumpet-shaped base in the end. They were collected from a junk station in Xianyang of Shaanxi Province.

Preserved in Shaanxi Museum of Medical History

華

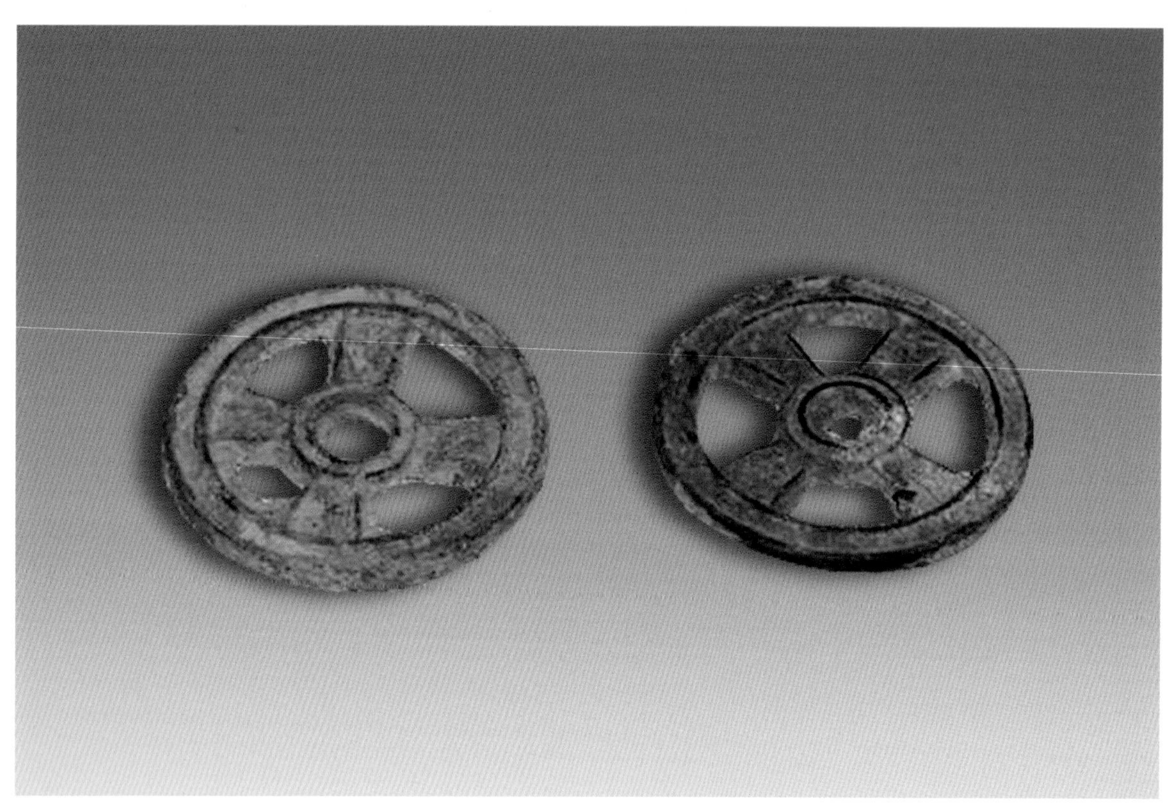

铜车饰

汉

铜质

直径 3.8 厘米，重 50 克

车轮形状。车饰部件。完整无损。

陕西医史博物馆藏

Copper Carriage Decoration

Han Dynasty

Copper

Diameter 3.8 cm/ Weight 50 g

The collections are in the shape of wheels. They are decorative parts for carriage and undamaged.

Preserved in Shaanxi Museum of Medical History

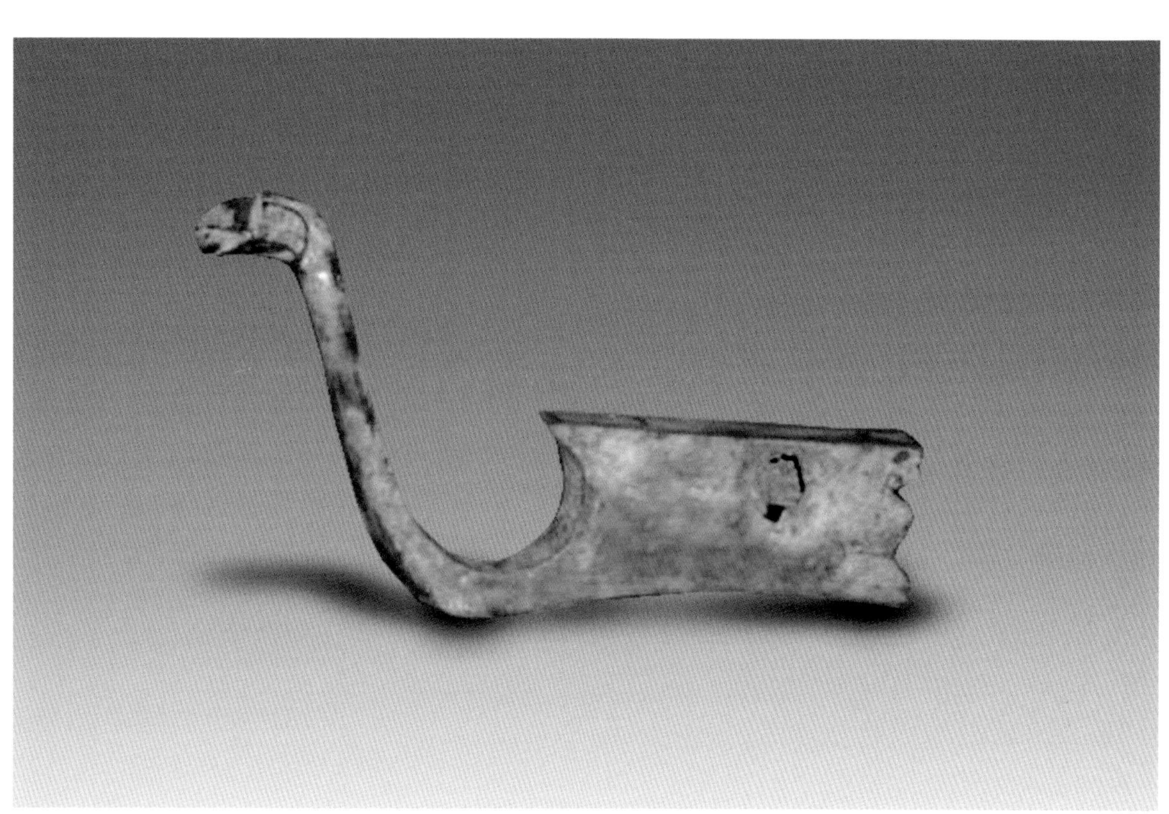

铜车饰

汉

铜质

长 22.5 厘米，宽 3 厘米，底径 14.5 厘米，重 600 克

骆驼头状，身为长方形，尾巴有一孔。车饰。腹有二小孔。陕西省咸阳市征集。

陕西医史博物馆藏

Copper Carriage Decoration

Han Dynasty

Copper

Length 22.5 cm/ Width 3 cm/ Bottom diameter 14.5 cm/ Weight 600 g

This collection is a decorative component for carriage. It is camel-shaped with a hole in its tail part. The body part is rectangular with two holes in it. It was collected from Xianyang of Shaanxi Province.

Preserved in Shaanxi Museum of Medical History

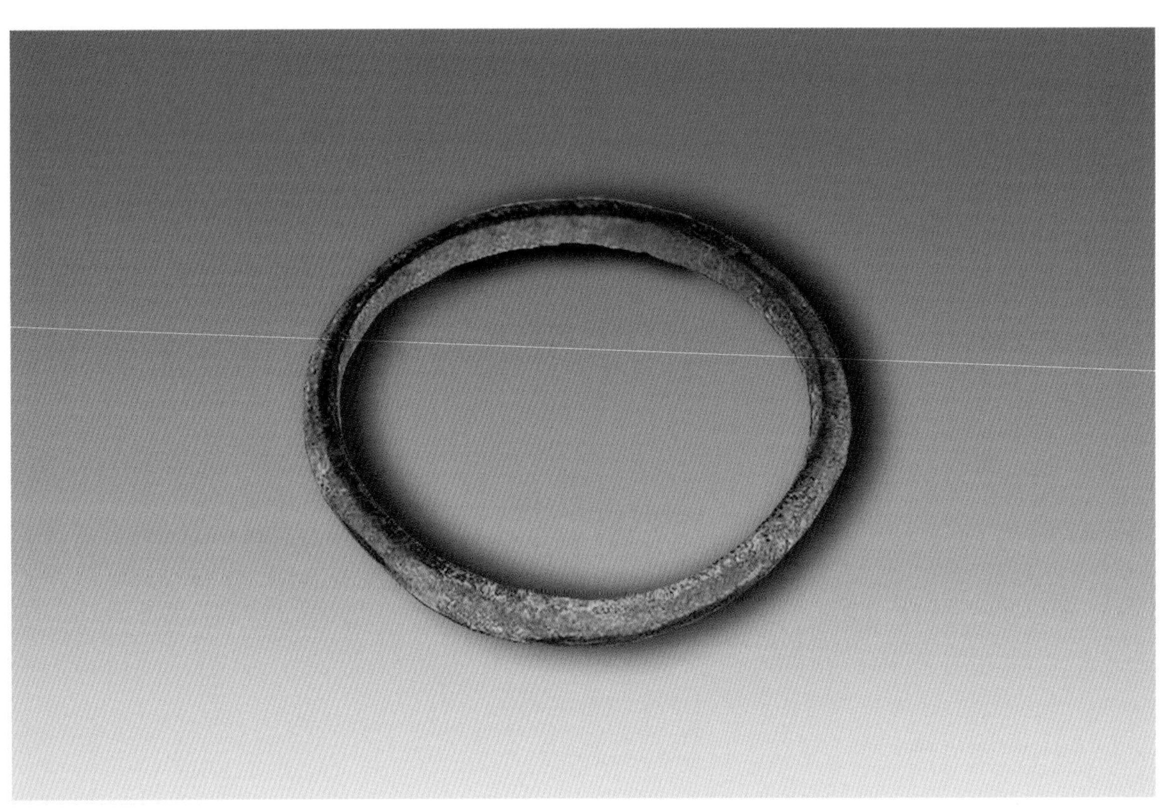

铜车环

汉

铜质

直径 6 厘米，重 30 克

圆环状。车饰部件。完整无损。

陕西医史博物馆藏

Copper Carriage Ring

Han Dynasty

Copper

Diameter 6 cm/ Weight 30 g

This ring, undamaged and circular, is a decorative component for carriage.

Preserved in Shaanxi Museum of Medical History

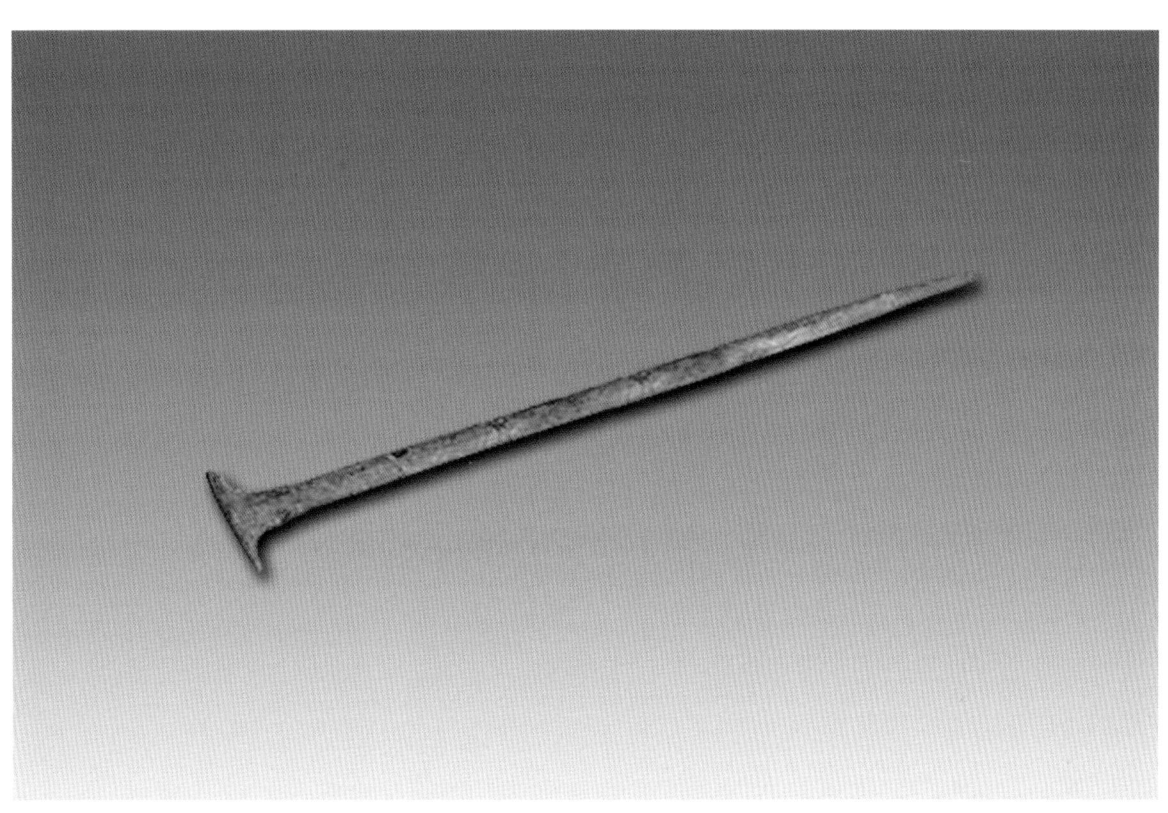

铜尖器

汉

铜质

长 21.7 厘米，头宽 4 厘米

锥状，一端为尖形，一端为平形。用途不详，完整无损。陕西中医药大学蒋志坚老师捐赠。

陕西医史博物馆藏

Copper Pointed Instrument

Han Dynasty

Copper

Length 21.7 cm/ Head diameter 4 cm

This instrument, in the shape of an awl, is pointed at one end and flat at the other. Its usage is unknown. It is intact and undamaged. It was donated by Jiang Zhijian, a teacher in Shaanxi University of Chinese Medicine.

Preserved in Shaanxi Museum of Medical History

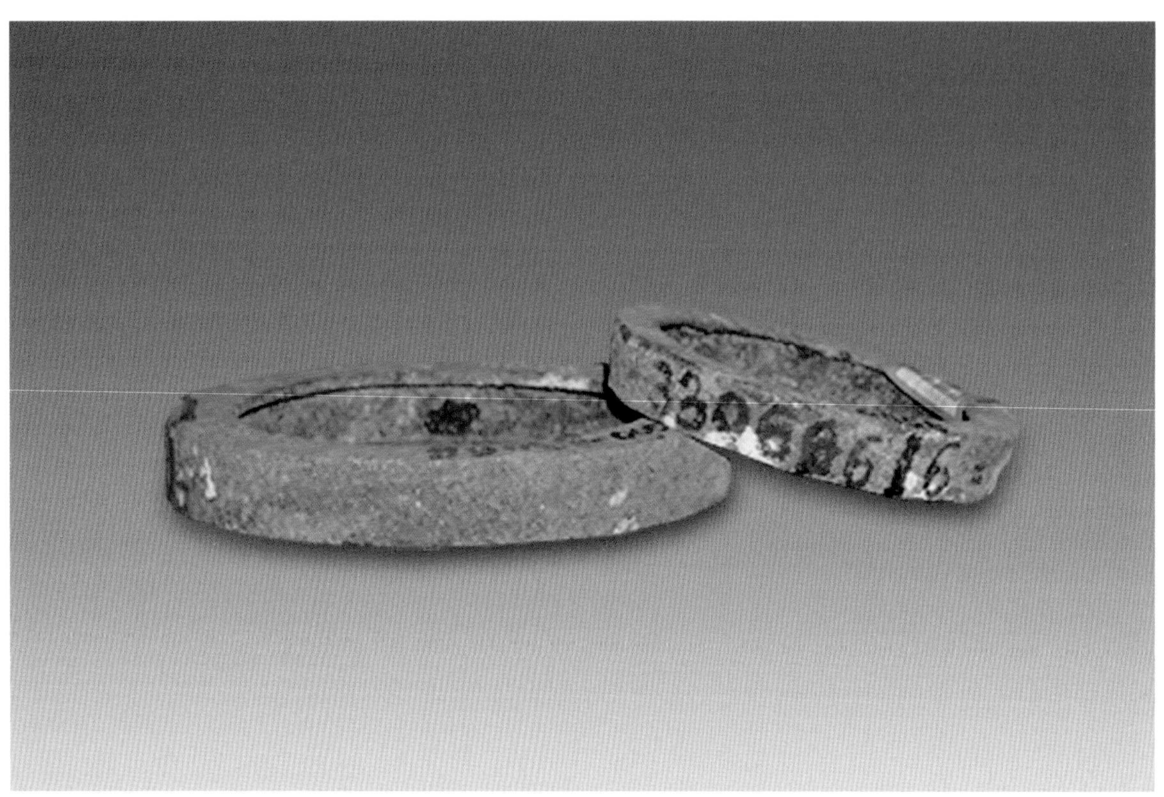

铜器物口

汉

铜质

口径 11.5 厘米，底径 11.5 厘米，通高 7.8 厘米，重 300 克

Copper Vessel Rims

Han Dynasty

Copper

Cup Diameter 11.5 cm/ Bottom Diameter 11.5 cm/ Height 7.8 cm/ Weight 300 g

圆圈状，一个大圈，一个小圈。完整无损。陕西省西安市边家村征集。

陕西医史博物馆藏

The rims, intact and undamaged, are Circular. One is small and the other is big. They were collected from Bianjia Village in Xi’an of Shaanxi Province.

Preserved in Shaanxi Museum of Medical History

華

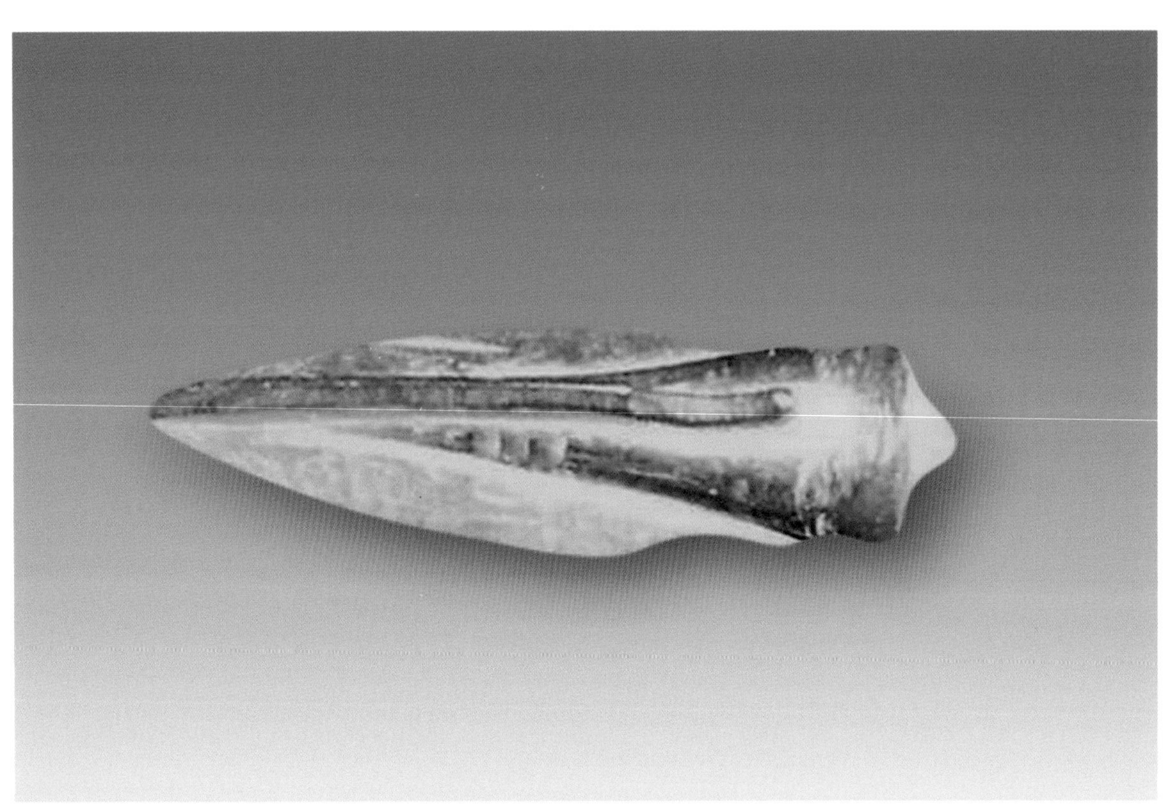

铜箭镞

汉

铜质

长 3.6 厘米，重 8 克

Copper Arrowhead

Han Dynasty

Copper

Length 3.6 cm/ Weight 8 g

三棱形。兵器。完整无损。内蒙古自治区东胜征集。

陕西医史博物馆藏

The arrowhead is a trigonous weapon. It is intact and undamaged. It was collected from Dongsheng District of Inner Mongolia Autonomous Region.

Preserved in Shaanxi Museum of Medical History

華

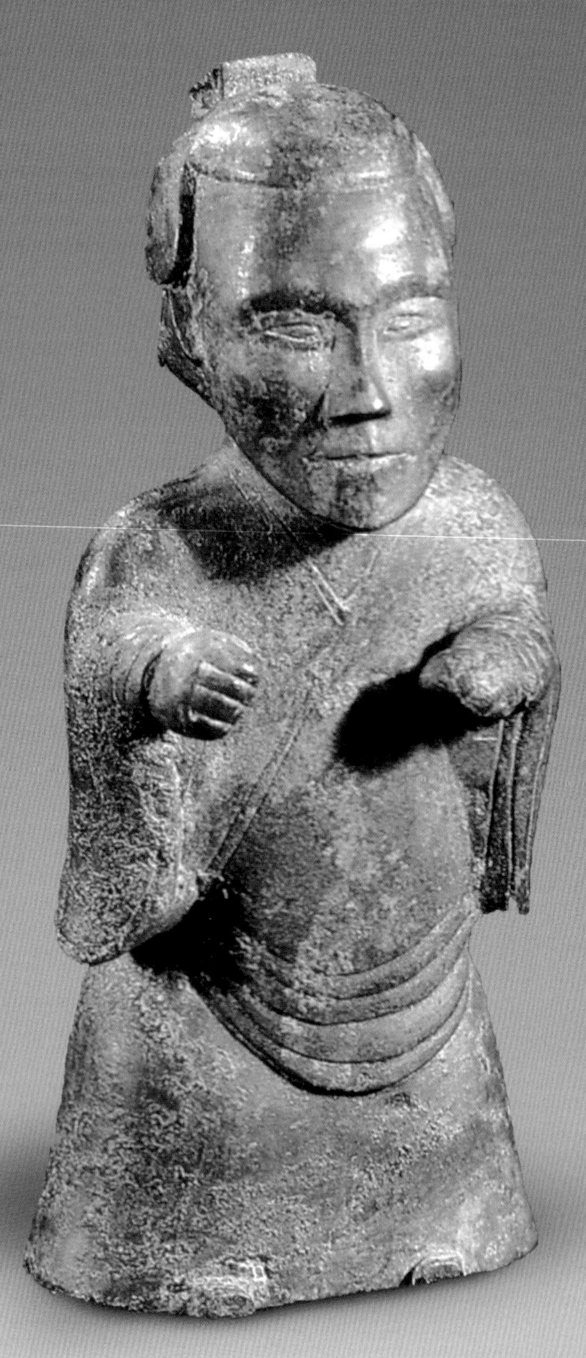

铜人俑

西汉

铜质

高 15.4 厘米

作立姿，高鼻，尖下颏，脑后挽发髻，上覆“缁撮”类小冠。身着交领右衽长衣，宽袖，两短臂抬起作持物状，下身短。

河北博物院藏

Bronze Figurine

Western Han Dynasty

Copper

Height 15.4 cm

The figurine is in the standing posture with a high nose and sharp chins. The hair bun overlying with a small black cloth-made crown is pulled at the back of the head. The figurine wears cross collar left lapel with full sleeves. The two short arms uplift for holding objects. The lower part of the body is short.

Preserved in Hebei Museum

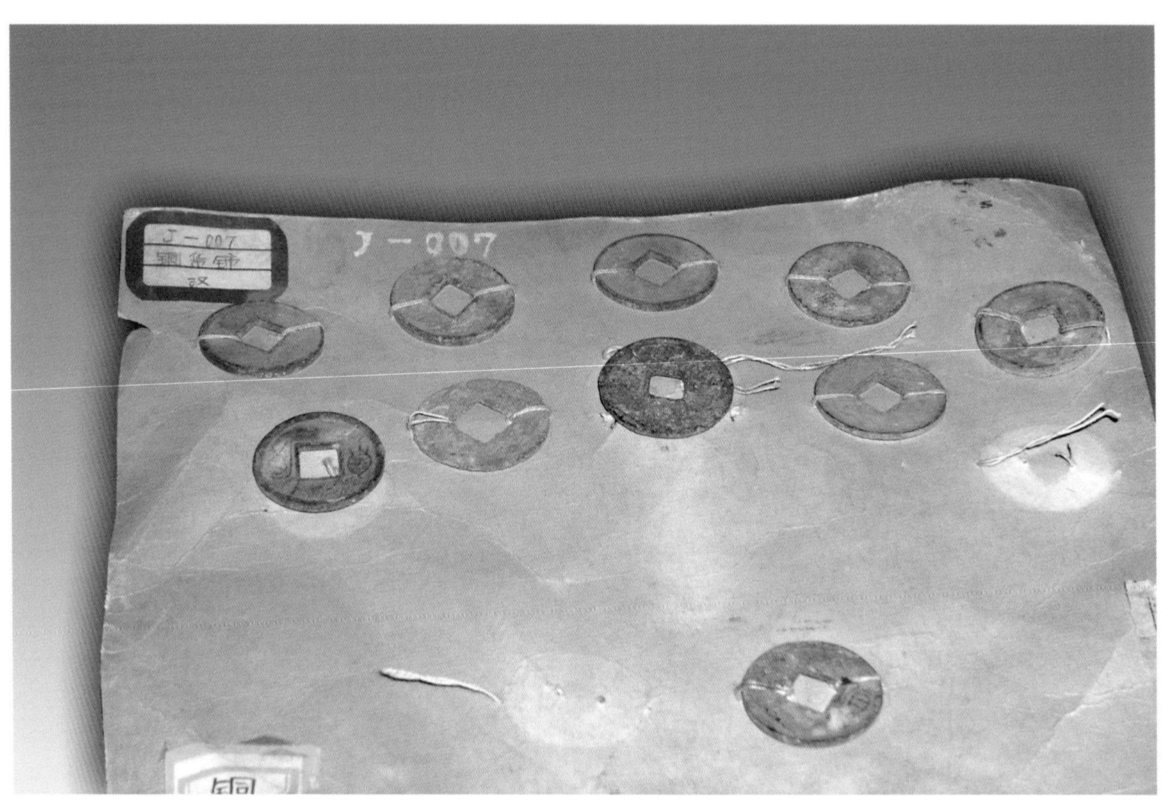

铜货币

汉代

铜质

直径 2.4 厘米，重 10 克

圆钱。货币。完整无损。陕西省博物馆调拨。

陕西医史博物馆藏

Copper Coins

Han Dynasty

Copper

Diameter 2.4 cm/ Weight 10 g

These coins, undamaged, are a round currency allotted from Shaanxi History Museum.

Preserved in Shaanxi Museum of Medical History

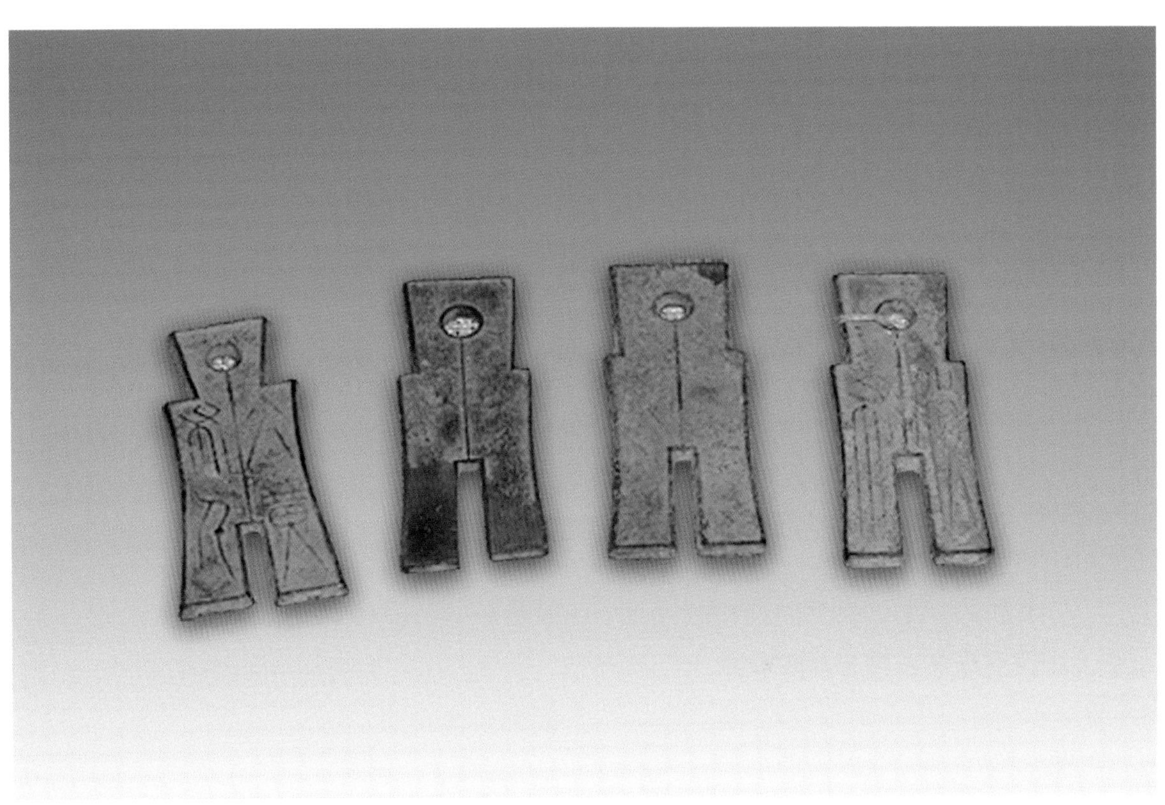

铜货币

新莽

铜质

长 6 厘米，宽 2.1 厘米，重 100 克

刀状。货币。完整无损。

陕西医史博物馆藏

Copper Coins

Xinmang period

Copper

Length 6 cm/ Width 2.1 cm/ Weight 100 g

The coins, undamaged, are in the shape of a knife.

Preserved in Shaanxi Museum of Medical History

華

索 引

（馆藏地按拼音字母排序）

Index

Preserved in Hanjiang District Administration Committee of Cultural Relics

Preserved in Hebei Museum

Preserved in Cultural Relics Institute of Hebei Province

Preserved in Henan Museum

Preserved in Henan Provincial Institute of Cultural Heritage and Archaeology

Preserved in Hunan Provincial Museum

Preserved in Shanxi Provincial Institute of Archaeology

Preserved in Pingshuo Archaeological Team of Shanxi Province

Preserved in Youyu Museum of Shanxi Province

Preserved in Chunhua Cultural Center of Shaanxi Province

Preserved in Shaanxi Provincial Institute of Archaeology

Preserved in Shaanxi History Museum

Preserved in Shaanxi Museum of Medical History

Preserved in Shaanxi History Museum

Preserved in Shanghai Museum

Preserved in Shanghai Museum of Traditional Chinese Medicine

Preserved in Shaoxing Museum

Preserved in the Capital Museum

Preserved in Tianchang Museum

Preserved in Xi'an Municipal Institute of Archaeology and Cultural Relics Protection

Preserved in Museum of the Western Han Dynasty Mausoleum of King Nanyue

Preserved in Yangzhou Museum

Preserved in Yangzhou Archaeological Team

Preserved in Yizheng Museum

Collected by Zhang Yazong

Preserved in Zhejiang Provincial Museum

Preserved in National Museum of China

Preserved in Chinese Medical Association/Museum of Chinese Medicine History, Shanghai University of Traditional Chinese Medicine

Preserved in Chongqing Museum

参考文献

[1] 李经纬 . 中国古代医史图录 [M]. 北京：人民卫生出版社，1992.

[2] 傅维康，李经纬，林昭庚 . 中国医学通史：文物图谱卷 [M]. 北京：人民卫生出版社，2000.

[3] 和中浚，吴鸿洲 . 中华医学文物图集 [M]. 成都：四川人民出版社，2001.

[4] 上海中医药博物馆 . 上海中医药博物馆馆藏珍品 [M]. 上海：上海科学技术出版社，2013.

[5] 西藏自治区博物馆 . 西藏博物馆 [M]. 北京：五洲传播出版社，2005.

[6] 崔乐泉 . 中国古代体育文物图录：中英文本 [M]. 北京：中华书局，2000.

[7] 张金明，陆雪春 . 中国古铜镜鉴赏图录 [M]. 北京：中国民族摄影艺术出版社，2002.

[8] 文物精华编辑委员会 . 文物精华 [M]. 北京：文物出版社，1964.

[9] 谭维四 . 湖北出土文物精华 [M]. 武汉：湖北教育出版社，2001.

[10] 常州市博物馆 . 常州文物精华 [M]. 北京：文物出版社，1998.

[11] 镇江博物馆 . 镇江文物精华 [M]. 合肥：黄山书社，1997.

[12] 贵州省文化厅，贵州省博物馆 . 贵州文物精华 [M]. 贵阳：贵州人民出版社，2005.

[13] 徐良玉 . 扬州馆藏文物精华 [M]. 南京：江苏古籍出版社，2001.

[14] 昭陵博物馆，陕西历史博物馆 . 昭陵文物精华 [M]. 西安：陕西人民美术出版社，1991.

[15] 南通博物苑 . 南通博物苑文物精华 [M]. 北京：文物出版社，2005.

[16] 邯郸市文物研究所 . 邯郸文物精华 [M]. 北京：文物出版社，2005.

[17] 张秀生，刘友恒，聂连顺，等 . 中国河北正定文物精华 [M]. 北京：文化艺术出版社，1998.

[18] 陕西省咸阳市文物局 . 咸阳文物精华 [M]. 北京：文物出版社，2002.

[19] 安阳市文物管理局 . 安阳文物精华 [M]. 北京：文物出版社，2004.

[20] 深圳市博物馆 . 深圳市博物馆文物精华 [M]. 北京：文物出版社，1998.

[21]《中国文物精华》编辑委员会 . 中国文物精华（1993）[M]. 北京：文物出版社，1993.

[22] 夏路，刘永生 . 山西省博物馆馆藏文物精华 [M]. 太原：山西人民出版社，1999.

[23] 文物精华编辑委员会 . 文物精华 [M]. 文物出版社，1957.

[24] 山西博物院，湖北省博物馆 . 荆楚长歌：九连墩楚墓出土文物精华 [M]. 太原：山西人民出版社，2011.

[25] 刘广堂，石金鸣，宋建忠 . 晋国雄风：山西出土两周文物精华 [M]. 沈阳：万卷出版公司，2009.

[26] 沈君山，王国平，单迎红 . 滦平博物馆馆藏文物精华 [M]. 北京：中国文联出版社，2012.

[27] 张家口市博物馆 . 张家口市博物馆馆藏文物精华 [M]. 北京：科学出版社，2011.

[28] 浙江省文物考古研究所 . 浙江考古精华 [M]. 北京：文物出版社，1999.

[29] 故宫博物院 . 故宫雕刻珍萃 [M]. 北京：紫禁城出版社，2004.

[30] 故宫博物院紫禁城出版社 . 故宫博物院藏宝录 [M]. 上海：上海文艺出版社，1986.

[31] 首都博物馆 . 大元三都 [M]. 北京：科学出版社，2016.

[32] 新疆维吾尔自治区博物馆 . 新疆出土文物 [M]. 北京：文物出版社，1975.

[33] 王兴伊，段逸山 . 新疆出土涉医文书辑校 [M]. 上海：上海科学技术出版社，2016.

[34] 刘学春 . 刍议医药卫生文物的概念与分类标准 [J]. 中华中医药杂志，2016，31（11）:4406-4409.

[35] 上海古籍出版社 . 中国艺海 [M]. 上海：上海古籍出版社，1994.

[36] 紫都，岳鑫 . 一生必知的 200 件国宝 [M]. 呼和浩特：远方出版社，2005.

[37] 谭维四 . 湖北出土文物精华 [M]. 武汉：湖北教育出版社，2001.

[38] 张建青 . 青海彩陶收藏与鉴赏 [M]. 北京：中国文史出版社，2007.

[39] 银景琦 . 仡佬族文物 [M]. 南宁：广西人民出版社，2014.

[40] 廖果，梁峻，李经纬 . 东西方医学的反思与前瞻 [M]. 北京：中医古籍出版社，2002.

[41] 梁峻，张志斌，廖果，等 . 中华医药文明史集论 [M]. 北京：中医古籍出版社，2003.

[42] 郑蓉，庄乾竹，刘聪，等 . 中国医药文化遗产考论 [M]. 北京：中医古籍出版社，2005.